Thyrotropin

Thyrotropin

Ultrasensitive TSH measurement in clinical research and diagnostics

Edited by
G. Leb · A. Passath · O. Eber · H. Höfler

Walter de Gruyter
Berlin · New York 1987

Prof. Dr. med. Georg Leb
Medizinische Universitätsklinik Graz
Auenbrugger Platz 15 · A-8036 Graz

Dr. med. Alois Passath
Medizinische Universitätsklinik Graz
Auenbrugger Platz 15 · A-8036 Graz

Prof. Dr. med. Otto Eber
Krankenhaus der Barmherzigen Brüder
Bergstraße 27 · A-8020 Graz

Dr. med. Heinz Höfler
Patholog. Anatomisches Institut der Universität Graz
Auenbrugger Platz 25 · A-8036 Graz

This book contains 124 illustrations and 85 tables

CIP-Kurztitelaufnahme der Deutschen Bibliothek

Thyrotropin : ultrasensitive TSH measurement in clinical research and diagnostics / ed. by G. Leb ... Berlin ; New York : de Gruyter, 1987.
ISBN 3-11-011017-2
NE: Leb, Georg [Hrsg.]

Library of Congress Cataloging in Publication Data

Thyrotropin : ultrasensitive TSH measurement in clinical research and diagnostics.
Includes indexes.
1. Thyrotropin− −Analysis. 2. Radioimmunoassay.
I. Leb. G. [DNLM: 1. Thyrotropin− −physiology− −congresses. WK 515 T5498]
QP572.T55T48 1987 616.07'56 87-8964
ISBN 0-89925-209-5 (U.S.)

Preface

The development of new methods for the ultrasensitive determination of thyrotropin has recently led to a number of new findings concerning the pathophysiology of thyroid-stimulating hormone (TSH) secretion. The second symposium on thyrotropin in Graz aims to summarize the state-of-the-art knowledge in this field, and to discuss the implications of the new findings for the clinical diagnosis of thyroid disorders.

The first section of this book surveys current basic research projects on the normal and pathologic biosynthesis of thyrotropin-releasing hormone (TRH) and TSH. The influence of central nervous system disorders and peripheral hormones on the hypothalamic and pituitary secretion of TRH and TSH is also examined. Fundamental studies with ultrasensitive techniques have demonstrated a close association between the thyroid hormone concentrations in the serum and TSH secretion, both in euthyroid patients and those with thyroid disorders. Furthermore, a number of groups have reported unanimously that the TSH increase after TRH stimulation is related in a polynomial function to the basal TSH level. The expected TSH surge after TRH administration can thus be predicted by the basal TSH level.

A further section is about the technique of ultrasensitive TSH determinations. The present results indicate that non-isotopic methods with the same sensitivity as the radioimmunoassay will become increasingly available. A number of albeit easily recognizable non-thyroidal conditions can influence the serum thyrotropin level and lead to misinterpretation of test results.

The studies presented here on the diagnostic applications of the ultrasensitive methods consider the question of how far their widespread use could supplant other tests of thyroid function, and in which circumstances this would diminish diagnostic accuracy. Ultrasensitive techniques now make it possible to distinguish hyperthyroid and euthyroid values by the basal TSH level, thus making the TRH test superfluous in most cases. Only in patients with borderline TSH concentrations and equivocal clinical findings is TRH stimulation still necessary. Guidelines defining these borderline cases are given for the individual tests. Normal TSH values rule out a disturbance of thyroid function with a high degree of accuracy. When determined by ultrasensitive methods, the TSH value is more useful for the exclusion or first diagnosis of thyroid disorders than are the free or total thyroid hormone levels. It can thus be recommended as a screening procedure. The free and, if necessary, the combined thyroid hormone concentrations can be used to determine the degree of the disorder and to follow its course.

The final chapter of this book is concerned with the structure of the TSH receptor. It also deals with the controversial subject of the clinical relevance of TSH-receptor antibodies for the autoimmune diseases of the thyroid, including the development of goiter.

The wide range of new findings about the central regulation of TSH secretion seems to make a broader and more subtle differentiated diagnosis necessary in special cases. On the other hand, as clinical and practice-oriented physicians, our efforts must be directed towards an improved and also simplified and standardized diagnostic capability of functional thyroid disorders – not least because of the cost explosion in medical diagnostics. The editors hope that this book is a step toward that goal.

March 1987 *Georg Leb*

Contents

III TSH in non-thyroidal illness

IV TSH in clinical diagnostics

I Regulation of TSH-secretion

Biosynthesis of Thyrotropin releasing hormone

R. H. Goodman, G. Mandel

The idea that the thyroid is controlled, at least in part, by neuronal influences has a long history. Early clinical observations that thyrotoxicosis is occasionally preceeded by episodes of psychic stress and that states of thyroid hormone excess are associated with symptoms and signs of increased sympathetic tone may have provided the first suggestion of a neural-thyroid connection. It is now clear that these clinical observations were misleading. Our current understanding of the neural control of thyroid function is the result of a series of more basic investigations of the hypothalamic-pituitary-thyroid axis.

Harris and colleagues, studying the function of pituitary glands grafted into various regions of the brain, first established the concept of a "thyrotropic" region of the hypothalamus. Subsequent experiments, using electrolytic lesions, defined the thyrotropic regions of the hypothalamus more precisely. These studies indicated that lesions in an area between the paraventricular nucleus of the hypothalamus and the median eminence blunt the secretion of thyroid stimulating hormone (TSH) from the pituitary. Electrolytic lesions destroy neuronal pathways as well as nuclei, however, and subsequent experiments involving electrical stimulation of specific brain regions improved our concept of the thyrotropic functions of the hypothalamus. Although it became clear that stimulation of the hypothalamus influences thyroid activity through an effect on the pituitary, the mechanism of this pathway was unknown.

The concept of a thyrotropin releasing factor was first proposed thirty years ago by Shibusawa. A few years later, Schrieber demonstrated that purified extracts of bovine hypothalamus stimulated TSH secretion from cultured pituitary cells. The chemical character of thyrotropin releasing hormone (TRH) was not determined until 1968, however, by the laboratories of Guillemin and Schally. The localization of TRH by immunohistochemistry confirmed the earlier physiological studies identifying the thyrotropic regions of the hypothalamus within the paraventricular nucleus.

Although TRH was the first of the hypophysiotropic factors to be chemically characterized, studies of TRH biosynthesis within the hypothalamus have been particularly problematic. In large part, the difficulties in studying TRH production are due to the small size of the molecule (three amino acids) and the low concentration of the peptide in hypothalamic tissues. Both of these factors

Thyrotropin

virtually preclude attempts to study TRH biosynthesis by the conventional approach of pulse-labeling with radioactive amino acids. By analogy with other neuropeptides however, it has long been believed that TRH is initially synthesized as a high molecular weight precursor, pre-proTRH. This precursor would undergo two types of proteolytic cleavage. The first cleavage would remove the signal region to generate proTRH. The prohormone would then be cleaved and further post-translationally modified to form the bioactive tripeptide, pyroGlu-His-Pro-amide.

A powerful approach to characterizing neuropeptide precursors is through recombinant DNA techniques. By isolating and sequencing the appropriate cDNA, one can deduce the structure of the precursor. In general, neuropeptide cDNAs can be isolated using oligonucleotide primers representing all of the possible codons predicted from a known amino acid sequence. The small size of the TRH sequence and the large number of codons that can specify the amino acids Glu-His-Pro precludes this approach however.

Recently, a novel cloning system has been developed that circumvents the need to use oligonucleotide primers. In this system, known as "expression-cloning," cDNAs are expressed in bacteria as fusion proteins linked at their amino terminus to the bacterial enzyme β-galactosidase. Individual cDNA molecules are detected immunochemically, using antisera to the proteins of interest. Using the lambda gt11 bacteriophage expression system, one can efficiently screen several million bacteriophage plaques, making it possible to isolate extremely rare cDNA clones. We chose to use this system to isolate the cDNA encoding pre-proTRH.

Because bacteria do not perform many of the post-translational modifications that are accomplished by specialized eukaryotic cells, antisera used to screen an expression library must not depend on any particular modifications such as amidation, glycosylation, or phosphorylation. In particular, antisera to the TRH molecule, in which two of the three amino acids are post-translationally modified, would not recognize the unmodified precursor protein produced in a bacteriophage expression library. We reasoned that an antiserum directed against the prohormone, rather than against TRH itself, would be an ideal reagent for screening a lambda gt11 library. Jackson, et al. raised such an antiserum to the synthetic peptide, Cys-Lys-Arg-Gln-His-Pro-Gly-Lys-Arg-Cys, presumed to represent a portion of the TRH precursor. The Lys-Arg sequences in the peptide were chosen as likely cleavage sites in the prohormone, Gln represents the precursor for pyroGlu, and the Gly residue was positioned adjacent to the Pro that is amidated in mature TRH. The flanking Cys residues were added to permit cyclization of the peptide, thereby favoring the generation of mid-portion directed antisera. One of the antisera raised against the synthetic peptide reacted with neurons in the parvocellular subdivision of the paraventricular nucleus and in the lateral hypothalamus, regions known to produce TRH. This antisera was used to screen a rat hypothalamic lambda gt11 library for the cDNA encoding the TRH precursor.

The lambda gt11 vector contains a unique cloning site near the carboxy-terminus of the β-galactosidase gene. Complimentary DNA molecules are inserted into this site using standard recombinant DNA techniques. When the cDNAs are inserted in the correct reading frame and orientation, the recombinant phage synthesize fusion proteins that contain, at their amino terminus, a portion of the β-galactosidase molecule, and at their carboxy terminus, a protein encoded by the cDNA. To screen a lambda gt11 cDNA library, a lawn of bacteria is infected with the recombinant phage. Bacteria infected by an individual phage appear as clear areas (plaques) in the otherwise confluent lawn. The proteins from the plaques are transfered to nitrocellulose filters and probed with antisera to the protein of interest.

```
                                                       TCCTTGGATTCGGGAGTATTGCAAACTCTAC
    CCAGCCAGTTTGCACTCTTCAGCTCAGCATCTTGGAAAGCTCTGCAGAGTCTCCACTTCGCAGACTCCAGG 102

    ATG CCG GGA CCT TGG TTG CTG CTG GCT CTG GCT TTG ATC TTC ACC CTA ACT GGT
  1 Met-Pro-Gly-Pro-Trp-Leu-Leu-Leu-Ala-Leu-Ala-Leu-Ile-Phe-Thr-Leu-Thr-Gly
    -----------------------------------------------------------------------
    ATC CCT GAA TCC TGC GCC TTG CCG GAG GCA GCC CAG GAG GAA GGT GCA GTG ACT 210
    Ile-Pro-Glu-Ser-Cys-Ala-Leu-Pro-Glu-Ala-Ala-Gln-Glu-Glu-Gly-Ala-Val-Thr
    ----------------------------
    CCT GAC CTT CCT GGC CTG GAG AAT GTT CAG GTC CGG CCA GAA CGT CGA TTC TTG
 37 Pro-Asp-Leu-Pro-Gly-Leu-Glu-Asn-Val-Gln-Val-Arg-Pro-Glu-Arg-Arg-Phe-Leu

    TGG AAA GAC CTC CAG CGG GTG AGA GGG GAC CTC GGT GCT GCC TTA GAC TCC TGG 318
    Trp-Lys-Asp-Leu-Gln-Arg-Val-Arg-Gly-Asp-Leu-Gly-Ala-Ala-Leu-Asp-Ser-Trp

    ATC ACA AAA CGC CAG CAT CCA GGC AAA AGG GAG GAG GAG GAA AAA GAC ATT GAA
 73 Ile-Thr-Lys-Arg-Gln-His-Pro-Gly-Lys-Arg-Glu-Glu-Glu-Glu-Lys-Asp-Ile-Glu

    GCT GAA GAG AGG GGA GAC TTG GGA GAA GGG GGA GCC TGG AGA CTC CAC AAA CGA 426
    Ala-Glu-Glu-Arg-Gly-Asp-Leu-Gly-Glu-Gly-Gly-Ala-Trp-Arg-Leu-His-Lys-Arg

    CAG CAC CCC GGC CGA CGT GCC AAC CAG GAC AAG TAT TCA TGG GCA GAT GAG GAG
109 Gln-His-Pro-Gly-Arg-Arg-Ala-Asn-Gln-Asp-Lys-Tyr-Ser-Trp-Ala-Asp-Glu-Glu

    GAC AGT GAC TGG ATG CCA CGG TCC TGG TTA CCA GAT TTC TTT CTG GAT TCC TGG 534
    Asp-Ser-Asp-Trp-Met-Pro-Arg-Ser-Trp-Leu-Pro-Asp-Phe-Phe-Leu-Asp-Ser-Trp

    TTC TCA GAT GTC CCC CAA GTC AAG CGG CAG CAC CCT GGC AGG CGA TCC TTC CCC
145 Phe-Ser-Asp-Val-Pro-Gln-Val-Lys-Arg-Gln-His-Pro-Gly-Arg-Arg-Ser-Phe-Pro

    TGG ATG GAG TCT GAT GTC ACC AAG AGG CAA CAT CCA GGC CGG AGG TTC ATA GAT 642
    Trp-Met-Glu-Ser-Asp-Val-Thr-Lys-Arg-Gln-His-Pro-Gly-Arg-Arg-Phe-Ile-Asp

    CCC GAG CTC CAA AGA AGC TGG GAA GAA AAA GAG GGA GAG GGT GTC TTA ATG CCT
181 Pro-Glu-Leu-Gln-Arg-Ser-Trp-Glu-Glu-Lys-Glu-Gly-Glu-Gly-Val-Leu-Met-Pro

    GAG AAA CGC CAG CAT CCT GGC AAA AGG GCA TTG GGT CAT CCC TGT GGG CCC CAG 750
    Glu-Lys-Arg-Gln-His-Pro-Gly-Lys-Arg-Ala-Leu-Gly-His-Pro-Cys-Gly-Pro-Gln

    GGG ACT TGT GGT CAA ACA GGC CTG CTC CAG CTT CTA GGT GAC CTG AGC AGG GGT
217 Gly-Thr-Cys-Gly-Gln-Thr-Gly-Leu-Leu-Gln-Leu-Leu-Gly-Asp-Leu-Ser-Arg-Gly

    CAG GAG ACC CTG GTG AAG CAA AGC CCA CAA GTG GAA CCC TGG GAC AAG GAA CCT 858
    Gln-Glu-Thr-Leu-Val-Lys-Gln-Ser-Pro-Gln-Val-Glu-Pro-Trp-Asp-Lys-Glu-Pro

    CTG GAG GAG TAAGGCCAGAGTCAGGCTTTAGGTCTAGGATGATGTAAGCCCTGTATTCCCTATCCTGT
253 Leu-Glu-Glu ***

    TCCCTTCACTAGCTGTCCTCTCTTAGATGCTAACCCTGGGCCCTCTGTACATCGTCCACCCAAACCCCTTC 997
    CTTACCGACTTCAGAGACTTTAGAAAGCCAGTCAGGAAGTTAAAACCCTACTTATCCCTTCA[illegible]AGGGG
    GTGGGAGTCACACCCCTTCAGCACTGGCCAAGATGGTTCTTTC[illegible]ACC[illegible]AAG[illegible]ACCTC[illegible]TCAGAAAG
    GAAGGGTAGAATTGAAATGTTTTGGTGTTAAAACTTCTGTAATCTGCCCCATGTGG[illegible]AAGA[illegible]TGACCTGGT
    ATAGCTTCAGCGCATCCTCCAAGGTTGGGGTCCCTGAGCAGTTTGGGAGATGTTTAGATATG[illegible] 1201
    TGGGGGGTCGCATCTTGTATATAACCCTGCTCTTGGGAAT
```

Fig. 1

Eight immunopositive phage were detected with the proTRH antisera. One of the major problems with the lambda gt11 cloning system is the detection of false positives however. This problem generally arises because the antisera used are not sufficiently specific and detect epitopes on multiple proteins. Ideally, the procedure used to confirm the identity of immunopositive bacteriophage should rely on non-immunological criteria.

We made use of the well-characterized anatomy of the hypothalamic TRH system to confirm the identity of the immunopositive bacteriophage. We reasoned that a cDNA encoding the authentic TRH precursor should hybridize to mRNA found only in TRH neurons. The recently developed technique of *in situ* hybridization histochemistry allows one to detect specific populations of mRNA in tissue slices. Consequently, we used *in situ* hybridization to determine whether any of the positive bacteriophage detected TRH neurons. The cDNA from one of the bacteriophage that we identified with the proTRH antisera also detected TRH neurons in the *in situ* hybridization assays. The nucleotide sequence of this cDNA was determined.

As shown in fig. 1, the sequence of the cDNA encoded a protein of 255 amino acids (molecular weight 29,247). The amino terminus of this protein is extremely hydrophobic, suggesting that it represents a signal sequence. The sequence Gln-His-Pro-Gly occurs five times in the molecule. In each instance, this sequence is flanked by pairs of basic amino acids, suggesting that five TRH molecules can be generated from the precursor. The structure of the TRH precursor is similar, therefore, to that of other neuropeptides such as enkephalin and FRMF-amide. With the exception of the repeated TRH sequences, there is not very much homology between the rat TRH precursor and the amphibian precursor characterized by Kreil and co-workers.

The isolation of the rat proTRH cDNA should greatly facilitate future studies of TRH biosynthesis. The cDNA can be used in hybridization assays to quantitate the levels of TRH mRNA in specific brain regions and to determine the effects of neurotransmitters, growth factors, and thyroid hormone itself on TRH biosynthesis. It should eventually be possible to determine precisely how the TRH gene is regulated. Antisera to non-TRH portions of the precursor will help elucidate the complex post-translational processing of proTRH and may be useful in determining whether this post-translational processing is also regulated. The small size of the TRH molecule should no longer be a limitation to studies of TRH biosynthesis.

Acknowledgements

We thank our collaborators R. Lechan, P. Wu, I. M. D. Jackson, S. Cooperman, H. Wolfe, and H. Hofler for their invaluable contributions to this project. This work was supported by grants from the National Institutes of Health and the Medical Foundation, Inc.

Hormonal regulation of Thyrotropin gene expression

W. W. Chin

Introduction

Thyrotropin (TSH) is the major regulator of thyroid gland growth and function in mammals and lower species. It interacts with its specific receptor on the plasma membrane of thyroid follicular cells to induce the production of thyroid hormones (TH). The TH produced by the thyroid gland then act on many tissues to regulate metabolic functions. Of special note, TH also act on the TSH-producing cell or thyrotrope located in the anterior pituitary gland to inhibit both the release and synthesis of TSH. This long-distance regulatory loop is a classic example of negative-feedback control of endocrine function [1].

TSH is a complex molecule consisting of two different components that are associated in a non-covalent manner. The components are termed α and TSHβ subunits. Each subunit is composed of a polypeptide backbone to which is attached carbohydrate moieties. Also, each subunit is folded in an intricate way using multiple disulfide links to permit the eventual formation of the functional heterodimer. Inasmuch as the structure of TSH is complex, it is easy to imagine that the biosynthetic pathway for TSH is also complicated. The α and TSHβ subunits are encoded by separate genes located on different chromosomes [2, 3]. Each subunit gene is transcribed in the thyrotrope to yield separate messenger RNAs (mRNA) which are translated in the cytoplasm of the thyrotrope. The translational products are rapidly altered via important co-translational steps. First, the N-terminal leader sequence is cleaved from the subunit precursor – a typical step in the production of most secretory and membrane proteins. The leader or signal sequence characteristically contains 20–30 amino acids with a hydrophobic core. This structure enables several cytoplasmic components to interact with the newly synthesized product to guide it into the endoplasmic reticulum where it may be sorted to membrane or vesicular addresses. Second, even before the completion of translation of each subunit, carbohydrate moieties are added to the protein backbone. The sugar groups are added to asparagine residues located in a specific amino acid sequence nest within the backbone. Next, these partially processed and immature glycosylated peptides undergo further multiple processing steps including [1] intrasubunit folding utilizing the

Thyrotropin

cysteine residues, [2] maturation of carbohydrate molecules, [3] dimerization, and [4] transport to secretory vesicles in their passage through the Golgi complex. This mature TSH is then stored in the endocrine secretory granule of the thyrotrope until its release is stimulated by various hypothalamic factors [4]. It is now evident that hormones such as TH and thyroid-releasing hormone (TRH) as well as other factors may regulate the synthesis of TSH at any or all of the steps just described. Our laboratory, over the last five years, has focused on the regulation of TSH synthesis at the pre-translational level. In particular, we have isolated and characterized the genes and cDNAs which encode the α and TSHβ subunits and have begun to examine the effects of various hormones on subunit gene expression. We have shown that TH and other hormones regulate the synthesis of TSH by the thyrotrope in large part at the transcriptional and post-transcriptional levels.

TSH subunit cDNAs and genes

In order to measure steady-state levels of subunit mRNAs and the rates of transcription of subunit genes, we required molecular probes for these nucleic acids. Several years ago, we set out to isolate complementary DNAs (cDNAs) representing the α and TSHβ mRNAs in mouse and rat. We utilized recombinant DNA technology in order to obtain cDNAs encoding the α and TSHβ subunits in mouse and rat [5–8]. Typical TSH subunit cDNAs and their corresponding RNA structures are shown in fig. 1. The sizes of the unique α and TSHβ mRNAs

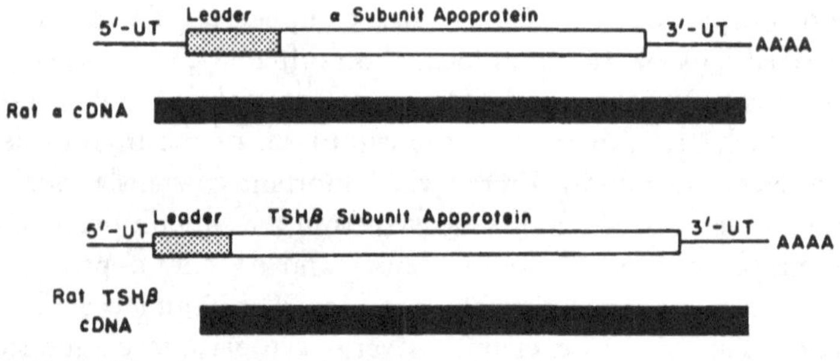

Fig. 1 The structure of mRNAs and cDNAs encoding the subunits of rat TSH. The top line in each section represents the mRNA encoding the α and TSHβ subunits in schematic form. The open box represents the portion of the RNA which encodes the protein precursor with the solid lines to the left and right representing the 5'- and 3'-untranslated regions of the mRNAs, respectively. The open box contains the precursor which is divided into two regions. The shaded region represents the leader peptide, 24 amino acids in α and 20 amino acids in TSHβ with structures typical of those found in secretory polypeptide precursors. The larger open box represents the subunit apoprotein. The solid box beneath each mRNA represents a typical cDNA used in some of the experiments described in this manuscript [5, 7].

are ~800 and ~700 bases, respectively. In addition, the genes encoding the subunits have also been isolated and characterized. The α subunit gene is > 9 – 10 Kb and contains 4 exons, and the TSHβ subunit gene is ~5 Kb and contains 3 exons [9, 10]. They have been localized to different chromosomes: α on chromosome 6 and chromosome 7 in man and mouse, respectively, and TSHβ on chromosomes 1 and 3 in man and mouse, respectively [11 – 13]. In sum, the subunits are encoded by single genes located on separate chromosomes.

Hormonal regulation of TSH subunit expression

We have determined the effect of various hormones, in particular thyroid hormones (TH), on the biosynthesis of TSH at the pre-translational level. We have determined the levels of α and TSHβ mRNAs in thyrotropic tissues in mouse and rat using nucleic acid hybridization techniques. In brief, tissues *in vivo* or *in vitro* were homogenized in guanidinium thiocyanate, a chaotropic denaturant, and the homogenate layered over a cesium chloride cushion. The homogenate was centrifuged at 100,000 xg for 8 – 18 hours in order to pellet total pituitary gland or thyrotropic RNA. These total RNAs were then subjected to Northern blot analysis using labeled α and TSHβ cDNAs of the rat and/or mouse. In general, 5 – 10 µg of total pituitary or thyrotropic tumor RNA were separated by agarose gel electrophoresis and RNAs were transferred to nitrocellulose filter paper. The RNAs were fixed to this paper and then hybridized to various labeled probes at high stringency. Using the DNA probe in excess, we could effectively quantitate the levels of α and TSHβ mRNAs using this technique. Several experimental protocols were used to evaluate the effects of thyroid hormones on TSH subunit mRNAs in rat pituitary glands as well as mouse thyrotropic tumor and pituitary tissue. First, subunit mRNAs in pituitary glands of normal and hypothyroid rats were examined. After two weeks of treatment with propylthiouracil (0.05% (wt/vol) in ad lib drinking water) or three weeks post-surgical thyroidectomy, the α (fig. 2) and TSHβ (fig. 3) mRNAs increased ~4 – 6-fold, and 7 – 10-fold, respectively [14]. Second, the effects of TH on TSH biosynthesis in a mouse thyrotropic tumor was explored. The mouse thyrotropic tumor, TtT97, is a transplantable pituitary neoplasm which was developed by Jacob Furth in the early 1950's. These tumors, derived from a special mouse strain, produce ample amounts of TSH that are regulated by TH and TRH. The growth of these tumors is dependent on a hypothyroid host mouse. In the first experiment, the hypothyroid mice bearing the TtT97 were injected with T3 (10 µg/100 g bw/d) and the time-course of effect of TH on α and TSHβ mRNAs was determined. The plasma TSH in these animals decreased sharply as anticipated from previous work. In addition, α and TSHβ mRNAs also decreased sharply but with the

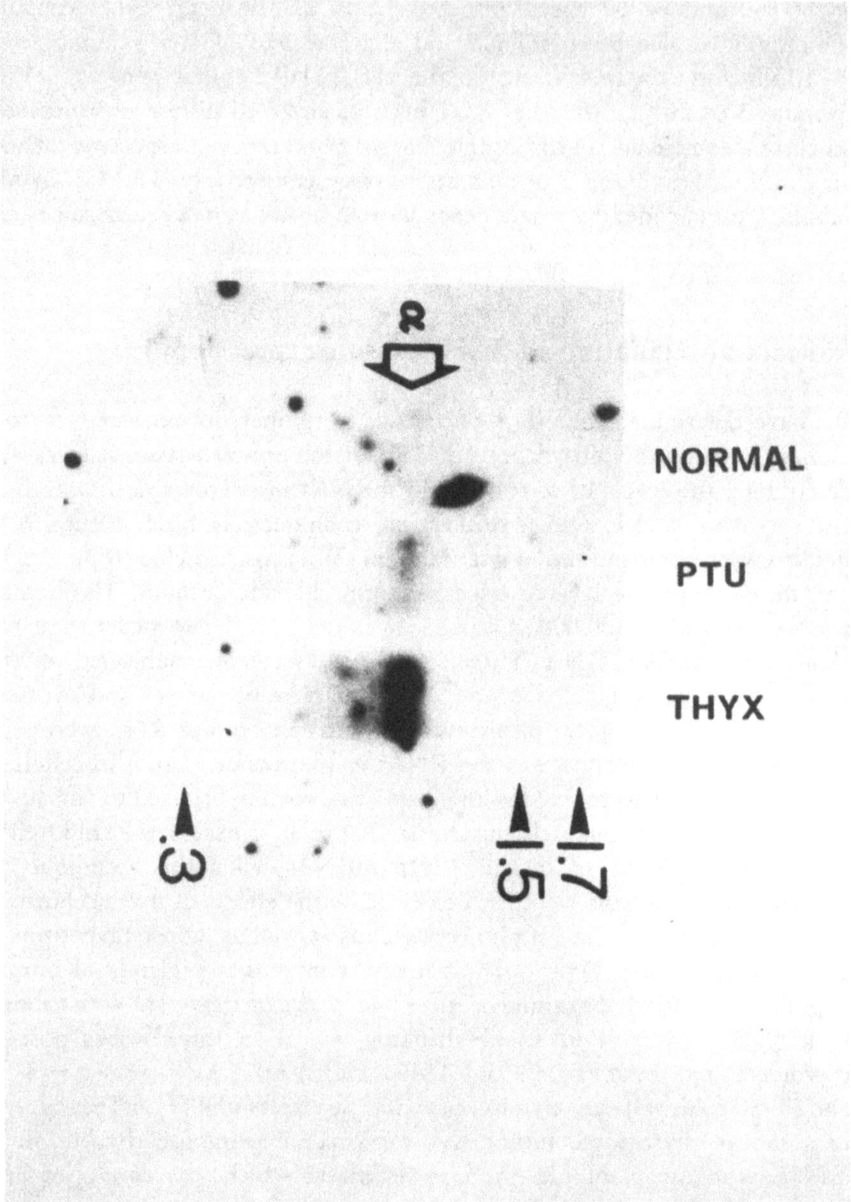

Fig. 2 Northern blot analysis of total rat pituitary RNA in normal and hypothyroid animals: α mRNA. Total RNA (10 μg) from the anterior pituitary glands of normal and hypothyroid (either propylthiouracil [0.05%]) in drinking water for two weeks (PTU) or three weeks post-surgical thyroidectomy (THYX) were subjected to agarose gel electrophoresis and Northern blot analysis using [^{32}P]-labeled α cDNA [5]. The blots were hybridized and washed under stringent conditions and the resultant blot subjected to autoradiography. The arrow points to a 800 base size mRNA representing the α subunit mRNA in the rat pituitary gland. (Modified from Chin et al. [7] with permission.)

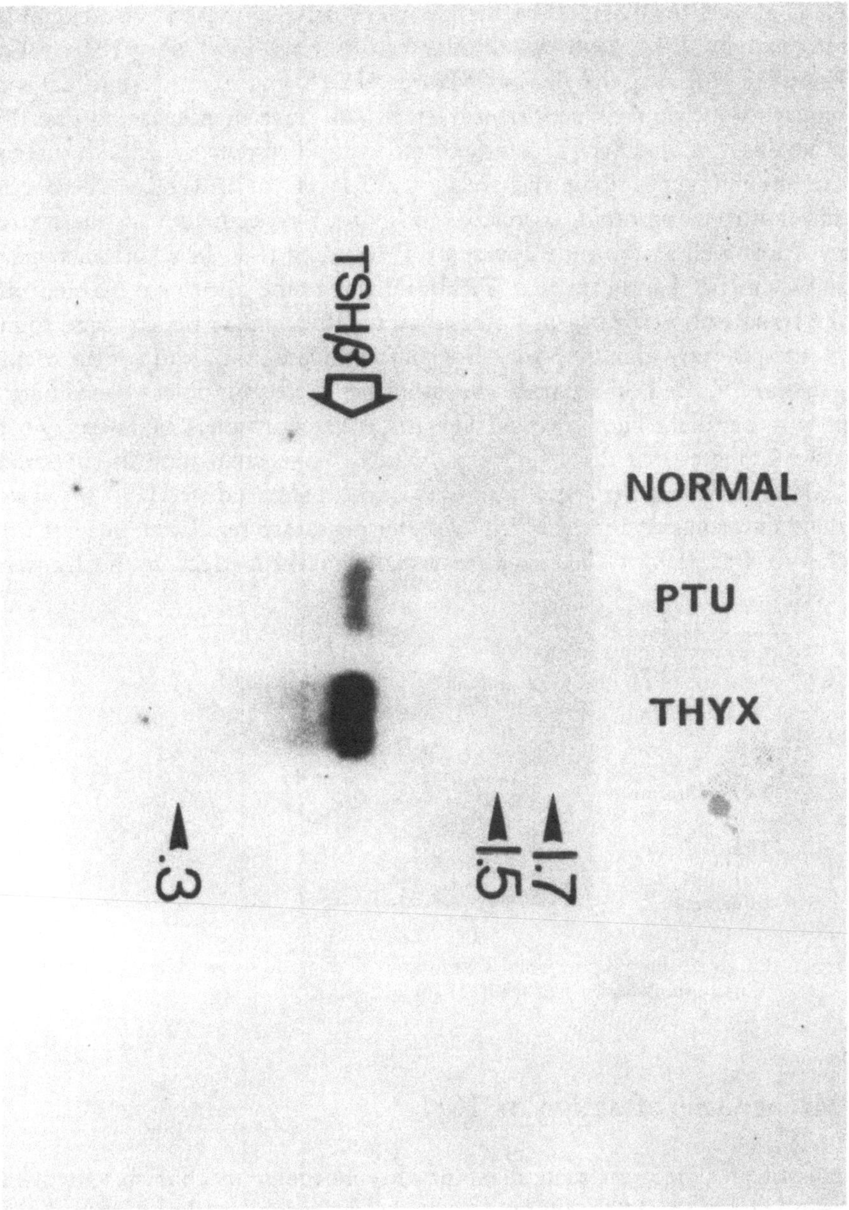

Fig. 3 Northern blot analysis of mRNA encoding TSHβ in normal and hypothyroid animals: TSHβ mRNA. The Northern blot used for fig. 2 was stripped of the α subunit cDNA and rehybridized with labeled cDNA encoding TSHβ subunit [7] and subjected to Northern blot analysis. The autoradiogram of such a study is shown. The arrow points to the TSHβ mRNA in the rat which is ~700 bases in size. (Modified from Chin et al. [7] with permission.)

effect greater for TSHβ. The changes were rapid so that the effect on TSHβ was maximal by 1–2 days [8]. Similar results have been observed by Gurr and Kourides [14] and Croyle and Maurer [15]. Using a transcriptional assay and mouse thyrotropic tissue, Shupnik et al. [16] have demonstrated that T3 at the same doses caused even greater and more rapid responses of the transcription of the subunit genes than the steady-state levels of mRNAs. These effects, in addition to being rapid, correlated well with the occupancy of nuclear receptors by T3 as well as the time course of T3 binding [17]. In addition, the results as shown in fig. 4 indicate that TRH and dopamine also have marked effects on the transcriptional rates of both subunits [18]. Similar results were found using mouse pituitary glands. Thus, these data indicate that although the α and TSHβ genes are located on separate chromosomes the regulation is coordinate but not strictly parallel. The effect of TH and other hormones on these two genes is always greatest for the TSHβ gene which is consistent with the hypothesis that TSHβ determines the actually amount of the TSH produced [19, 20]. In summary, these data suggest that the TSH subunit genes are regulated, at least in part, at the pre-translational level with especially marked effect at the transcriptional level.

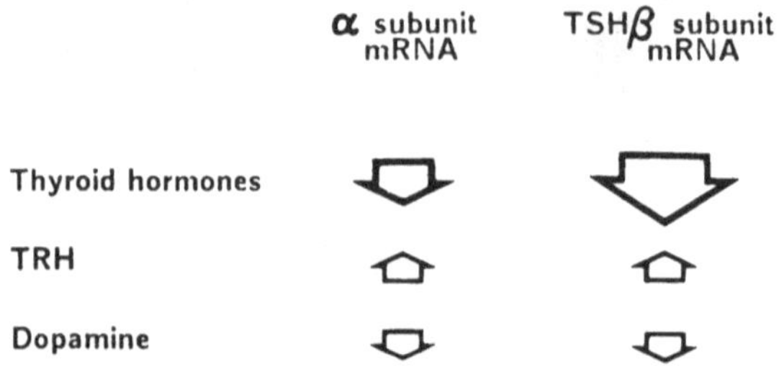

Fig. 4 Effects of thyroid hormones, thyrotropin-releasing hormone (TRH), and dopamine on the transcriptional activity of the TSH subunit genes.

Mechanisms of action of TSH

It is of great interest to understand the molecular mechanisms involved in the regulation of the TSH subunit genes by TH. The availability of well characterized TSH subunit genes will enable us, using recombinant DNA molecular biology techniques, to dissect structure-function relationships of various subunit gene promoter regions and thyroid-hormone regulation. Similar studies have recently been performed using the rat growth hormone gene by several groups [21, 22]. These studies indicate that there is a region in the 5′-flanking region close to the promoter of the rat growth hormone gene which is necessary for the thyroid hormone response. Similar studies are underway to identify possible regulatory elements as shown in fig. 5 which may mediate the thyroid hormone effects in the TSH system.

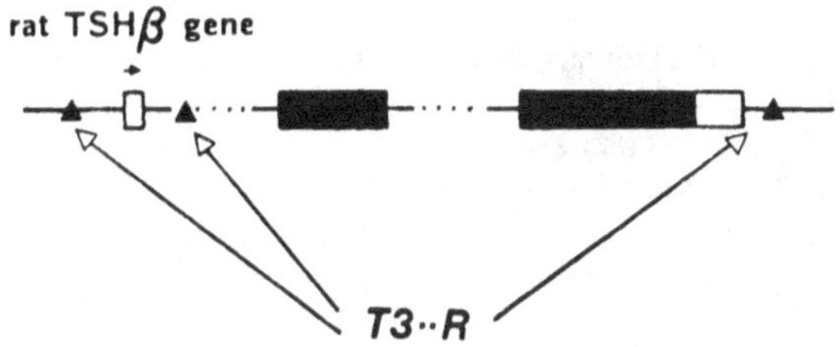

Fig. 5 Effect of T3-nuclear-receptor complex on the gene encoding the TSHβ subunit. Thyroid hormones decrease the transcriptional activity of the TSHβ gene. Although the molecular mechanisms involved in this process are not yet clarified, potential sites of thyroid hormone interaction include the 5′-flanking, intronic, and 3′-flanking regions (Δ). The rat TSHβ gene, in schematic form, is shown. The boxes represent the three exons (open: untranslated regions; and black: coding regions). The small solid arrow indicates the start of transcription [9].

Prospects

Thus, over the last several years, we have learned a great deal about the structure of the genes and mRNAs which encode the separate subunits of TSH. We have also learned that the regulation of synthesis of TSH is, in large part, manifested at the pre-translational level. In fact, the regulation of TSH synthesis at the transcriptional level is marked with evidence to suggest that this effect is direct and independent of protein synthesis. Such information provides hope that we will be able to understand better the molecular mechanisms involved in the interaction of T3-nuclear receptor complexes with TSH subunit genes. These subunit genes along with the possible advent of thyroid hormone receptor protein derived from molecular cloning provide hope that we may soon be able to understand in great detail the biophysical nature of nuclear T3 receptor and specific DNA target complexes. We look forward to such advances with great anticipation.

Acknowledgements

I wish to thank Drs. Margaret A. Shupnik, Frances E. Carr, Douglas S. Ross, Susan L. Naylor, Joel F. Habener and E. C. Ridgway for their major contributions to this work. In addition, I would like to thank N. Patterson for her secretarial assistance in this manuscript.

References

[1] Hershman, J. M., A. E. Pekary: In: The Pituitary Gland (Imura, H., ed.) pp. 149 – 166. Raven Press, New York 1985.
[2] Pierce, J. G., T. F. Parsons: Annu. Rev. Biochem. **50** (1981) 465 – 495.
[3] Chin, W. W.: In: The Pituitary Gland (Imura, H., ed.), pp. 164 – 184. Raven Press, New York 1985.
[4] Chin, W. W.: In: Secretory Tumors of the Pituitary Gland (Black, P. M. et al., ed.), pp. 327 – 342. Raven Press, New York 1984.
[5] Godine, J. E., et al.: J. Biol. Chem. **257** (1982) 8368 – 8371.
[6] Chin, W. W., et al.: Proc. Natl. Acad. Sci. USA **78** (1981) 5329 – 5333.
[7] Chin, W. W., et al.: Biochem. Biophys. Res. Commun. **128** (1985) 1152 – 1158.
[8] Chin, W. W., et al.: Endocrinology **116** (1985) 873 – 878.
[9] Chin, W. W., et al.: (personal communication).
[10] Carr, F. E., et al.: 9th Int. Thyroid Cong., Sao Paulo, Brazil, Abstract No. 13 (1985).
[11] Naylor, S. L., et al.: Somatic Cell Genet. **9** (1983) 757 – 770.
[12] Kourides, I. A., et al.: Proc. Natl. Acad. Sci. USA **81** (1984) 517 – 519.
[13] Naylor, S. L., et al.: Som. Cell. Genet. (in press).
[14] Gurr, J. A., I. A. Kourides: J. Biol. Chem. **258** (1983) 10208 – 10211.
[15] Croyle, M. L., R. A. Maurer: DNA **3** (1984) 231 – 236.
[16] Shupnik, M. A., et al.: J. Biol. Chem. **260** (1985) 2900 – 2903.
[17] Shupnik, M. A., et al.: Endocrinology **117** (1985) 1940 – 1946.
[18] Shupnik, M. A., et al.: The Endocrine Society Abstracts, 68th Annual Mtg, Anaheim, CA. (1986).
[19] Chin, W. W., et al.: J. Biol. Chem. **256** (1981) 3059 – 3066.
[20] Weintraub, B. D., et al.: J. Biol. Chem. **255** (1980) 5715 – 5723.
[21] Crew, M. D., S. R. Spindler: J. Biol. Chem. **261** (1986) 5018 – 5022.
[22] Casanova, J., et al.: J. Biol. Chem. **260** (1985) 11744 – 11748.

Regulation of Thyrotropin secretion and its derangements*

G. Faglia, P. Beck-Peccoz, G. Piscitelli, G. Medri

Introduction

A well-balanced action of stimulatory and inhibitory factors regulates the proper secretion of TSH from the pituitary: circulating thyroid hormone exert a dominant inhibitory action, while TRH has a powerful stimulatory effect. Recent investigations have demonstrated that dopamine, somatostatin, and corticosteroids on one hand, and norepinephrine and estrogens on the other hand, contribute to inhibitory or stimulatory control of TSH secretion, respectively. In addition, very recent evidence has been given that, under particular circumstances, TSH may vary its biological activity. Thus, hypothalamic-pituitary lesions, or alterations of TSH regulatory mechanisms, or modifications of TSH bioactivity may result in disorders of thyroid function. Although rare, these disorders should be recognized as their management differs from that of conventional hyper- or hypothyroidism.

Regulation of Thyrotropin secretion

In recent years, basic and clinical research on the regulation of TSH secretion has rapidly expanded (see [1–2]). The aim of this section is to focus on aspects particularly pertinent to diagnostic and therapeutical approaches utilized in patients with clinical disorders primarily related to alterations of TSH secretion.

TSH is a glycoprotein hormone of approximately 28,000 daltons composed of two dissimilar noncovalently bound subunits (alpha and beta). The alpha-subunit is virtually identical to that of other glycoprotein hormones LH, FSH, and hCG [3], while the beta-subunit confers biological specificity. Both individual subunits are devoid of biological activity [4]. They are synthesized independently in the thyrotrophs, where undergo subsequent glycosylation, and then are assembled to form complete TSH molecule prior to secretion [5, 6]. Only very minute

* This work has been partially supported by CNR, Special Project Oncology, contract n° 85.02148.44.115.04912, and by founds from Ministero della Pubblica Istruzione, Rome, Italy.

amounts of alpha and beta subunits are secreted in the free form and are measurable in the peripheral blood [7]. Conformational changes of TSH molecule due to alterations in glycosylation can affect its biological activity [8].

The main regulatory factor of TSH secretion is the dominant inhibitory action of thyroid hormone directly at the pituitary level. Very small changes in circulating thyroid hormone levels reciprocally affect both basal and TRH-stimulated serum TSH levels [9]. This very sensitive negative feedback is presumed to be mainly exerted via the intrapituitary conversion of T4 into T3 by 5′-monodeiodase, as the TSH suppressive effect of T4 is abolished by the blockade of 5′ monodeiodination by iopanoic acid [10]. T3 is believed to suppress TSH secretion by inducing the formation of a transferable substance [11] and by reducing the number of TRH receptors on thyrotrophs [12]. There is evidence that T3 also exerts a direct negative feedback on the hypothalamus [13].

The other major regulator of TSH secretion is the tripeptide TRH which is synthesized by peptidergic neurons, transferred into the basal hypothalamus and median eminence by axonal transport [14], and then to the anterior pituitary via the hypophyseal portal blood flow. TRH binds to specific receptors on thyrotroph plasma membrane and stimulates the release and synthesis of TSH chiefly through a rise in cytoplasmic free calcium concentration resulting from the activation of a TRH-dependent calcium channel [15] and release of calcium from other intracellular compartments [16], and through the hydrolysis of phosphatidylinositol [17].

Several other factors contribute to the control of TSH. Though minor, they may have important influences under particular conditions. The inhibitory effect of dopamine on TSH secretion has been well documented in physiological and pathological conditions: DA infusion [18], L-DOPA [19], or bromocriptine [20] administration lower basal and TRH-stimulated TSH levels in normals and hypothyroid patients, while DA receptor blocking agents increase serum TSH [21].

Somatostatin infusion has also been shown to inhibit basal and TRH-stimulated TSH levels in normal subjects [22] and in hypothyroid patients [23]. Conversely, the administration of antisomatostatin antisera to intact animals increases TSH response to cold stress [24].

Therefore, there is evidence for a physiological inhibitory role of TSH secretion of both dopamine and somatostatin that suggests their potential use in the treatment of hyperthyroidism due to inappropriate secretion of thyrotropin.

Glucocorticoid administration is known to lower basal and TRH-stimulated serum TSH [25], while estrogens and contraceptives seem to enhance serum TSH response to TRH [26, 27].

The possible role of catecholamines, serotonin, histamine, gamma-aminobutirric acid, opioids, melatonin, and prostaglandins as modulators of TSH secretion has been studied less extensively with conflicting results. Hence, as their physiological role is not yet well understood, they have not been employed for the study of primary disorders of TSH secretion.

Central hyperthyroidism

With the term "central hyperthyroidism" we define hyperthyroidism due to excessive thyrotropic stimulation of the thyroid gland by pituitary TSH. This syndrome is also referred to as "inappropriate secretion of thyrotropin" or "TSH-induced hyperthyroidism". Since the introduction of specific radioimmunoassay for TSH, it has become clear that the large majority of hyperthyroid patients showed suppressed TSH secretion, as thyroid hyperfunction is depending on thyroid overstimulation by thyroid-stimulating immunoglobulins (i. e. Graves' disease) or thyroid autonomy (i. e. autonomous hyperfunctioning uni- and multinodular goiter). By contrast, a small group of patients with thyrotoxicosis had inappropriately high serum TSH levels suggesting some derangement in thyrotropin regulation. Patients with central hyperthyroidism typically show signs and symptoms of hyperthyroidism, recurrent goiter, absence of ophthalmopathy and acropachy, high levels of circulating free thyroid hormones, in face of elevated or unsuppressed (within the "normal range") serum TSH.

Central hyperthyroidism is believed to be a rare clinical syndrome. However, although the number of case reports is rapidly expanding, its prevalence is presumably underestimated. In fact, TSH is generally not measured in hyperthyroid patients and most routine TSH assays are unable to discriminate suppressed from unsuppressed TSH. The very recent introduction of ultrasensitive immunoradiometric or immunochemiluminescent methods for TSH assay [28, 29] and reliable direct and absolute methods for the measurement of serum free thyroid hormone concentration [30], and their use as "first line" thyroid function tests [28, 31] will probably lead to the recognition of many other cases of central hyperthyroidism. These assays also will facilitate the distinction from other conditions that may be confused with TSH-induced hyperthyroidism (tab. 1). In fact, ultrasensitive TSH assay methods are able to clearly distinguish suppressed from unsuppressed TSH levels. Furthermore, they are unaffected by the presence of circulating either heterophilic antibodies (anti-rabbit or anti-bovine immunoglobulins) or anti-TSH antibodies – which often causes overestimation of serum TSH concentration by conventional RIA methods – (tab. 2) [31], and do not show crossreactions with circulating alpha and beta TSH subunits. The measurement of free thyroid hormones allows the distinction of patients with central

Table 1 Conditions that may be confused with central hyperthyroidism

1. Methodological interferences:
   a) Circulating anti-rabbit IgG antibodies
   b) Circulating anti-bovine TSH antibodies
   c) Circulating anti-iodothyronine autoantibodies
2. Alterations in thyroid hormone transport:
   a) Increase in serum binding proteins
   b) Familial dysalbuminemic hyperthyroxinemia
3. Inhibition of the conversion of T4 into T3:
   a) Idiopathic
   b) Nonthyroidal illnesses
   c) Drugs (amidoarone, iodinated contrast agents)
4. Others:
   a) L-T4 treated hypothyroid patients
   b) Neonatal period

Table 2 Reliability of immunoradiometric TSH assay in sera from hyperthyroid patients with either heterophilic or anti-TSH antibodies in which conventional radioimmunoassay gave misleading results

Antibodies (case n*)	TSH (IRMA) (μU/ml)	TSH (RIA)* (μU/ml)	F-T4 (pmol/l)	F-T3 (pmol/l)
Heterophilic				
(1)	< 0.07	5.2	42.5	19.8
(2)	< 0.07	4.4	26.4	14.8
(3)	< 0.07	4.2	25.6	9.7
Anti-TSH				
(4)	< 0.07	25.3	22.4	18.5
(5)	< 0.07	45.0	10.4	25.0
Normal range	0.15 – 6.0	< 0.5 – 7.0	9 – 20	3.8 – 8.9

*Bound: free separation carried out by second antibody.

hyperthyroidism from those with elevated total thyroid hormone levels due to quantitative or qualitative alterations of thyroid hormone transport proteins, or to the presence of circulating anti-iodothyronine autoantibodies [30].

It is worth mentioning that in about a fourth of patients with central hyperthyroidism, TSH levels do not exceed the "normal range". In some of these cases evidence for the secretion of TSH with enhanced biological activity has been given. In one patient we demonstrated that immunoreactive TSH (basal level: 1.2 μU/ml) partially prepurified by immunoaffinity chromatography showed a significantly higher biological activity, and had a smaller apparent molecular size than normal TSH [32]. In another patient with serum TSH level of 7.0 μU/ml, Bevan et al. [33] found a 4-fold increase in biological activity by cytochemical bioassay.

Although there are several potentially pathogenetic mechanisms able to cause TSH overproduction (outlined in tab. 3, according to the classification recently proposed by Brenner-Gati and Gershengorn [34] with minor modifications), only TSH excess due to pituitary TSH-secreting tumors (Class I A1 and I A2) and nonneoplastic pituitary hypersecretion of TSH due to selective pituitary resistance to thyroid hormone suppression (Class II A1) have been documented so far as clinical entities.

Table 3 Classification of central hyperthyroidism

Features	Class	Available cases
Neoplastic central hyperthyroidism	I A	76
Not associated with hypersecretion of other anterior pituitary hormones	I A1	49
Associated with hypersecretion of other anterior pituitary hormones	I A2	27
with GH hypersecretion	I A2a	19
with PRL hypersecretion	I A2b	7
with LH/FSH hypersecretion	I A2c	1
with ACTH hypersecretion*	I A2d	
Nonneoplastic central hyperthyroidism	II	36
Defective suppression of TSH secretion	II A	36
by thyroid hormones ("pituitary resistance")	II A1	36
by somatostatin*	II A2	
by dopamine*	II A3	
by other suppressors*	II A4	
Excessive stimulation of TSH secretion*	II B	
by TRH*	II B1	
by other stimulators*	II B2	

*Not yet documented in any report.

Neoplastic pituitary hypersecretion of TSH

Clinical aspects

To date 69 cases of neoplastic pituitary hypersecretion of TSH have been reported [32–94]. In addition, we recently observed another patient and received biological material and clinical informations of other 6 patients from different Centers (tab. 4). However, not all the patients described have been completely studied or are clearly classifiable. For example, the study by Wollesen et al. [67], is confined to radiological aspects, the patient described by Chanson et al. [70]

Table 4 Patient profile of 7 cases with neoplastic, and of 8 cases of nonneoplastic central hyperthyroidism (not yet published)

Author	Age	Sex	Previous therapy	Goiter	Sella alterat.	FT4 pmol/l	FT3 pmol/l	TSH μU/ml	alpha-subunit ng/ml	a:TSH molar ratio
Neoplastic										
Class I A1										
1. Bevan	60	F	MMI	–	yes	20.0	2.5	19.0	–	–
			131-I			4.3	2.8	118.6	4.8	0.2
			L-T4							
2. De Filippis	–	M	–	–	yes	82.8	34.8	11.8	6.9	3.6
3. Murat	58	F	ThyX	yes	yes	15.7	8.5	17.0	4.7	1.7
			MMI							
			131-I							
4. Pinchera	41	F	–	–	yes	46.5	16.7	4.5	1.8	2.4
Class I A2a										
5. Faglia	32	M	None	yes	yes	24.3	14.6	2.8	2.6	5.7
6. Bertoli	50	M	ThyX	yes	yes	34.9	15.0	2.7	3.5	8.0
			HyX							
			TCT							
Class I A2b										
7. Murat	60	F	MMI	no	yes	*16.9	*7.2	3.3	*10.2	*17.4
			Brc							
Nonneoplastic										
Class II A1										
1. Gruters	9	F	MMI	yes	no	24.4	34.7	#21.6	#1.2	0.3
2. Pinchera	28	F	–	yes	no	28.9	9.6	1.6	0.6	2.3
3. Pinchera	51	F	–	–	no	28.3	12.2	4.6	–	–
4. Faglia	29	F	MMI	yes	no	10.1	6.4	182.0	2.5	0.1
			ThyX							
5. De Filippis	–	F	–	–	no	15.8	9.7	23.0	0.6	0.2
6. De Filippis	50	F	–	–	no	23.3	12.3	8.8	0.9	0.6
7. Eber	34	F	MMI	yes	no	24.2	12.5	16.7	0.9	0.3
8. Wendel	5	F	–	–	–	49.0	22.2	1.0	–	–

* During bromocriptine treatment, # sample 30 min after TRH.
MMI = methimazole, 131-I = radioiodine, ThyX = thyroidectomy, Brc = bromocriptine.

presumably had a feedback tumor, and those described by Koide et al. [94] and by Scanlon et al. [73] were euthyroid and their diagnosis mainly based on histopathological aspects. Furthermore, in Brenner-Gati and Gershengorn's report [34] the case quoted from Carlson et al. [86] is the same as the one previously reported by Hill et al. [53], and the cases quoted from Emerson and Utiger [57, 58] and Connell et al. [62] are listed in the Class II A (nonneoplastic pituitary hypersecretion of TSH), while their classification is uncertain, and they probably should be classified as I A (pituitary tumors).

Clinical aspects, diagnostic procedures and therapeutic approaches will be described taking all the available data together.

Contrary to conventional hyperthyroidism, there is no preferential distribution among sexes (43 women, 33 men). The age range was 17 – 69 years. At the time of the study 38 of 63 had received previous treatments with antithyroid drugs, radioiodine, thyroid surgery alone or in combination; 4 patients were on thyroid hormone replacement therapy, and 10 patients had previous pituitary surgery or radiotherapy. Goiter was reported in 43 of 52 cases and frequently had recurred after subtotal thyroidectomy or radioiodine therapy. Exophthalmos occurred very seldom [35, 52, 60, 79, 92]; in two patients it was unilateral and in one of them caused by orbital invasion by the pituitary tumor [52]. Acropachy was never observed (tab. 5).

Table 5 Clinical and biochemical profile of patients with central hyperthyroidism

	Neoplastic (n = 76)	Nonneoplastic (n = 37)
Age (range)	17 – 69	4 – 80
Sex (F/M)	43/33	28/8
Goiter*	43/52	22/23
Sella alterations*	61/66	0/37
Exophthalmos*	5/76	0/37
Acropachy*	0/76	0/37
TSAb, TBI, or LATS*	1/26	1/11
TSH μU/ml (range)	1.2 – 480	1.0 – 182
alpha-subunit, ng/ml (range)	0.5 – 105	0.5 – 7.7
alpha-subunit : TSH molar ratio (range)	0.5 – 98	0.08 – 4.4
alpha-subunit : TSH molar ratio > 1*	35/38	5/20

* Presence of the sign/reported cases.

Hyperthyroidism was usually mild. In 2 cases [50, 86], tumoral inappropriate secretion of TSH was not accompanied by overt clinical hyperthyroidism in spite of high serum thyroid hormone levels, suggesting the coexistence of a peripheral resistance to thyroid hormone action. Two patients did not show any elevation in circulating thyroid hormone levels [73, 94]; in one of them, serum TSH was definitely high [94], suggesting a reduced biological activity of the secreted TSH.

Autoantibodies to thyroid antigens were generally not detectable. In particular, thyroid-stimulating immunoglobulins (TSI) were present in only 1 patient [60] who developed Graves' disease after pituitary surgery and irradiation. Another patient [35] had positive thyroid binding immunoglobulins (TBI), but undetectable TSI [38].

In some patients clinical manifestations of pituitary tumor (visual field defects, proptosis, headache) or partial hypopituitarism (amenorrhea, hypogonadism) frequently were the presenting symptoms. Nineteen patients with associated acromegaly [32, 37, 49, 53, 77 – 88, and two unpublished cases], and 7 with hyperprolactinemia [89 – 93 and one unpublished case] all showed typical signs and symptoms of GH or PRL excess, while one patient with associated TSH and FSH hypersecretion [94] did not show any disturbance referable to FSH excess.

Alterations of the sella profile at plain radiograms were present in all patients except five [57, 62, 63, 74, 86]. In one of them a tumor was subsequently demonstrated by pneumoencephalography [86], in one a microadenoma was detected at high resolution computed tomography [63], and in another one [74] at surgical exploration of the sella.

Hormonal studies

Serum TSH levels layed in a very wide range (1.2 – 480 μU/ml) and did not appear correlated with the severity of hyperthyroidism suggesting possible variations in TSH biological activity. TSH-β was generally within the normal range or slightly elevated, while disproportionately high alpha-subunit levels were present in most cases, resulting in an alpha-subunit: TSH molar ratio greater than 1 in 35 of 38 cases. The finding of alpha-subunit: TSH molar ratio in some cases as high as 98 (that means that the tumor secreted 98-fold more alpha-subunit than TSH) rises the question of whether some of these tumors actually are alpha-subunit secreting adenomas with associated TSH hypersecretion.

Table 6 Dynamic secretory testing in patients with central hyperthyroidism (Data are expressed as responsive/tested patient)

	Neoplastic (n = 76)	Nonneoplastic (n = 37)
TRH	17/66	31/31
ADA*	1/12	4/4
ATD*	14/20	9/11
T3	6/38	25/25
CS*	11/12	15/15
DAA*	7/31	6/6
SRIF	3/12	1/1

* ADA: antidopaminergic drugs, ATD: antithyroid drugs, CS: corticosteroids, DAA: dopamine agonists.

The regulatory control of TSH secretion is usually lost in patients with central hyperthyroidism due to pituitary TSH-secreting adenomas (tabs. 6, 7). The large majority of patients were unresponsive to TRH stimulation (49 of 66) and to T3 suppression (32 of 38). However, some of TRH responsive patients showed very sluggish responses [59, 73, 76], and one was on antithyroid treatment when tested [48]. In this last case TSH could have been released from normal thyrotrophs no longer suppressed by thyroid hormone excess. Only in 3 patients TSH elevation after TRH was associated to TSH suppression by T3 [55, 56, 76], suggesting that, exceptionally, some TSH-secreting adenomas are not completely

Table 7 TSH and *alpha-subunit* response to stimulatory and inhibitory tests, in 6 patients with neoplastic and 4 with nonneoplastic central hyperthyroidism (unpublished)

	Stimulatory tests		Inhibitory tests		
Authors	TRH	ADA*	T3	CS*	DAA*
Neoplastic					
Class I A1					
1. Bevan	no	no	no	–	no
	no	*no*	–	–	*no*
2. De Filippis	no	no	no	–	–
	no	*no*	–	–	–
3. Murat	no	no	no	yes	no
	no	*no*	*no*	*no*	*no*
Class I A2a					
5. Faglia	no	no	no	–	no
	no	*no*	*no*	–	*no*
6. Bertoli	no	no	no	–	no
	no	*no*	*no*	–	*no*
Class I A2b					
7. Murat	no	–	no	–	no
	yes	–	*no*	–	*no*
Nonneoplastic					
Class II A1					
1. Gruters	yes	–	yes	yes	–
	–	–	*yes*	*yes*	–
2. Pinchera	yes	yes	yes	–	yes
	yes	–	*yes*	–	–
3. Pinchera	yes	–	yes	–	–
	yes	–	*yes*	–	*no*
4. Faglia	yes	yes	yes	–	yes
	yes	*yes*	*yes*	–	*yes*

* ADA: antidopaminergic drugs, CS: corticosteroids, DAA: dopamine agonists.

autonomous. The reduction in serum thyroid hormone levels induced by antithyroid drug administration caused TSH to rise in 14 of 20 patients tested, probably reflecting a response of nontumorous thyrotrophs. Dopamine agonists were unable to suppress TSH secretion in 24 of 31 patients, and dopaminergic disinhibition by receptor blockers did not cause any TSH increase in 11 of 12 cases, while in the patient described by Chanson et al. [70] there was a paradoxical TSH increase after L-dopa. Somatostatin infusion was effective in reducing serum TSH levels in 3 of 12 cases, and corticosteroid administration induced a clear decrease in serum TSH in 11 of 12 patients. Smallridge et al. [81] reported that prednisone administration was able to inhibit TSH, but not alpha-subunit secretion in two patients, and claimed that this dissociated response may have diagnostic value. However, although this finding was confirmed in another patient (Murat, personal communication, tab. 7), this was not the case in other 4 patients [32, 37, 44, 58].

Growth hormone secretion dynamics in patients with central hyperthyroidism associated with acromegaly, although investigated in a small number of patients, has revealed variable patterns of response. Smallridge et al. [81] reported that in one acromegalic woman the secretion of TSH, alpha-subunit, GH, and PRL were unresponsive to TRH when the patient was hyperthyroid, while TRH-responsive when she became hypothyroid on antithyroid drugs. Lamberg et al. [85] described a patient with very variable responses of TSH and GH to TRH-stimulation carried out on several occasions. In that patient GH and TSH were not reduced by long-term bromocriptine administration, while both hormones were inhibited by somatostatin infusion. In one acromegalic patient [32] alpha-subunit responses to dynamic tests paralleled those of GH rather than those of TSH: after TRH administration TSH did not increase, while GH and alpha subunit showed a marked increment. The same pattern of response was observed when TRH was injected during somatostatin infusion, and when sulpiride was administered during dopamine infusion. Two other patients we studied did not increase TSH, alpha-subunit, or GH after the three above mentioned tests.

In patients with central hyperthyroidism associated with hyperprolactinemia the two hormones may behave differently, probably reflecting differences in tumor cell receptors. Horn et al. [89] reported no increase in TSH and PRL levels after TRH adminstration and a significant suppression of both hormones by dopaminergic agonists. In two patients, described by Werner et al. [92], PRL, but not TSH, was stimulated by TRH and inhibited by L-dopa. One patient (Murat, personal communication, tab. 7) did not increase TSH, alpha-subunit, or PRL after TRH administration.

Hypothalamic deafferentation by the impingement of an expanding tumor, might explain the slightly high serum PRL levels found in some patients. In fact in some of them no lactotrophs were found into the excised tumor [34, 59, 73].

Morphological studies

TSH-secreting adenomas are characteristically chromophobic or basophilic with variable cytoplasmatic PAS positivity. At electron microscopy examination the salient features include the presence of well developed Golgi apparatus and RER, and very abundant mitochondria. The secretory granules are very small (80 – 180 nm) and lined up along the cytoplasmatic membranes [55, 56, 84, 91].

TSH and other anterior pituitary hormone associated hypersecretions are generally due to mixed tumors. Very recently, utilizing the double gold immunostaining technique, we described in a pituitary tumor surgically removed from a patient with acromegaly and central hyperthyroidism [32] the presence of secretory granules positive for both GH and alpha-subunit in the majority of the adenomatous cells, while few cells were positive for TSH-β as well as for GH and alpha-subunit. However, specific immunostaining for GH was detected in TSH-secreting tumors causing [84, 85] or not [51, 55] acromegaly, and immunostaining with specific anti-TSH and anti-PRL antisera was observed not only in TSH-secreting tumors associated to hyperprolactinemia [89], but also in the presence of normal levels of serum PRL [55, 91].

In vitro studies

In vitro studies have been carried out in a limited number of patients. Yovos et al. [52] reported that TRH was unable to stimulate TSH release from cultured tumor cells, while in another study [61] in vitro TSH secretion from tumoral thyrotrophs was stimulated by TRH, not affected by T3 and inhibited by dopamine. Dopaminergic receptors were identified on cell membranes from a TSH-secreting adenoma [70].

The few available data concerning mixed adenomas suggest a wide variability of responsiveness to different stimuli *in vitro*. Lamberts et al. [87] reported that TSH and GH secretion by cultured cells from a TSH/GH-secreting adenoma were stimulated by TRH and GnRH, but unaffected by bromocriptine. TSH release was inhibited both by T3 and dexamethasone. In a TSH/PRL-secreting tumor Jaquet et al. [93] observed a significant inhibition of the two hormones by T3 and bromocriptine and a lack of effect of TRH on TSH release.

We recently reported *in vitro* hormone secretion studies in one pure TSH-secreting adenoma [69]. In short term incubation of tissue fragments, the TSH adenoma secreted large amount of TSH, alpha-subunit and TSH-β, which were inhibited by dopamine in a dose dependent manner. However, dopamine was more effective in inhibiting TSH and TSH-β than alpha subunit (−53%, −55%, and −19%, respectively, at DA 10^{-7} M). In the same tumor similar results were obtained with somatostatin: in fact, SRIF (10^{-7} M) suppressed TSH and TSH-β by about 40% and alpha-subunit by 13%. In this adenoma, SRIF inhibited adenylate cyclase activity in a dose dependent manner, while dopamine did not affect adenylate cyclase activity, suggesting different intracellular mechanisms involved in the control of TSH secretion by the two agents. We also studied *in vitro* hormone secretion in two TSH- and GH-secreting adenomas. These tumors released large amounts of TSH, TSH-β, alpha-subunit and GH which were inhibited by DA and SRIF in one case and unaffected in the other one (tab. 8). In both cases a good correlation between *in vivo* and *in vitro* responsiveness to DA and SRIF was observed.

Table 8. Effects of SRIF and DA on hormone release (per mg prot. in 30 min) from 2 cultured TSH/GH-secreting pituitary adenomas

	baseline	SRIF 10^{-7} M	DA 10^{-7} M
Case 1			
TSH (μU)	19.3 ± 3.1	7.2 ± 1.0*	7.0 ± 1.2*
alpha-subunit (ng)	66.3 ± 5.0	40.1 ± 3.0*	45.0 ± 2.8*
GH (ng)	4.1 ± 0.9	1.8 ± 0.3*	2.0 ± 0.5*
Case 2			
TSH (μU)	5.0 ± 1.0	5.0 ± 1.5	4.9 ± 1.0
alpha-subunit (ng)	28.2 ± 6.2	29.2 ± 2.0	30.2 ± 5.0
GH (ng)	10.4 ± 1.2	9.8 ± 2.0	10.1 ± 1.5

* $P < 0.01$

Treatment

Most patients with neoplastic TSH-induced hyperthyroidism received therapies directed to the thyroid gland in order to control thyroid hyperfunction. However, conventional treatments may cause TSH to rise and presumably favor tumor expansion, while the obvious goal of the therapy of neoplastic central hyperthyroidism is to normalize TSH secretion.

Pituitary surgery or irradiation or both have been extensively used. Nineteen out of 62 patients were cured by pituitary surgery, although 3 patients required two operations [59, 61, 63]. Two patients of 5 who had radiotherapy as the initial treatment were cured [35, 36]. Other 7 patients of 17 unsuccessfully operated upon were cured by radiant therapy [37, 39, 44, 59, 71, 81, 87]. Thus, from the available data, the success rate appears to be about 33% with surgery and 41% with combined surgical and radiant therapy.

Although most patients were unresponsive to acute administration of dopaminergic agents, longterm bromocriptine treatment was tried in 13 cases: clinical improvement and reduction of TSH and thyroid hormone level occurred in 3 patients [62, 66, 76].

Table 9 Effects of somatostatin analog SMS 201-995 (100 µg s.c., t.i.d. for 5 days) on serum TSH, alpha-subunit, free-T4 and free-T3 levels in 2 patients with neoplastic (cases 1 and 2) and 2 with nonneoplastic (cases 3 and 4) central hyperthyroidism

Hormone	Case	Baseline	Day 1	Day 2	Day 3	Day 4	Day 5
TSH	1.	2.0	0.8	0.4	0.3	0.3	0.2
(µU/ml)	2.	4.3	1.0	1.1	0.9	0.9	1.4
	3.	4.5	1.7	1.4	1.8	1.6	2.4
	4.	32.2	26.4	27.2	27.8	29.8	17.0
alpha-subunit	1.	2.8	0.9	0.5	0.7	0.5	0.4
(ng/ml)	2.	1.1	0.8	0.5	0.2	0.2	0.3
	3.	1.1	1.2	1.7	0.9	1.0	0.8
	4.	2.4	2.3	1.9	2.4	2.6	2.9
F-T4	1.	40.1	41.7	20.4	23.2	20.2	16.4
(pmol/l)	2.	23.7	25.2	21.0	18.8	19.2	14.9
	3.	20.1	19.0	17.1	14.2	14.5	12.5
	4.	14.0	14.2	13.8	16.0	15.5	16.5
F-T3	1.	21.0	15.6	6.6	7.6	6.8	6.9
(pmol/l)	2.	11.7	8.9	6.3	4.8	4.5	2.8
	3.	9.8	7.4	5.1	5.1	5.2	4.8
	4.	9.8	8.8	8.6	7.3	8.8	8.7

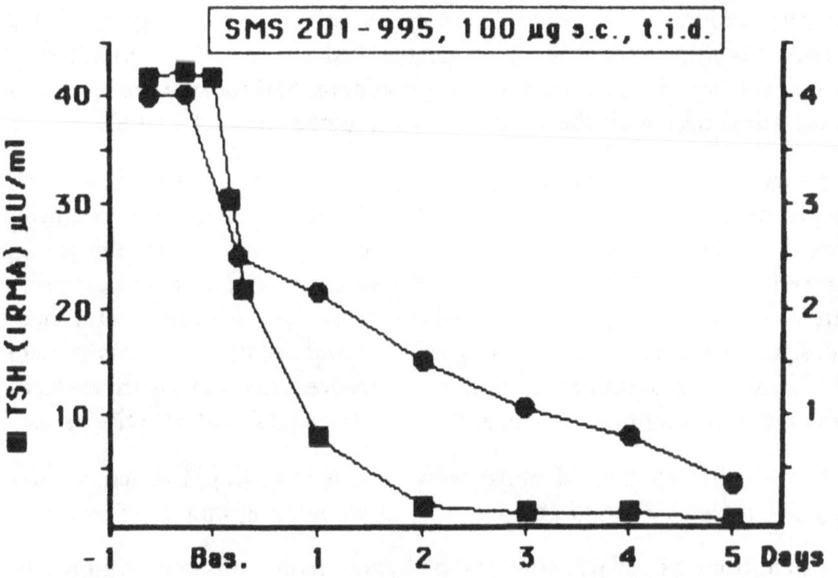

Fig. 1 Effect of long-acting somatostatin analogue SMS 201-995 on serum TSH and alpha-subunit levels in one patient with TSH-secreting pituitary adenoma.

We recently administered the long-acting somatostatin analogue SMS 201-995 (100 μg s.c., t.i.d. for 5 consecutive days) to 2 patients unsuccessfully treated by pituitary surgery. A marked decrease in serum TSH, alpha-subunit, and thyroid hormone levels occurred, which was evident after the first injection and persisted throughout the whole period of treatment (tab. 9). SMS 201-995 also provoked a dramatic fall in TSH and alpha-subunit levels in another patient who previously underwent total thyroidectomy and was on L-T4 replacement therapy (fig. 1). If these preliminary results will be confirmed in a larger number of cases and for more prolonged periods of treatment, long-acting somatostatin analogues will represent a valid therapeutic tool for the management of patients with neoplastic central hyperthyroidism.

Nonneoplastic pituitary hypersecretion of TSH

Clinical aspects

Clinical features of 28 patients with nonneoplastic TSH-induced hyperthyroidism have been reported so far [95 – 111]. In addition we received biological material and clinical informations concerning 7 other patients from several Centers in Europe, and observed directly another one case (tabs. 4 and 7). Differently from Brenner-Gati and Gershengorn [34], we excluded the patients reported by Emerson and Utiger [57, 58] and Connel et al. [62], as they presumably had a pituitary tumor, and the case described by Salmeron De Diego et al. [99] who showed features compatible with generalized peripheral resistance to thyroid hormone. Clinical aspects, diagnostic procedures and therapeutic approaches will be described taking all the available data together (tabs. 5 and 6).

Although the disease appears to be more frequent in women than in men, the female : male ratio (about 2 : 1) is quite different from the one in conventional hyperthyroidism (about 5 : 1). Some cases occurred in the same family, suggesting a genetic disease [101, Pinchera, De Filippis, personal communication]. At the time of the study 20 patients had received previous treatment with antithyroid drugs, radioiodine, or thyroid surgery. Thyroid enlargement was present in 22 of 23 cases and a history of goiter recurrence after partial thyroidectomy or radioiodine was frequent. None of the patient had ophthalmopathy or acropachy.

Autoantibodies to thyroid antigens were generally not detected. In particular only one patient [97] had positive thyroid stimulating immunoglobulins.

No alterations of sella profile nor of hypothalamic-pituitary region have been documented at radiological examination in patient with nonneoplastic central hyperthyroidism.

Hormonal studies

Basal serum TSH levels varied widely (1.0 – 182 μU/ml) and did not appear correlated with either the severity of the hyperthyroid state or the concentration of circulating thyroid hormones, suggesting possible variations of biological activity. TSH-β levels were within the normal range or slightly elevated. Generally, alpha-subunit was in the normal range resulting in an alpha-subunit: TSH molar ratio < 1. The only exceptions were 5 patients [105, 108, 109] and 1 unpublished cases listed in table 4).

TSH response to TRH was qualitatively normal in all (31/31) patients, but frequently exaggerated. TSH was lowered by T3 administration in all (25/25) cases. However, TSH secretion was not fully suppressed in several cases, and, contrary to normal subjects, TSH response to TRH persisted during T3 administration [100]. A clear TSH elevation was caused in 9 of 11 patients by antithyroid drug-induced reduction of circulating thyroid hormone. Dopamine agonist lowered serum TSH levels in all the patients tested (6/6), while dopaminergic disinhibition by specific receptor blockers elicited a marked TSH increase in 4 of 4 patients tested ([104,111] and 2 unpublished cases shown in table 7). This last finding suggests that in these patients the central dopaminergic tone may be enhanced [111]. Somatostatin infusion caused TSH to fall in the only 1 patient tested. Serum TSH was lowered by glucocorticoid administration in all (15/15) patients.

Treatment

The therapeutical approach to patients with nonneoplastic central hyperthyroidism is still debated. Conventional treatments for controlling hyperthyroidism are merely palliative. Furthermore, therapies directed to the thyroid gland cause TSH to rise and carry the potential risk that thyrotroph hyperplasia may progress to tumor.

Although TSH secretion is reduced by glucocorticoid administration, we do not recommend longterm corticosteroid treatment that may cause the appearance of cushigoid features and hypothalamic-pituitary-adrenal axis suppression.

There are no reports concerning propranolol administration that theoretically might ameliorate the cardiac function and hyperthyroidism by reducing the peripheral conversion of T4 into T3, probably without affecting TSH secretion.

Bromocriptine has been reported to normalize TSH secretion in 1 [107] of 11 cases [103 – 108, 111, and 4 unpublished cases]. In our hands it was ineffective in controlling TSH secretion in one case, as an escape occurred after an initial decrease of serum TSH [104].

The etiopathogenetic hypothesis that the reduced sensitivity to thyroid hormone at the pituitary level [95] might be mediated by impaired intrapituitary conversion of T4 into T3, and the finding that T3 administration is able to decrease TSH secretion, prompted Roesler et al. [101] to treat 3 patients with a single morning dose of 25 – 50 μg T3. This treatment was able to reduce TSH secretion and to ameliorate hyperthyroidism. However, serum T3 concentration was frankly above the normal range for 6 – 8 hr a day after T3 ingestion, maintaining a mild hyperthyroid state.

We recently reported [104] very favorable results by administering the sodium salt of 3,5,3′-triiodothyroacetic acid (TRIAC) to one patient. This compound, a natural metabolite of T3, is practically free of peripheral metabolic activity, but exerts a potent inhibitory action at the pituitary level. After our first observation, a dramatic fall in serum TSH levels followed by diminution of circulating thyroid hormones and full remission of clinical conditions has been reported in other two cases [108, 109] and observed in 2 unpublished patients (tab. 10).

Table 10 Effect of TRIAC administration on serum TSH, free-T4 and free-T3 levels in 5 patients with nonneoplastic central hyperthyroidism

Case	Ref. [ ]	Dose (mg/day)	Duration (weeks)	Goiter size reduct.	*TSH (μU/ml) Before	*TSH (μU/ml) During	*F-T4 (pmol/l) Before	*F-T4 (pmol/l) During	*F-T3 (pmol/l) Before	*F-T3 (pmol/l) During
1.	[104]	2.1	(160)	+ +	14.0	5.0	25.5	14.1	13.8	7.1
2.	[108]	2.8	(2)	?	10.9	< 1.0	23.8	3.0	–	–
3.	unpubl.	2.1	(58)	+ +	180.0	14.0	–	–	–	–
4.	[109]	3.0	(3)	+ +	12.9	4.0	45.6	16.0	21.5	6.5
5.	unpubl.	2.1	(25)	+ + +	3.0	0.2	28.3	13.1	13.4	4.9

* Determinations made in our Laboratory.

As somatostatin is a well known physiological inhibitor of TSH secretion, we carried out a short-term therapeutic trial by adminstering the novel long-acting somatostatin analogue SMS 201 – 995 (100 μg s.c., t.i.d. for 5 days) to 2 patients (tab. 9). In one of them serum TSH levels promptly fell by 45 – 70% and circulating FT4 and FT3 normalized, while in the other one serum TSH remained elevated during the first 4 days of treatment and decreased by 47% only on the last day of treatment.

Conclusions

The number of patients with central hyperthyroidism has increased in recent years, and will probably continue to expand thanks to the routinary use of the new ultrasensitive and highly specific methods of TSH and free thyroid hormone assay as first line tests in hyperthyroidism. Inappropriate secretion of TSH should be suspected in all patients showing elevated levels of free thyroid hormones and unsuppressed TSH. The clinical importance of discriminating this syndrome from conventional hyperthyroidism is evident, as their management is different.

The radiological study of the sella region, including high resolution computed tomography, and the investigation of TSH responsiveness to stimulatory (TRH) and inhibitory (T3) stimuli are of great help in differentiating TSH-induced hyperthyroidism due to TSH-secreting pituitary adenomas (generally unresponsive) from nonneoplastic disorder (generally responsive).

As in patients with TSH-secreting pituitary adenomas, alpha-subunit is hypersecreted, the finding of an alpha-subunit : TSH molar ratio greater than 1 will favor the diagnosis of neoplastic central hyperthyroidism. However, attention should be payed to the possible contribution of LH and FSH, the alpha-subunit of which is identical to that of TSH, in enhancing alpha-subunit levels. In this respect, the absolute alpha-subunit levels should be compared to appropriate normal control groups matched for age and sex, and the alpha-subunit : TSH molar ratio should be recalculated after estrogen-induced gonadotropin suppression in patients who are in the menopause.

Pituitary surgery, followed by pituitary irradiation in case of surgical failure represents the therapy of choice for patients with TSH-secreting pituitary adenomas. An additional approach could be bromocriptine chronic administration. Preliminary very promising results have been obtained administering the novel long-acting somatostatin analogue SMS 201-995.

The administration of low dose once a day T3, or of thyroid hormone derivatives with strong inhibitory effect on TSH secretion, but poor peripheral thyromimetic activity (e. g. TRIAC) seems to be a valid therapeutic approach in nonneoplastic TSH-induced hyperthyroidism.

Central hypothyroidism

Partial thyroid atrophy and reduced secretion of thyroid hormones result from lack of stimulation by TSH of an otherwise intrinsically normal thyroid gland. This condition is currently termed "central hypothyroidism" and may occur as a consequence of anatomical or functional abnormalities of the anterior pituitary ("pituitary hypothyroidism" or "secondary hypothyroidism"), the hypothalamus ("hypothalamic hypothyroidism" or "tertiary hypothyroidism") or both.

Undetectable or low-normal serum TSH levels in association with low serum concentrations of thyroid hormones, absence of antithyroid autoantibodies, and adequate responsiveness of the thyroid gland to exogenous TSH administration are typical of both pituitary and hypothalamic hypothyroidism. Serum TSH response to TRH has been assumed to be a useful criterion for the distinction of the two forms: absent or impaired TSH responses have been considered characteristic of pituitary hypothyroidism, whereas positive (and frequently delayed or exaggerated and/or prolonged) TSH responses have been considered indicative of hypothalamic hypothyroidism. Moreover, normal or even slightly high serum levels of immunoreactive TSH, associated with exaggerated responses to TRH have been frequently found in hypothyroid patients with hypothalamic hypothyroidism, and evidence has recently been provided that secretion of biologically inactive TSH occurs in these patients.

Central hypothyroidism is frequently accompanied by decreased secretion of other anterior pituitary hormones.

Although central hypothyroidism is a rare clinical entity, its recognition is of clinical importance as replacement therapy with thyroid hormone alone is inadequate for correction of other associated hormone deficiencies. In particular, thyroid hormone treatment carries the risk of causing acute adrenocortical failure in the case of associated ACTH deficiency.

Clinical aspects

As different hypothalamic and/or pituitary disorders may underlie central hypothyroidism, the resulting clinical features may be overshadowed by manifestations of gonadal, adrenocortical and somatotropic insufficiency, the extreme situation being overt panhypopituitarism. In this context, the severity of hypothyroidism may widely vary: from a mild subclinical disorder to severe myxedema, but generally, hypothyroidism is more commonly mild. Although essentially similar to those of primary thyroid failure, there are several features which help to distinguish central from primary hypothyroidism. The skin is pale and cool, but not as coarse and dry, as in primary hypothyroidism, the texture of hair is thinner, the enlargement of the tongue is absent, the coarseness of the voice less pronounced, and the heart tends to be small.

Pituitary adenomas are the most frequent causes of central hypothyroidism, accounting for about 50% of the cases in several large series [112 – 114]. Various degrees of central (either "pituitary" or "hypothalamic") hypothyroidism may result from compression of nontumorous portion of the pituitary, involvement of the pituitary stalk and hypothalamus by suprasellar extension of the adenoma, and interference with portal blood flow.

Craniopharingyoma is a relatively frequent cause of central hypothyroidism, especially in the younger age group. In a recent series, 13 of 20 patients with craniopharyngioma had central hypothyroidism and 6 had abnormal TSH response to TRH [117]. Meningiomas, glyomas, breast or lung carcinoma deposits in the pituitary or hypothalamus, may also cause central hypothyroidism. If not present initially, central hypothyroidism may result from surgical therapy or irradiation [118] of pituitary, or parasellar, or hypothalamic tumors, or in patients submitted to pituitary surgery or stalk section for other diseases (such as breast carcinoma or diabetic retinopathy [119, 120], or to external radiotherapy for tumors of nasopharinx or paranasal sinues [121, 122]. Postpartum pituitary necrosis (Sheehan's syndrome) [123], pituitary necrosis due to other causes [119], or hypothalamic lesions consequent to severe head injuries [124 – 126], hypophysitis [127], granulomatous lesions [128], histiocytosis [129], and hemochromatosis [130] may also result in central hypothyroidism. Central hypothyroidism has also been described in patients with pituitary aplasia or hypoplasia [131], and in familial panhypopituitarism [132]. Idiopathic hypopituitarism is a relatively frequent cause of central hypothyroidism. In a recent series [133] 26 of 105 patients with TSH deficiency had idiopathic hypopituitarism. Birth trauma is probably implicated as etiological factor because of the frequent occurrence of breech or vacuum extraction delivery in the history of these patients [134].

Isolated TSH deficiency has been reported in several cases [135 – 138], sometimes associated with pseudohypoparathyroidism [139].

Functional alterations in TSH secretion have been observed in a number of situations. Transient central hypothyroidism may occur in euthyroid subjects after withdrawal of prolonged thyroid suppression treatment with thyroid hormones [140 – 142], or in patients operated upon for toxic uninodular goiter. Prolonged treatment with hGH for pituitary dwarfism may result in reversible central hypothyroidism, presumably mediated by reactive somatostatin hypersecretion [143]. The extremely low levels of circulating thyroid hormones found in critically ill patients receiving dopamine have been partially attributed to the suppressive effect of dopamine on pituitary TSH secretion.

Hormonal studies

This chapter will be confined to studies concerning the hypothalamic-pituitary-thyroid function, with particular emphasis on biologically inactive TSH.

Measurement of free thyroid hormones has shown that serum free-T4 levels are clearly in the hypothyroid range in almost all patients with central hypothyroidism, while free-T3 levels may often be within the normal range [133].

Basal serum TSH concentration are inappropriately low with respect to the decreased serum thyroid hormone levels, and are undetectable or in the low normal range in the majority of patients [144 – 152]. However, in a remarkable proportion of cases serum TSH is in the upper normal range or slightly elevated

[113–115, 153–155], though it fails to reach the concentrations which are commonly found in patients with primary hypothyroidism having a comparable reduction of serum T4. This finding could not be explained by the coexistence of hypothalamic-pituitary defect and primary thyroid failure as these patients showed an adequate response to exogenous TSH [115, 155] and had no evidence of thyroid autoimmunity [115]. Therefore, it has been suggested that in such patients hypothyroidism may result from the secretion of thyrotropin with reduced biological activity [113–115, 152–157].

The study of TSH response to TRH has shown that patients with central hypothyroidism may exhibit different types of response with respect to the magnitude of TSH increase (absent, impaired, normal, or exaggerated) and to the pattern of the response curve (regular, delayed, or prolonged) [115]. However, a clearcut difference between patients with hypothalamic or pituitary anatomical lesions cannot be found. In fact, although absent or impaired TSH responses occur more frequently in patients with pituitary lesions [112, 115, 147, 148, 149], these also occur in some cases with hypothalamic disorders without apparent pituitary involvement [114, 150]. Conversely, normal or even exaggerated TSH response with delayed or prolonged response curve are usually exhibited by hypothyroid patients with hypothalamic disorders [115, 150–152, 158, 159], but are also found in patients with documented primary pituitary disease with no apparent hypothalamic involvement [113, 114, 117, 150, 153]. In other words, the pattern of TSH response to TRH reflects more a functional setting than the site of anatomical lesion. It should be noted that some euthyroid patients with hypothalamic pituitary disorders also show abnormal TSH responses to TRH. Whether these abnormal responses may be predictive of subsequent development of central hypothyroidism still remains to be ascertained [112, 113, 153].

As before mentioned, the finding of slightly elevated serum immunoreactive TSH has raised the hypothesis that some patients may secrete TSH with reduced biological activity. In support to this hypothesis we showed that in 25 patients with central hypothyroidism and normal or increased TSH responses to TRH, the T3 response to endogenous thyrotropin after TRH administration was significantly lower than in euthyroid patients [160]. Furthermore, two independent groups of workers [115, 161] found that serum thyrotropin from a total of seven patients with idiopathic hypothalamic hypothyroidism showed reduced biological activity as assessed by cytochemical bioassay [162]. These results were recently confirmed and extended in other 7 patients by measuring the adenylate cyclase stimulating activity of immunoreactive TSH, pre-purified by immunoaffinity chromatography, on human thyroid membrane preparation. The bioactivity to immunoreactivity ratio (B/I) was less than 0.2 in six patients and 0.9 in one, in contrast to the ratios (4.5 ± 1.2) in 4 patients with primary hypothyroidism [163] (fig. 2). The diminished biological activity has been demonstrated to result

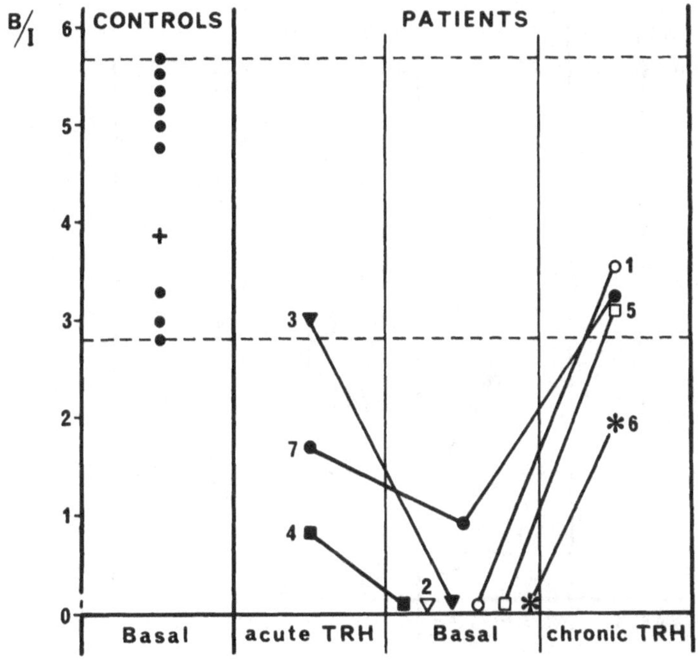

Fig. 2 Bio- to immuno-reactivity ratio of immunopurified serum TSH, before and after acute or chronic TRH administration, in 7 patients with hypothalamic hypothyroidism.

from a failure of TSH to interact with plasma membrane receptor. In fact, no radioreceptor-binding activity of immunopurified TSH was found in 4 patients. The radioreceptor-binding activity to immunoreactivity ratio (R/I) was less than 0.15, in contrast to that (1.7 ± 0.8) in 6 controls with primary hypothyroidism [163] (fig. 3).

The molecular basis for such reduced biological activity has not yet been elucidated. A defect in the glycosylation of TSH moleculate could be implicated, as differences in the biological activity of certain forms of bovine and mouse TSH have been reported to be associated with variations in their carbohydrate composition [8]. It has been suggested that TRH is necessary to produce TSH of full biological potency [155, 163, 164], as indicated by the finding of normalized B/I and R/I ratios in sera from patients with hypothalamic hypothyroidism and bioinactive TSH after the administration of TRH for several weeks [163], accompanied by an increase in serum thyroid hormone concentration [163, 164]. Therefore, the secretion of bioinactive TSH could be due to the lack of TRH. We have recently reported that patients with central hypothyroidism and bioinactive TSH had an excess of circulating TSH-β [164] resulting in a TSH-β : alpha-subunit molar ratio higher than in normal and primary hypothyroid controls,

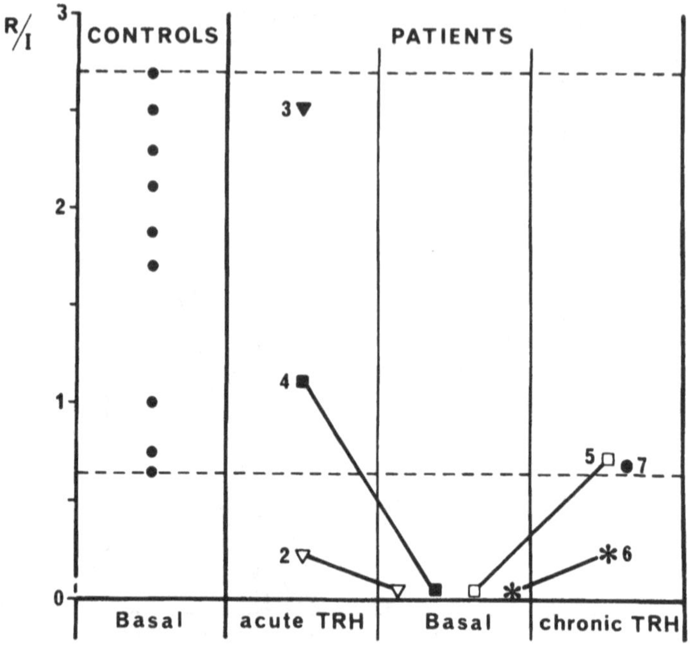

Fig. 3 Radioreceptor to immuno-reactivity ratio of immunopurified serum TSH, before and after acute or chronic TRH administration, in 7 patients with hypothalamic hypothyroidism.

which normalized after TRH administration for several weeks. Hence, the question may be raised of whether this reflects some abnormality in assembling TSH molecule that might be corrected by TRH administration.

No major alterations of bioinactive TSH apparent molecular size after Sephadex G 100 gel-filtration have been reported [115]. However, we recently reconsidered whether more refined chromatographic studies would have revealed any molecular abnormality. We carried out gel-filtration studies utilizing Superose 6B columns followed by a re-chromatography of the collected peak fractions on Ultrapac TSK G 2000 SW. By this procedure bioinactive TSH peak appeared frankly anticipated with respect to standard TSH and TSH from patients with primary thyroid failure [165] (fig. 4). Interestingly, this abnormality disappeared in sera from chronically TRH treated patients.

Taken together, the data obtained after chronic TRH administration suggest that TRH regulates not only the secretion of TSH, but also its specific and conformational features required for hormone action.

The immunoreactive TSH of these patients has been shown to respond like normal TSH to agents known to modulate TSH secretion at the pituitary or hypothalamic level. In fact, basal and TRH stimulated TSH were completely

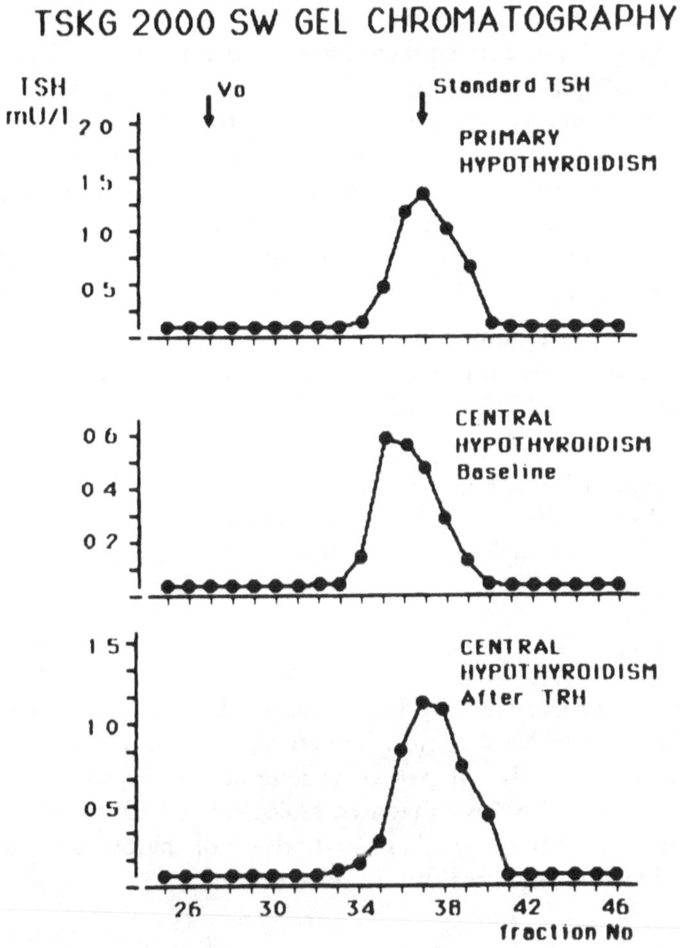

Fig. 4 Normalization of serum TSH elution pattern after chronic TRH administration in hypothalamic hypothyroidism.

suppressed by T3 and blunted by dexamethasone or dopaminergic agents [115]. However, in some cases TSH did not increase after dopaminergic blockade by domperidone, suggesting that a dopamine defect may contribute to the slight elevation of basal TSH [166]. This last finding may be of interest considering that, in patients with hypothalamic-pituitary disorders, a defect of other hypothalamic factors controlling TSH secretion may also be involved.

Treatment

The therapy of central hypothyroidism is directed at the restoration of euthyroidism and the correction of any hypofunction of the other endocrine glands resulting from anterior pituitary hormone deficiencies. There is general consensus that replacement therapy with L-thyroxine should be started with low doses and then progressively increased up to 1.8 – 2.2 μg/Kg body weight and adjusted according to its peripheral effects and measurement of serum thyroid hormone concentration. Contrary to primary thyroid failure, the estimation of serum TSH is not a useful guideline for adjusting thyroid hormone dosage. In patients with impaired hypothalamic-pituitary-adrenal axis, L-thyroxine therapy should not be given before a full replacement corticosteroid treatment is initiated, because of the possible precipitation of an adrenal crisis.

There are no reasons for treating patients with central hypothyroidism with bovine TSH, in view of its cost, scanty supply, possible allergic reactions, development of anti-bovine TSH antibodies, and requirement for intramuscular administration.

In patients with hypothalamic hypothyroidism, treatment with oral TRH has been demonstrated to be effective [163, 164] in short-term trials. However, the possibility of inducing thyrotroph receptor desensitization with long-term therapy should be considered.

Conclusions

In recent years many progresses have been done in the knowledge of central hypothyroidism. They have been of great interest not only on clinical, but also on pathophysiological grounds. Of particular interest are the recent findings concerning the secretion of TSH with reduced biological activity and the notion that TRH regulates not only the synthesis and release of thyrotropin, but also its conformational features required for hormone action.

Acknowledgments

We are indebted to the National Pituitary Agency (NIADDK, Bethesda, Md. USA) for the gift of TSH-β and alpha-subunit and related antisera, and Dr. E. Del Pozo (Sandoz Ltd. Basel, Switzerland) for the gift of SMS 201-995. We also thank Prof. A. Pinchera (University of Pisa, Italy), Dr. A. Bertoli (Catholic University, Rome, Italy), Dr. A. Gruters (Free University of Berlin), Dr. A. Murat (University of Nantes, France), Dr. J. S. Bevan (Oxford, U.K.), Dr. V. De Filippis (Ospedale Mauriziano, Torino Italy), Dr. O. Eber (University of Graz, Austria), and Dr. U. Wendel (University of Düsseldorf, FRG), for sending us biological specimens from their patients.

References

[1] Morley, J. E.: Neuroendocrine control of thyrotropin secretion. Endocr. Rev. 2 (1981) 396 – 436.

[2] Hershman, J. M., A. E. Pekary: Regulation of thyrotropin secretion. In: The pituitary gland (H. Imura, ed.), pp. 149 – 188, Raven Press, New York 1985.

[3] Fiddes, J. C., H. M. Goodman: The gene encoding the common alpha subunit of the four human glycoprotein hormones. J. Mol. Appl. Genet. **1** (1981) 3–18.
[4] Pekonen, F., B. D. Weintraub: Thyrotropin receptors and bovine thyroid membranes: two types with different affinities and specificities. Endrocrinology **105** (1979) 352–359.
[5] Kourides, I. A., N. C. Vamvakopoulos, G. M. Maniatis: mRNA-directed biosynthesis of alpha- and beta subunits of thyrotropin, J. Biol. Chem. **254** (1979) 11106–11110.
[6] Weintraub, B. D., B. S. Stannard, D. Linnekin, et al.: Relationship of glycosilation to the novo thyroid stimulating hormone biosynthesis and secretion by mouse pituitary tumor cells. J. Biol. Chem. **255** (1980) 5715–5723.
[7] Kourides, I. A., B. D. Weintraub, E. C. Ridgway, et al.: Pituitary secretion of free alpha and beta subunit of human thyrotropin in patients with thyroid disorders. J. Clin. Endocrinol. Metab. **40** (1975) 872–885.
[8] Joshi, L. R., B. D. Weintraub: Naturally occurring forms of thyrotropin with low bioactivity and altered carbohydrate content act as competitive antagonists to more bioactive forms. Endocrinology **113** (1983) 2145–2154.
[9] Snyder, P. J., R. D. Utiger: Inhibition of thyrotropin response to thyrotropin-releasing hormone by small quantities of thyroid hormones. J. Clin. Invest. **5** (1972) 2077–2084.
[10] Larsen, P. R., T. E. Dick, B. P. Markovitz, et al.: Inhibition of intrapituitary thyroxine to 3,5,3' triiodothyronine conversion prevents the acute suppression of thyrotropin release by thyroxine in hypothyroid rats. J. Clin. Invest. **64** (1979) 117–128.
[11] Melmed, S., J. Park, J. M. Hershman: Triiodothyronine induces a transferable factor which suppresses TSH secretion in mouse thyrotropic tumor cells. Biochem. Biophys. Res. Commun. **98** (1981) 1022–1028.
[12] Gershengorn, M. C.: Bihormonal regulation of the thyrotropin-releasing hormone receptor in mouse pituitary thyrotropic tumor cells in culture. J. Clin. Invest. **62** (1978) 937–943.
[13] Belchetz, P. E., G. Gredley, D. Bird, et al.: Regulation of thyrotropin secretion by negative feedback on tri-iodothyronine on the hypothalamus. J. Endocrinol. **76** (1978) 439–448.
[14] Palkovits, M., R. L. Eskay, M. J. Brownstein: The course of thyrotropin-releasing hormone fibers to the median eminence in rats. Endocrinology **110** (1982) 1526–1534.
[15] Gershengorn, M. C.: Thyrotropin-releasing hormone. Mol. Cell. Biochem. **45** (1981) 163–179.
[16] Snyder, G., Z. Naor, C. P. Fawcett, et al.: Action of thyrotropin-releasing hormone on mammotrophs and thyrotrophs. Am. J. Physiol. **241** (1981) E298–304.
[17] Rebecchi, M. J., R. Kolesnick, M. C. Gershengorn: Thyrotropin-releasing hormone stimulates rapid loss of phosphatidylinositol and its conversion to 1,2 diacylglycerol and phosphatidic acid in rat mammotropic pituitary cells. J. Biol. Chem. **258** (1983) 234–258.
[18] Besses, G. S., G. N. Burrow, S. W. Spaulding, et al.: Dopamine infusion acutely inhibits the TSH and prolactin responses to TRH. J. Clin. Endocrinol. Metab. **41** (1975) 985–988.
[19] Rapoport, B., S. Refetoff, V. S. Fang, et al.: Suppression of serum thyrotropin (TSH) by L-dopa in chronic hypothyroidism: Interrelationships in the regulation of TSH and prolactin secretion. J. Clin. Endocrinol. Metab. **36** (1973) 256–262.
[20] Miyai, K., T. Onishi, M. Hosokawa, et al.: Inhibition of thyrotropin and prolactin secretion in primary hypothyroidism by 2-Br-alpha-ergocryptine. J. Clin. Endocrinol. Metab. **39** (1974) 391–394.
[21] Scanlon, M. F., B. R. Smith, R. Hall: Thyroid-stimulating hormone: Neuroregulation and clinical applications. Clin. Sci. **55** (1978) 1–10, 129–138.
[22] Siler, T. M., S. S. C. Yen, W. Vale, et al.: Inhibition by somatostatin on the release of TSH induced in man by thyrotropin-releasing factor. J. Clin. Endocrinol. Metab. **38** (1974) 742–745.
[23] Lucke, C., B. Hoeffken, A. Von zur Muehlen: The effect of somatostatin on TSH levels in patients with primary hypothyroidism. J. Clin. Endocrinol. Metab. **41** (1975) 1082–1084.

[24] Ferland, L., F. Labrie, M. Jobin, et al.: Physiological role of SRIF in the control of GH and TSH secretion. Biochem. Biophys. Res. Commun. **68** (1976) 149–156.

[25] Faglia, G., C. Ferrari, P. Beck-Peccoz, et al.: Reduced plasma thyrotropin response to thyrotropin-releasing hormone after dexamethasone administration in normal subjects. Horm. Metab. Res. 5 (1973) 289–292.

[26] Faglia, G., P. Beck-Peccoz, C. Ferrari, et al.: Enhanced plasma thyrotropin response to thyrotropin-releasing hormone following oestradiol administration in man. Clin. Endocrinol. (Oxf.) 2 (1973) 207–210.

[27] Ramey, J. N., G. N. Burrow, R. J. Polackwich, et al.: The effect of oral contraceptive steroids on the response of TSH to TRH. J. Clin. Endocrinol. Metab. **40** (1975) 712–714.

[28] Martino, E., G. Bambini, L. Bartalena, et al.: Human serum thyrotropin measurement by ultrasensitive immunoradiometric assay as first line test in the evaluation of thyroid function. Clin. Endocrinol. (Oxf.) **24** (1986) 141–148.

[29] Weeks, I., M. Sturgess, K. Siddle, et al.: A high sensitivity immunochemiluminometric assay for human thyrotropin. Clin. Endocrinol. (Oxf.) **20** (1984) 489–496.

[30] Beck-Peccoz, P., P. B. Romelli, M. G. Cattaneo, et al.: Evaluation of free thyroxine methods in the presence of iodothyronine-binding autoantibodies. J. Clin. Endocrinol. Metab. **58** (1984) 736–739.

[31] Beck-Peccoz, P., G. Piscitelli, G. Medri, et al.: Thyroid test strategy. Lancet **1** (1985) 1456.

[32] Beck-Peccoz, P., G. Piscitelli, S. Amr, et al.: Endocrine, biochemical, and morphological studies of a pituitary adenoma secreting growth hormone, thyrotropin (TSH), and alpha-subunit: Evidence for secretion of TSH with increased bioactivity. J. Clin. Endocrinol. Metab. **62** (1986) in press.

[33] Bevan, J. S., M. M. Esiri, N. Loveridge, et al.: TSH secreting pituitary adenoma: Case report, characterization of TSH and tumor cell perifusion. J. Endocrinol. **104** Suppl. (1985) 51.

[34] Brenner-Gati, L., M. C. Gershengorn: Thyroid-stimulating hormone-induced hyperthyroidism. In: The pituitary gland (Imura, H., ed.), pp. 467–500, Raven Press, New York 1985.

[35] Jailer, J. W., D. A. Holub: Remission of Graves disease following radiotherapy of a pituitary neoplasm. Am. J. Med. 28 (1960) 497–500.

[36] Hamilton, C. R. jr., L. C. Adams, F. Maloof: Hyperthyroidism due to thyrotropin-producing pituitary chromophobe adenoma: N. Engl. J. Med. **238** (1970) 1077–1080.

[37] Kourides, I. A., E. C. Ridgway, B. D. Weintraub, et al.: Thyrotropin-induced hyperthyroidism: Use of alpha and beta subunit levels to identify patients with pituitary tumors. J. Clin. Endocrinol. Metab. **43** (1977) 575–581.

[38] Kourides, I. A., F. Pekonen, B. D. Weintraub: Absence of thyroid-binding immunoglobulins to patients with thyrotropin-mediated hyperthyroidism. J. Clin. Endocrinol. Metab. **51** (1980) 271–274.

[39] Mornex, R., M. Tommasi, M. Cure, et al.: Hyperthyroidines associeés à un hypopituitarisme au cours de l'évolution d'une tumeur hypophysaire secrétant TSH. Ann. Endocrinol. (Paris) **33** (1972) 390–396.

[40] Hrubesch, M., K. Boeckel, H. Vorsberg, et al.: Hyperthyreose durch TSH produzierendes chromophobes Hypophysenadenom. Verh. Dtsch. Ges. Inn. Med. **78** (1972) 1529–1532.

[41] Faglia, G., C. Ferrari, V. Neri, et al.: High plasma thyrotropin levels in two patients with pituitary tumor. Acta Endocrinol. (Copenh.) **69** (1971) 649–658.

[42] Reschini, E., G. Giustina, L. Cantalamessa, et al.: Hyperthyroidism with elevated plasma TSH levels and pituitary tumor: Study with somatostatin. J. Clin. Endocrinol. Metab. **43** (1976) 924–927.

[43] O' Donnel, J., D. R. Hadden, J. A. Weaver, et al.: Thyrotoxicosis recurring after surgical removal of thyrotropin-secreting pituitary tumor. Proc. R. Soc. Med. **66** (1973) 441–442.

[44] Tolis, G., C. Bied, G. Bertrand, et al.: Pituitary hyperthyroidism: Case report and review of the literature. Am. J. Med. **64** (1978) 177–181.
[45] Afrasiabi, A., L. Valenta, G. Gwinup: A TSH secreting pituitary tumor causing hyperthyroidism: Presentation of a case and review of the literature. Acta Endocrinol. (Copenh.) **92** (1979) 448–454.
[46] Waldhäusl, W., P. Bratusch-Marrain, P. Nowotny, et al.: Secondary hyperthyroidism due to thyrotropin hypersecretion: Study of pituitary tumor morphology and thyrotropin chemistry and release. J. Clin. Endocrinol. Metab. **49** (1979) 879–887.
[47] Benoit, R., B. E. Pearson-Murphy, F. Robert: Hyperthyroidism due to a pituitary TSH-secreting tumour with amenorrohoea-glactorrhoea. Clin. Endocrinol. (Oxf.) **12** (1980) 11–19.
[48] Salti, I. S., N. Nuwayri-Salti, R. A. Bergman, et al.: Thyrotropin-secreting pituitary tumors: A cause of hyperthyroidism. J. Neurol. Neurosurg. Psychiatry **43** (1980) 1141–1145.
[49] Gershengorn, M. C.: Inappropriate secretion of thyroid-stimulating hormone: Description and classification. In: Weintraub, B. D.: (mod) Inappropriate secretion of thyroid-stimulating hormone. Ann. Int. Med. **95** (1981) 340–344.
[50] Takano, K., M. Kogawa, T. Tsushima, et al.: A TSH-secreting pituitary tumor accompanied by high stature. Presentation of a case and review of the literature. Endocrinol. Jpn. **28** (1981) 215–223.
[51] Cravioto, H., T. Fukaya, E. Zimmerman, et al.: Immunohistochemical and electron-microscopic studies of functional and nonfunctional pituitary adenomas including one TSH secreting tumor in a thyrotoxic patient. Acta Neuropath. (Berl.) **53** (1981) 281–292.
[52] Yovos, S. J. G., J. M. Falko, T. M. O' Dorisio, et al.: Thyrotoxicosis and thyrotropin-secreting pituitary tumor causing unilateral exophthalmos. J. Clin. Endocrinol. Metab. **53** (1981) 338–343.
[53] Hill, S., J. Falko, C. Wilson, et al.: Thyrotropin-producing pituitary adenomas. J. Neurosurg. **57** (1982) 515–519.
[54] Smith, C. E., R. C. Smallridge, R. C. Dimond, et al.: Hyperthyroidism due to a thyrotropin-secreting pituitary adenoma: Studies of thyrotropin and subunit secretion. Arch. Intern. Med. **142** (1982) 1709–1711.
[55] Gharib, H., P. Carpenter, B. Scheithauser, et al.: The spectrum of inappropriate pituitary thyrotropin secretion associated with hyperthyroidism. Mayo Clin. Proc. **57** (1982) 556–563.
[56] Mashiter, K., S. Van Noorden, R. Fahlbusch, et al.: Hyperthyroidism due to TSH secreting pituitary adenoma: Case report, treatment and evidence for adenoma TSH by morphological and cell culture studies. Clin. Endocrinol. (Oxf.) **18** (1983) 473–483.
[57] Emerson, C. H., R. D. Utiger: Hyperthyroidism and excessive thyrotropin secretion. N. Engl. J. Med. **287** (1972) 328–333.
[58] Mihailovic, V., M. S. Feller, I. A. Kourides, et al.: Hyperthyroidism due to excess thyrotropin secretion: Follow-up studies. J. Clin. Endocrinol. Metab. **50** (1980) 1135–1138.
[59] Barbarino, A., L. De Marinis, C. Anile, et al.: Normal pituitary function and reverse after selective transsphenoidal removal of a thyrotropin-producing pituitary adenoma. Metabolism **29** (1980) 739–744.
[60] Azukizawa, M., S. Morimoto, K. Miyai, et al.: TSH-producing pituitary adenoma associated with Graves' disease. In: Thyroid Research VIII (Stockigt, J. R., S. Nagataki, eds.), pp. 645–648, Australian Academy Sciences, Canberra 1980.
[61] Filetti, S., B. Rapoport, D. C. Aron, et al.: TSH and TSH-subunit production by human thyrotropic tumour cells in monolayer culture. Acta Endocrinol. (Copenh.) **99** (1982) 224–231.
[62] Connell, S., D. C. McCruden, D. L. Davies, et al.: Bromocriptine for inappropriate thyrotropin secretion. Ann. Intern. Med. **96** (1982) 251–252.
[63] Kellet, H. A., A. H. Wyllie, B. A. B. Dale, et al.: Hyperthyroidism due to thyrotropin-secreting microadenoma. Clin. Endocrinol. (Oxf.) **19** (1983) 57–65.

[64] De Rosa, G., S. M. Corsello, S. Della Casa, et al.: Graves' disease with pituitary adenoma and elevated plasma TSH levels. In: Advances on Thyroid hormones (Carpi, L., ed.), pp. 213 – 224, E.T.S., Pisa 1983.
[65] Savastano, S., B. Merola, N. Panza, et al.: Associazione di ipertiroidismo con sindrome amenorrea-galattorrea: descrizione di un caso clinico, Prime Giornate Italiane della Tiroide, p. 147, Napoli, 3 – 5 Novembre 1983.
[66] Stepanas, T. V., F. Lomas, R. L. G. Newcombe: Bromocriptine treatment of a TSH-secreting pituitary adenoma, Abs. 83, Meeting of Australian Society of Endocrinology 1983.
[67] Wollesen, F., T. Andersen, A. Karle: Size reduction of extrasellar pituitary during bromocriptine treatment. Quantitation of effect on different types of tumor. Ann. Intern. Med. **96** (1982) 281 – 286.
[68] Davies, R. R., R. E. Ferner, R. Ferry, et al.: Tunbridge, W. M. G.: TSH-secreting pituitary tumor. 1st Joint Meeting of British Endocrine Societies, Abs. 47, 1982.
[69] Spada, A., M. Bassetti, E. Martino, et al.: In vitro studies on TSH secretion and adenylate cyclase activity in a human TSH-secreting pituitary adenoma. Effects of somatostatin and dopamine. J. Endocrinol. Invest. **8** (1985) 193 – 198.
[70] Chanson, P., J. Orgiazzi, P. J. Derome, et al.: Paradoxical response of thyrotropin to L-dopa and presence of dopaminergic receptors in a thyrotropin-secreting pituitary adenoma. J. Clin. Endocrinol. Metab. **59** (1984) 542 – 546.
[71] Chiarini, V., E. Graziano, N. Cremonini, et al.: Ipertiroidismo associato a tumore ipofisario TSH-secernente. Seconde Giornate Italiane della Tiroide, Abs. 73, Padova, 25 – 27 Ottobre 1984.
[72] Kamoi, K., T. Mitsuma, H. Sato, et al.: Hyperthyroidism caused by a pituitary thyrotropin-secreting tumor with excessive secretion of thyrotropin-releasing hormone and subsequently followed by Graves' disease in a middle-aged woman. Acta Endocrinol. (Copenh.) **110** (1985) 373 – 382.
[73] Scanlon, M. F., S. Howells, J. R. Peters, et al.: Hyperprolactinaemia, amenorrhoea and galactorrhoea due to a pituitary thyrotroph adenoma. Clin. Endocrinol. (Oxf.) **23** (1985) 35 – 42.
[74] Gesundheit, N., P. A. Petrick, T. Taylor, et al.: Comparison of a pituitary TSH-secreting micro- versus macro-adenoma: clinical and biochemical features. 9th International Thyroid Congress, Abs. 112, 1 – 6 September 1985, Sao Paulo, Brazil.
[75] Montini, M., M. Salmoiraghi, M. D. Pagani, et al.: TSH-secreting pituitary macroadenoma: report of two cases. J. Endocrinol. Invest. **8**, Suppl. 3 (1985) 180.
[76] Gallone, G., O. Testori, S. Ratibondi, et al.: Efficacia della bromocriptina nella terapia di un adenoma ipofisario TSH secernente. Terze Giornate Italiane della Tiroide, Abs. 16, Torino 21 – 23 Novembre 1985.
[77] Lamberg, B. A., S. Ripatti, A. Gordin, et al.: Chromophobe pituitary adenoma with acromegaly and TSH-induced hyperthyroidism associated with parathyroid adenoma. Acta Endocrinol. (Copenh.) **60** (1969) 157 – 172.
[78] Linquette, M., P. Fossati, M. Decoulx, et al.: Adénomes thyréotropes. In: Les adénomes hypophysaires secrétants, pp. 155 – 168, Masson, Paris, 1971.
[79] Hamilton, C. R. jr., F. Maloof: Acromegaly and toxic goiter: Cure of hyperthyroidism and acromegaly by proton-beam partial hypophysectomy. J. Clin. Endocrinol. Metab. **35** (1972) 659 – 664.
[80] Sandler, R.: Recurrent hyperthyroidism in an acromegalic patient previously treated with proton-beam irradiation: Graves' disease as probable etiology based on follow-up observations. J. Clin. Endocrinol. Metab. **42** (1976) 165 – 168.
[81] Smallridge, R. C., L. Wartofsky, R. C. Diamond: Inappropriate secretion of thyrotropin: Discordance between the suppressive effect of corticosteroids and thyroid hormone. J. Clin. Endocrinol. Metab. **48** (1979) 700 – 705.

[82] Meinders, A. E., F. L. A. Willekens, C. A. E. Barends, et al.: Acromegaly and thyrotoxicosis induced by a GH and TSH-producing pituitary tumor which also contained prolactin. Neth. J. Med. **24** (1981) 136 – 144.

[83] Coculescu, M., A. Pop, A. L. Constantinovici, et al.: Mixed TSH- and HGH-secreting pituitary adenoma. Endocrinologie 20 (1982) 209 – 216.

[84] Saeger, W., D. Luedecke: Pituitary adenomas with hyperfunction of TSH. Virchows Arch. (Pathol. Anat.) **394** (1982) 255 – 267.

[85] Lamberg, B. A., R. Pelkonen, A. Gordin, et al.: Hyperthyroidism and acromegaly caused by a pituitary TSH and GH secreting tumor. Acta Endocrinol. (Copenh.) **103** (1983) 7 – 14.

[86] Carlson, H. A., J. A. Linfoot, G. D. Braunstein, et al.: Hyperthyroidism and acromegaly due to a thyrotropin- and growth hormone-secreting pituitary tumor. Am. J. Med. 74 (1983) 915 – 923.

[87] Lamberts, S. W. J., R. Oosterom, T. Verleun, et al.: Regulation of hormone release by cultured cells from a thyrotropin-growth hormone-secreting pituitary tumor. Direct inhibiting effects of 3,5,3′-triiodothyronine and dexamethasone on thyrotropin secretion. J. Endocrinol. Invest. 7 (1984) 313 – 317.

[88] Ishihara, A., H. Nasu, M. Hieda, et al.: A case of the pituitary tumor with combined hyperthyroidism and acromegaly – TSH and GH producing tumor –. 7th International Congress of Endocrinology, Quebec City, Abs. 1773, July 1 – 7, 1984.

[89] Horn, K., F. Erhard, R. Fahlbusch, et al.: Recurrent goiter, hyperthyroidism, galactorrhea and amenorrhea due to a thyrotropin and prolactin-producing pituitary tumor. J. Clin. Endocrinol. Metab. **43** (1976) 137 – 143.

[90] Baylis, P. H.: Case of hyperthyroidism due to chromophobe adenoma. Clin. Endocrinol. (Oxf.) 5 (1976) 145 – 150.

[91] Duello, T. M., N. S. Halmi: Pituitary adenoma producing thyrotropin and prolactin. An immunocitochemical and electron microscopic study. Virchows Arch. (Anat. Pathol.) **376** (1977) 255 – 265.

[92] Werner, S.: Human pituitary adenomas with hypersecretion of TSH and prolactin. Evidence that receptor sites for dopamine may be absent on TSH producing while present on prolactin producing cells. Horm. Metab. Res. **11** (1979) 452 – 453.

[93] Jaquet, P., J. Hassoun, P. Delori, et al.: A human pituitary adenoma secreting thyrotropin and prolactin: Immunohistochemical, biochemical, and cell culture studies. J. Clin. Endocrinol. Metab. **59** (1984) 817 – 824.

[94] Koide, Y., N. Kugai, S. Kimura, et al.: A case of pituitary adenoma with possible simultaneous secretion of thyrotropin and follicle-stimulating hormone. J. Clin. Endocrinol. Metab. **54** (1982) 397 – 403.

[95] Gershengorn, M. C., B. D. Weintraub: Thyrotropin-induced hyperthyroidism caused by selective pituitary resistance to thyroid hormone: A new syndrome of "inappropriate secretion of TSH". J. Clin. Invest. **56** (1975) 633 – 642.

[96] Elewaut, A., M. Mussche, A. Vermeulen: Familial partial target organ resistance to thyroid hormones. J. Clin. Endocrinol. Metab. **43** (1976) 575 – 581.

[97] Novogroder, M., R. Utiger, R. Boyar, et al.: Juvenile hyperthyroidism with elevated thyrotropin (TSH) and normal 24 hour FSH, LH, GH and prolactin secretory patterns. J. Clin. Endocrinol. Metab. **45** (1977) 1053 – 1059.

[98] Sato, T., K. Saida, Y. Suzuki, et al.: A case of the syndrome of inappropriate secretion of TSH. Endocrinol. Jpn. **26** (1977) 623 – 630.

[99] Salmeron De Diego, J., C. Alonso Rodriguez, A. Salazar Orlando, et al.: Syndrome of "inappropriate secretion" of thyroid-stimulating hormone by partial target organ resistance to thyroid hormones. Acta Endocrinol. (Copenh.) **97** (1977) 361 – 368.

[100] Spanheimer, R. G., R. S. Bar, T. C. Hayford: Hyperthyroidism caused by inappropriate thyrotropin hypersection: Studies in patients with selective pituitary resistance to thyroid hormone. Arch. Intern. Med. **142** (1982) 1283 – 1286.

[101] Roesler, A., Y. Lituin, C. Hage, et al.: Familial hyperthyroidism due to inappropriate thyrotropin secretion successfully treated with triiodothyronine, J. Clin. Endocrinol. Metab. **54** (1982) 76 – 82.

[102] Lantigua, R. A., P. Hinkle, P. Woolf, et al.: Inappropriate TSH secretion: Search for circulating inhibitors of thyroid hormone action. Clin. Res. **28** (1980) 626 A.

[103] Vance, M. L., W. S. Evans, M. O. Thorner, et al.: Pituitary resistance to thyroid hormones: Prolactin abnormalities and dopamine agonist therapy. Clin. Res. **30** (1980) 278 A.

[104] Beck-Peccoz, P., G. Piscitelli, M. G. Cattaneo, et al.: Successful treatment of hyperthyroidism due to non-neoplastic pituitary TSH hypersecretion with 3,5,3'-triiodothyroacetic acid (TRIAC). J. Endocrinol. Invest. **6** (1983) 217 – 223.

[105] Sarne, D. H., S. Refetoff: Clinical and pathological findings in a patient with pituitary resistance to thyroid hormone and an islet cell carcinoma. The Endocrine Society Program and Abstracts, 65th Annual Meeting, Abs. 446, June 8 – 10, 1983. San Antonio, Texas.

[106] Sriwatanakul, K., K. McCormick, P. Woolf: Thyrotropin (TSH)-induced hyperthyroidism: Response of TSH to dopamine and its agonists. J. Clin. Endocrinol. Metab. **58** (1984) 255 – 261.

[107] Takamatsu, J., T. Mozai, K. Kuma: Bromocriptine therapy for hyperthyroidism due to increased thyrotropin secretion. J. Clin. Endocrinol. Metab. **58** (1984) 934 – 936.

[108] Chiarini, V., E. Graziano, M. Cremonini, et al.: Ipertiroidismo da inappropriata secrezione di TSH: Primi risultati della terapia con TRIAC. Atti delle Terze Giornate Italiane della Tiroide, p. 18, Torino 21 – 23 Novembre 1985.

[109] Orgiazzi, J., X. Ducottet, Y. Barbier, et al.: Inappropriate TSH hypersecretion: Opposite effect of T4 and T3 on the thyrotrophs? Ann. Endocrinol. (Paris) **45** (1985) 89 A.

[110] Drucker, D., R. Jossè: Inappropriate TSH secretion with abnormal thyrotroph sensitivity to dopamine. Clin. Invest. Med. **8** (1985) 117 – 120.

[111] Magee, B., B. Sheridan, M. F. Scanlon, et al.: Inappropriate thyrotropin secretion, increased dopaminergic tone and preservation of the diurnal rhythm in serum TSH. Clin. Endocrinol. (Oxf.) **24** (1986) 209 – 215.

[112] Schalch, D. S., D. Gonzales-Barcena, A. J. Kastin, et al.: Abnormalities in the release of TSH in response to TRH in patients with disorders of the pituitary, hypothalamus and basal ganglia. J. Clin. Endocrinol. Metab. **35** (1972) 609 – 615.

[113] Faglia, G., P. Beck-Peccoz, C. Ferrari, et al.: Plasma thyrotropin response to thyrotropin-releasing hormone in patients with pituitary and hypothalamic disorders. J. Clin. Endocrinol. Metab. **37** (1973) 595 – 601.

[114] Snyder, P. J., L. S. Jacobs, M. M. Rabello, et al.: Diagnostic value of thyrotropin-releasing hormone in pituitary and hypothalamic disorders. Ann. Intern. Med. **81** (1974) 751 – 757.

[115] Faglia, G., L. Bitensky, A. Pinchera, et al.: Thyrotropin secretion in patients with central hyperthyroidism: Evidence for reduced biological activity of immunoreactive thyrotropin. J. Clin. Endocrinol. Metab. **48** (1979) 989 – 998.

[116] Hershman, J. H.: Hypothalamic and pituitary hypothyroidism. In: Bastenie, P. A., M. Bonnis, L. Vanhaelst (eds.): Recent Progress in Diagnosis and Treatment of Hypothyroid Conditions, Excerpta Medica, Amsterdam, 1980, pp. 40 – 49 (1980).

[117] Jenkins, J. S., C. G. Gilbert, V. Ang: Hypothalamic-pituitary function in patients with craniopharyngiomas. J. Clin. Endocrinol. Metab. **43** (1976) 394 – 399.

[118] Linfoot, J. A.: Alpha particle pituitary irradiation in the primary and post-surgical management of pituitary microadenomas. In: Pituitary Microadenomas (Faglia, G., M. A. Giovanelli, R. M. MacLeod, eds.), pp. 515 – 529, Academic Press, New York, 1980.

[119] Daniel, P. M., M. M. L. Prichard: Studies of the hypothalamus and the pituitary gland with special reference to the effects of the transection of the pituitary stalk. Acta Endocrinol. (Copenh.) **80**, Suppl. 201 (1975) 1 – .

[120] Dugger, G. S., J. J. Van Wyk, J. F. Newsome: The effect of pituitary stalk-section on thyroid function and gonadotropin hormone excretion in women with mammary carcinoma. J. Neurosurg. **19** (1962) 589 – 597.

[121] Naguib, A. S., A. Cangir, N. H. Maor, et al.: Effect of irradiation on hypothalamic-pituitary and thyroid function in patients with tumors of the head and neck. In: Recent Advances in the Diagnosis and Treatment of Pituitary Tumors (Linfoot, J. A., ed.), pp. 148 – 161, Raven Press, New York, 1979.

[122] Samaan, N. A., M. M. Bakdasm, J. B. Caderao, et al.: Hypopituitarism after external irradiation. Evidence for both hypothalamic and pituitary origin. Ann. Intern. Med. **83** (1975) 771 – 779.

[123] Singer, P. A., J. H. Mestman, P. R. Manning, et al.: Hypothalamic hypothyroidism secondary to Sheehan's syndrome. West J. Med. **120** (1974) 416 – 419.

[124] Pittman, J. A., E. D. Haigler, J. M. Hershman, et al.: Hypothalamic hypothyroidism. N. Engl. J. Med. **285** (1971) 844 – 845.

[125] Valenta, L. J., D. R. De Feo: Post-traumatic hypopituitarism due to a hypothalamic lesion. Am. J. Med. **68** (1980) 614 – 619.

[126] Woolf, P. D., D. S. Schalch: Hypothyroidism secondary to hypothalamic insufficiency. Ann. Intern. Med. **78** (1973) 88 – 97.

[127] Hendricks, S. A., B. M. Lippe, S. A. Kaplan, et al.: Hypothalamic atrophy with progressive hypopituitarism in an adolescent girl. J. Clin. Endocrinol. Metab. **52** (1981) 562 – 568.

[128] Stuart, C. A., F. A. Neelon, H. E. Lebovitz: Hypothalamic insufficiency: The cause of hypopituitarism in sarcoidosis. Ann. Intern. Med. **88** (1978) 589 – 595.

[129] Ezrin, C., R. Chaikoff, H. Hoffman: Panhypopituitarism caused by Hand-Schuller-Christian disease. Can. Med. Assoc. J. **89** (1963) 1290 – 1293.

[130] Peillon, F., J. Racadot: Modifications histopathologiques de l'hypophyse dans six cas d'hémochromatose. Ann. Endocrinol. (Paris) **39** (1972) 800 – 806.

[131] Steiner, M. W., J. D. Boggs: Absence of pituitary gland, hypothyroidism, hypoadrenalism and hypogonadism in a 17-year-old dwarf. J. Clin. Endocrinol. Metab. **25** (1964) 1591 – 1595.

[132] Parks, J. M., A. Tenore, A. M. Bongiovanni, et al.: Familial hypopituitarism with large sella turcica. N. Engl. J. Med. **298** (1978) 698 – 701.

[133] Faglia, G., P. Beck-Peccoz: Thyrotropin secretion in central hypothyroidism. In: Radioimmunoassay of Hormones, Proteins and Enzymes (Albertini, A., ed.), pp. 48 – 57, Excerpta Medica, Amsterdam 1980.

[134] Andler, W., H. Stolecke, U. Kohns: Thyroid function in children with growth hormone deficiency either idiopathic or caused by diseases of the central nervous system. Eur. J. Pediatr. **128** (1978) 273 – 279.

[135] Lee, H. B., C. Faiman: Isolated thyrotropin deficiency due to a pituitary tumor. Canad. Med. Assoc. J. **116** (1977) 520 – 524.

[136] Chandra, M., F. Lifshitz, P. Fort, et al.: Isolated thyrotropin deficiency in diabetes mellitus. Acta Endocrinol. (Copenh.) **84** (1977) 80 – 83.

[137] Boehm, T. M., R. C. Dimond, L. Wartofsky: Isolated thyrotropin deficiency with thyrotropin-releasing hormone induced TSH secretion and thyroidal reserve. J. Clin. Endocrinol. Metab. **43** (1976) 1041 – 1046.

[138] Job, J. C., J. Vassal, J. L. Chaussain, et al.: Hypothyroidie infantile par déficit isolée en hormone thyréotrope hypophysaire. Arch. Fr. Pediatr. **30** (1973) 61 – 67.

[139] Marks, S. J., J. M. Hershman, G. D. Aurbach: Thyroid dysfunction in pseudohypoparathyroidism. J. Clin. Endocrinol. Metab. **33** (1971) 822 – 828.

[140] Krugman, L. C., J. M. Hershman, I. J. Chopra, et al.: Patterns of recovery of the hypothalamic-pituitary-thyroid axis in patients taken off chronic thyroid therapy. J. Clin. Endocrinol. Metab. **41** (1975) 70–76.

[141] Vagenakis, A. G., L. E. Braverman, F. Azizi, et al.: Recovery of pituitary thyrotropic function after withdrawal of prolonged thyroid-suppression therapy. N. Engl. J. Med. **293** (1975) 681–683.

[142] Singer, P. A., J. T. Nicoloff, R. B. Stein, et al.: Transient TRH deficiency after prolonged thyroid hormone therapy, J. Clin. Endocrinol. Metab. **47** (1978) 512–518.

[143] Lippe, B. M., A. J. Van Herle, S. H. La Franchi, et al.: Reversible hypothyroidism in growth hormone-deficient children treated with human growth hormone. J. Clin. Endocrinol. Metab. **40** (1975) 612–618.

[144] Anderson, M. S., C. Y. Bowers, A. J. Kastin, et al.: Synthetic thyrotropin releasing hormone. N. Engl. J. Med. **285** (1971) 1279–1283.

[145] Berthézéne, F., R. Mornex, B. Chavier: A study of thyrotropin deficiencies by the combination of two tests of TSH function. J. Clin. Endocrinol. Metab. **38** (1974) 1068–1072.

[146] Faglia, G., P. Beck-Peccoz, B. Ambrosi, et al.: Prolonged and exaggerated elevations in plasma thyrotropin (hTSH) after thyrotropin-releasing factor (TRF) in patients with pituitary tumors. J. Clin. Endocrinol. Metab. **33** (1971) 999–1002.

[147] Foley, T. P. jr., J. Owings, J. T. Hayford, et al.: Serum thyrotropin response to synthetic thyrotropin-releasing hormone in normal children and in hypopituitary patients, J. Clin. Invest. **51** (1972) 2143–2150.

[148] Haigler, E. D., J. A. Pittman, jr., J. M. Hershman, et al.: Direct evaluation of pituitary thyrotropin reserve utilizing synthetic thyrotropin-releasing hormone. J. Clin. Endocrinol. Metab. **33** (1971) 573–581.

[149] Karlberg, B., S. Almqvist: Clinical experience with thyrotropin-releasing hormone (TRH) stimulation test in patients with thyroid, pituitary and hypothalamic disorders. Acta Endocrinol. (Copenh.) **72** (1973) 967–973.

[150] McLaren, E. H., S. Hendricks, B. L. Pimstone: Thyrotropin response to intravenous thyrotropin-releasing hormone in patients with hypothalamic and pituitary diseases. Clin. Endocrinol. (Oxf.) **3** (1974) 113–122.

[151] Otsuki, M., H. Mori, S. Bada, et al.: Effect of synthetic thyrotropin-releasing hormone in patients with hypothalamic-pituitary disorders. Acta Endocrinol. (Copenh.) **73** (1973) 233–239.

[152] Mitsuma, T., L. Shenkman, A. Suphavai, et al.: Hypothalamic hypothyroidism: Diminished thyroidal response to thyrotropin-releasing hormone. Am. J. Med. Sci. **265** (1973) 315–318.

[153] Patel, Y. G., H. G. Burger: Serum thyrotropin (TSH) in pituitary and/or hypothalamic hypothyroidism: Normal or elevated basal levels and paradoxical responses to thyrotropin-releasing hormone. J. Clin. Endocrinol. Metab. **37** (1973) 190–196.

[154] Woolf, P. D., L. S. Jacobs, R. Donofrio, et al.: Secondary hypopituitarism: Evidence for continuing regulation of hormone release. J. Clin. Endocrinol. Metab. **38** (1974) 71–76.

[155] Illig, R., M. Krawczynska, T. Torresani, et al.: Elevated plasma TSH and hypothyroidism in children with hypothalamic hypothyroidism. J. Clin. Endocrinol. Metab. **41** (1975) 722–728.

[156] Hall, R.: The immunoassay of thyroid stimulating hormone and its clinical applications. Clin. Endocrinol. (Oxf.) **1** (1972) 115–125.

[157] Krieger, D. T.: Glandular and organ deficiency associated with secretion of biologically inactive pituitary peptides. J. Clin. Endocrinol. Metab. **36** (1974) 964–975.

[158] Hall, R., B. J. Ormston, G. M. Besser, et al.: The thyrotropin-releasing hormone test in diseases of the pituitary and hypothalamus. Lancet **I** (1972) 759–763.

[159] Suter, S. N., S. L. Kaplan, M. L. Aubert, et al.: Plasma prolactin and thyrotropin response to thyrotropin-releasing factor in children with primary and hypothalamic hypothyroidism. J. Clin. Endocrinol. Metab. **47** (1978) 1015–1021.

[160] Faglia, G., C. Ferrari, A. Paracchi, et al.: Triiodothyronine response to thyrotropin-releasing hormone in patients with hypothalamic-pituitary disorders. Clin. Endocrinol. (Oxf.) **4** (1975) 585 – 590.

[161] Petersen, V. B., A. M. McGregor, P. E. Belchetz, et al.: The secretion of thyrotropin with impaired biological activity in patients with hypothalamic-pituitary diseases. Clin. Endocrinol. (Oxf.) **8** (1978) 397 – 402.

[162] Bitensky, L., J. Alaghband-Zadeh, J. Chayen: Studies on thyroid-stimulating hormone and the long-acting thyroid stimulating activity. Clin. Endocrinol. (Oxf.) 3 (1974) 363 – 374.

[163] Beck-Peccoz, P., S. Amr, M. M. Menezes-Ferreira, et al.: Decreased receptor binding of biologically inactive thyrotropin in central hypothyroidism. N. Engl. J. Med. **312** (1985) 1085 – 1090.

[164] Faglia, G., P. Beck-Peccoz, M. Ballabio, et al.: Excess of β-subunit of thyrotropin (TSH) in patients with idiopathic central hypothyroidism due to the secretion of TSH with reduced biological activity. J. Clin. Endocrinol. Metab. **56** (1983) 908 – 914.

[165] Ballabio, M., M. Nissim, N. Torno, et al.: Gel chromatography of circulating TSH in primary thyroid failure and in central hypothyroidism due to bioinactive TSH, J. Endocrinol. Invest. 8, Suppl. 1 (1985) 57.

[166] Faglia, G., P. Beck-Peccoz: Thyrotropin, thyrotropin beta and alpha-subunit secretion in central hypothyroidism. In: Pituitary Hormones and Related Peptides (Motta, M., M. Zanisi, F. Piva, eds.), pp. 353 – 364, Academic Press, London 1982.

TSH-Release and TSH-synthesis: two different effects of TRH

W. Tenschert, K. Schemmel

Introduction

First hints of the existance of a thyreotropic hormone were made by Ragowitsch [1] and Stieda [2] in 1890. Preparation and purification procedures were then reported by Ciereszko [3], Condliffe and Bates [4] and by Adams and Kennedy [5].

Several methods had to be developed in order to prove the specific influence of TSH to the thyroid gland. One of the most successfull applied bio-assays was described by Mc. Kenzie [6] in 1958, the most sensitive way of specific measurement of TSH is the radioimmunoassay which was developped by Odell and Utiger [7].

The chemical structure of TRH, a peptide hormone was unrevelled by Shally et al. in 1969. It was first supposed to influence only the release of TSH from the adenohypophysis, then Sinka and Meites [8] suggested that TRH it as well responsible for the synthesis of TSH in the pituitary β-cells.

The aim of this study was to investigate: First, whether the synthetic TRH is able to influence the functions of normal and T-4 suppressed pituitary glands of rats. Second, the changes of TSH serum levels of T-4 suppressed and non-suppressed animals under the influence of TRH. Third, the synthesis and release rate of TSH in the pituitary glands of T-4 treated and non pretreated rats, independence from time and dose application.

Methods and material

All investigations were carried out on 640 white Wistar rats, aged 5 to 7 weeks, weight between 180 and 250 grs.

In the pretreated period 40 µg T-4 or 0.9% NaCl-solution were injected intraperitonally to each group of 320 animals for 10 days.

The synthetic TRH was applied in a dosage of 5, 50, 100, 200, 400 µg also intraperitonally. The animals then were sacrificed after having taken blood

Thyrotropin

samples at time intervals of 5, 30 and 120 minutes. Blood samples were centrifuged in heparinezed vials and kept frozen at −20 °C until the radioimmunoassay was performed.

Pituitary glands were taken from each animal and stored after having crushing them in 0,05 mol phosphate buffer (pH 7.5) at −20 °C. The radioimmunoassay materials for rat TSH was provided by Dr. Parlowe, Univesity of Los Angeles, California. (NIAMDD Rat Pituitary Hormone Distribution.) All blood samples and pituitary homogenates for TSH measurement were investigated in triplicates. Standard curves are given in figure 1.

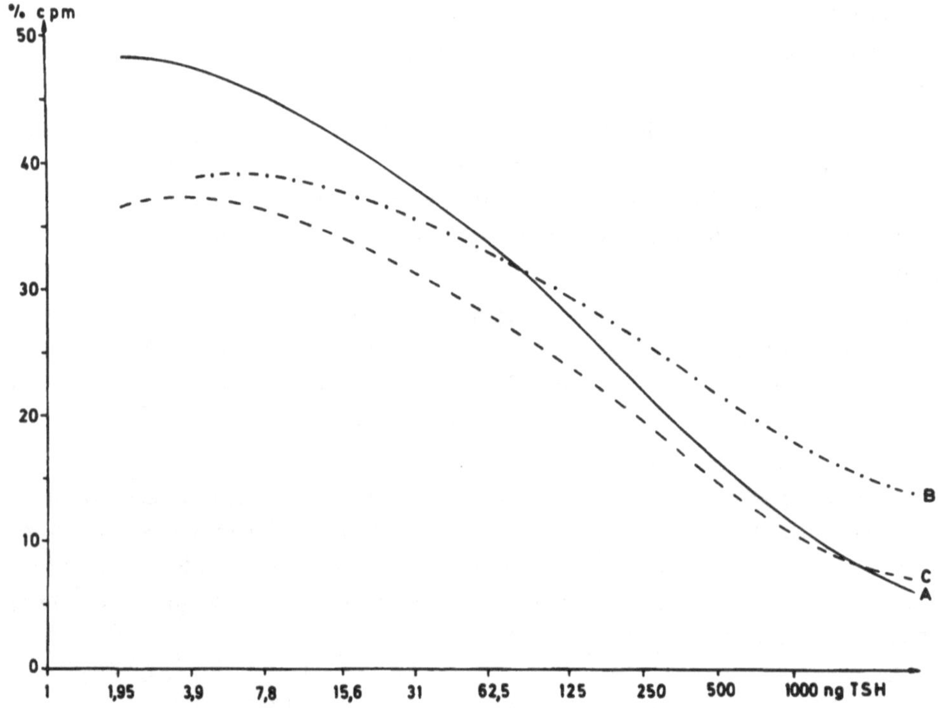

Fig. 1 Standard curves of the rat – TSH-RIA: plot A represents a standard curve in buffer solution, plot B represents the standard curve for all serum aliquots (T_4 pretreated and non-pretreated) and plot C represents the standard curve for the pituitary extracts.

The calculation of the results was made by a Diehl-alphatronic calculation program for radioimmunoassays, statistical analysis was performed by variation-analysis and by Tukey-test.

Results

After pretreatment and suppression of the regular pituitary function by 40 µg of T-4 given intraperitonally the physiological pituitary contence of TSH in test animals is significantly decreased compared to untreated animals. In untreated rats TSH contence was 3.720 ± 1.052 ng TSH/mg pituitary wet weight while the contence in T-4 treated animals was 10.4 ± 11.4 µg TSH/mg pituitary wet weight.

Also, the serum levels of TSH in T-4 pretreated animals were obviously lower compared to normal animals.

After stimulation by TRH in the applied dosage intraperitonally a dose-dependent increase of TSH serum levels was observed. The TSH maximum level was reached after 5 to 15 minutes, the increase rate for reaching the maximal level was nearly equal for each TRH dosage. The decrease of the TSH levels was observed in a time intervall of two hours at a dosage of 5 to 200 µg of TRH while the application of 400 µg TRH showed only a slight decrease of TSH-serum levels within 120 minutes (fig. 2).

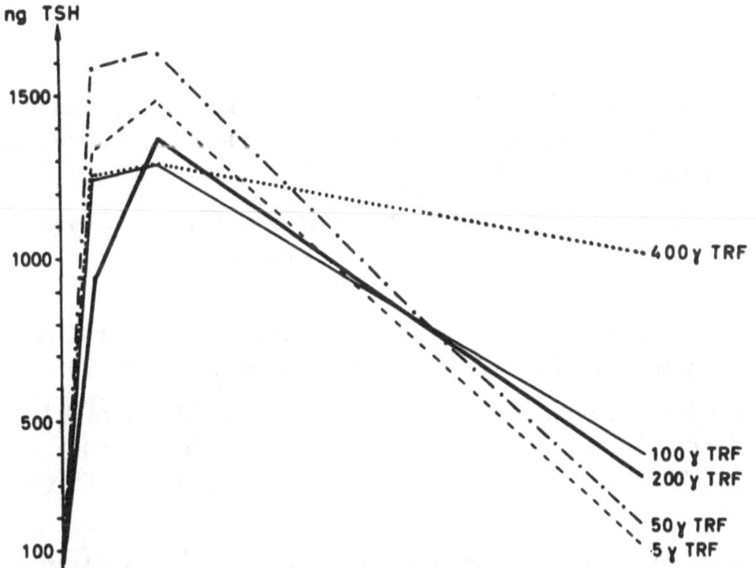

Fig. 2 Measurement of TSH-levels in serum of unpretreated rats after stimulation with different dosages of TRH (5 γ to 400 γ) and observation of the serum levels over a time period of 120 minutes.

In T-4 suppressed animals the increase of TSH synthesis and the TSH release is time delayed as well in the pituitary gland as in the peripheral blood. The maximum of TSH-synthesis is reached after 30 minutes, the release depends on the amount of previously synthezised hormone. In the peripheral blood different patterns of TSH levels are found at the time intervals of 15, 60 or 120 minutes.

The results of the study lead to the following conclusions: The peripheral blockade by T-4 does not influence the TSH-synthesis within the pituitary gland. There is a marked decrease in pituitary TSH content which is equalled immediatly by application of TRH. The main influence of TRH is the synthesis of TSH within the pituitary gland which is regulated by a short feed back mechanism. The peripheral serum levels of TSH are different, depending whether the animal was T-4 pretreated or not. In untreated animals TSH levels are dependent on the applied dosage of TRH and the time intervall.

The patterns of TSH contence in the pituitary glands of T-4 pretreated and untreated animals differ within the inital 30 minutes depending on the synthesis rate of TSH after recovering from the impoverishment during the T-4 pretreatment period. The measurement of TSH levels in the peripheral blood by radioimmunoassay is technically simple albeit it may not lead to conclusions concerning the rates of hormone synthesis or contence in the pituitary gland.

Discussion

As described previously by Reichlin et al. [9] our investigations showed that TSH levels in serum and TSH contence in the pituitary glands of rats can be measured by a radioimmunoassay.

The value of TSH levels in normal rat serum was 67.2 ± 42.8 ng/ml. The homogenates of the pituitary glands had a contence of 3.720 ± 1.052 ng TSH/ per mg wet weight.

As shown by Studer and Steiner [10] the application of 10 ng TRH leads of a significant increase of TSH as well in the pituitary as in the peripheral blood.

Investigations by Weisbecker et al. [11] showed that 250 µg of TRH were necessary to overwhelm a suppression of the pituitary gland which was set by application of 30 µg T-4. These investigations were done by the TSH bioassay of Mc. Kenzie.

Basing on these results the suppression of the rats was achieved by application of 40 µg T-4 for 10 days. This made us find TSH serum levels under the limit of measurement and a pituitary contence of 10.4 ± 11.4 ng TSH/mg wet weight.

Piva and Steiner [12] showed the LD-50 for TRH in Albino rats at 2.500 mg/kg body weight, this allowed us to choose a dosage of 400 µg TRH/animal without reaching the toxic limit. In accordance with other authors we saw the maximum of TSH-secretion in non-pretreated animals after 15 minutes in the peripheral blood and after 30 minutes in the pituitary glands.

Albeit the content of TSH in the pituitary glands was significantly different in the suppressed and in the non suppressed group before the injection of TRH, the synthesis ran on rapidly within the observed time. The different levels of TSH amounts converged in relation to time and application of the TRH dosage.

To our opinion the data reveal that TSH synthesis is a strong effect of TRH, which becomes more obvious when the pituitary gland is impoverished of TSH.

Both effects of TRH, release and synthesis, are related to different specific receptors on the pituitary β-cell, as investigations by Studer and Steiner [10] showed. The intact Pyroglutaminacid molecule seems to be responsible for the release, while synthesis is located at the histidin molecule.

The involvement of specific receptors is also shown by the results of Vale et al. [13], who found that the deminishing of calcium-ions decreased the effect of TRH on TSH.

As shown by Bowers et al. [14] TRH increases the generation of cyclic AMP in the pituitary cell.

Our results show that the pretreatment by T-4 makes the release of TSH less effective. Vale [13] could demonstrate that the addition of actomycin D neutralizes the T-4 suppression on TRH in vitro.

By drawing the conclusion of our results, we could demonstrate by in vivo investigation that TSH release and TSH synthesis are two different effects of TRH due to the different specific receptor sites of the pituitary cell.

Abstract

Thyreotropin releasing hormone (TRH) is known to act upon the negative feed back system of the adenohypophysis. The goal of this study was to investigate the extent of the influence of TRH on the release and synthesis of pituitary TSH, and furthermore, if they are independent, superimposed or time related.

Investigations were carried out in 640 Wistar rats, whereby a number of 320 animals were pretreated by daily injections of 40 μg T-4 over a period of 10 days and the same number of rats served as control group, treated with 0.9% NaCl solution.

After application of increasing doses of TRH (5 – 400 μg) the animals were sacrified and TSH-content of the pituitary glands and the coresponding TSH-Serum levels were measered by radioimmunoassay at different times.

Non suppressed animals, stimulated by TRH show a dose and time related increase in TSH serum levels with a maximum rate at 15 minutes, in T-4 suppressed animals the maximum stimulation effect of TSH synthesis in the pituitary gland is shown at 30 minutes and the increase of serum levels appeared time-delayed.

The data lead to following conclusions: TRH stimulates the release and synthesis of TSH. Pretreatment by T-4 makes the release of TSH less effective, while the synthesis seems not to be influenced. Hence, TSH synthesis should be regarded as the stronger and more constant effect of TRH.

References

[1] Ragowitsch, N.: Die Veränderungen der Hypophyse nach Entfernung der Schilddrüse. Beitr. path. Anat. **4** (1889) 453 – 469.

[2] Stieda, H.: Über das Verhalten der Hypophyse des Kaninchens nach Entfernung der Schilddrüse. Beitr. path. Anat. 7 (1890) 535 – 552.

[3] Ciereszko, L. S.: Preparation of pituitary thyrotropic hormone. I. Biol. Chem. **160** (1945) 585 – 592.

[4] Condliffe, P. G., R. W. Bates: Chromatography of thyroid stimulating hormone on carboxymethylcellulose. I. Biol. Chem. **223** (1956) 843 – 852.

[5] Adams, D. D., T. H. Kennedy: Measurement of the thyroid-stimulating hormone content of serum from hypothyroid and euthyroid people. I. Clin. Endocr. **28** (1968) 325 – 332.

[6] Mc. Kenzie, J. M.: The bio-assay of thyreotropin in serum. Endocr. **63** (1958) 372 – 382.

[7] Odell, W. D., J. F. Wilber, R. Utiger: Studies of thyrotropin physiology by means of radioimmunoassay. Recent Progr. Horm. Res. **23** (1967) 47 – 58.

[8] Sinka, D. K., J. Meites: Stimulation of pituitary thyrotropin synthesis and release by hypothalamic extract. Endocr. **80** (1961) 957 – 961.

[9] Reichlin, S., J. B. Martin, R. L. Boshaus, et al.: Measurement of TSH in plasma and pituitary of the rat by a radioimmunoassay utilizing bovine TSH: Effect of thyroidectomy or thyroxine administration on plasma TSH levels. Endocr. **82** (1970) 1022 – 1031.

[10] Studer, R. O., H. Steiner: Hypothalamische Releasing Hormone. Schweiz. Med. Wochenschr. **102** (1972) 1270 – 1275.

[11] Weisbecker, L., K. Schemmel, V. Mokmol, et al.: Die dosisabhängige Zunahme von TSH Aktivitäten unter (pyro)-Glu-His-Pro (NH-2) im Mc. Kenzie Assay, ihre Abhängigkeit von der Blockade mit Thyroxin sowie die potenzierende Wirkung von Vasopressin. In: Thyreotropin-Releasing-Hormon (F. A. Horster, ed.) pp. 45 – 48. Schattauer, Stuttgart 1972.

[12] Piva, F., H. Steiner: Bioassay and toxicology of TRH. Front. Horm. Res. **1** (1972) 11 – 21.

[13] Vale, W., R. Giullemin, R. Bergus: The hypothalamic hypophysotropic thyrotropin-releasing factor. Vitam. Horm. **29** (1971) 1 – 39.

[14] Bowers, C. J., A. V. Shally: In: Hypophysiotropic Hormones of the Hypothalamus (J. Meites, ed.). Williams & Wilkins, Baltimore 1970.

Feedback regulation and thyroid status evaluated by an ultrasensitive TSH-IRMA in euthyroidism and borderline hyperthyroidism

U. Loos, F. S. Keck, L. Duntas, E. F. Pfeiffer

Introduction

It is generally accepted that thyroid hormones, whose secretion is controlled by TSH, regulate TSH secretion via a feedback mechanism and thus ensure euthyroidism under physiological conditions [7]. Evaluation of serum concentration (SC) of TSH before and after TRH stimulation is considered to be the most sensitive discriminator of thyroid dysfunction because it amplifies minor changes in the peripheral thyroid status [8]. However, because of the limited sensitivity of radioimmunoassay (RIA), until recently, basal TSH-SC was believed to be incapable of discriminating between hyperthyroidism and euthyroidism, unless the RIA was technically improved [9, 10]. These problems should be solved by the new TSH determination using immuno-radiometricassay (IRMA) techniques, which, from a theoretical point of view, are so sensitive as to nearly detect even a single molecule of TSH. In this study, an ultrasensitive TSH-IRMA [5] has been evaluated with respect to SC of thyroid hormones in euthyroidism and borderline hyperthyroidism.

Material and methods

Ninety-nine clinically euthyroid, including 31 by laboratory data (TSH 0.05 – 0.5 µU/ml) borderline hyperthyroid, males (n = 34) and females (n = 65) were subjected to the following protocol: After an overnight fast, blood samples were collected between 8.00 and 8.30 a.m. for measurements of SC of following hormones: T_4-SC was determined by radioimmunoassay (Seralute T_4, Bayropharm), normal range: 4 – 12 µd/dl, T_3-SC was also estimated by radioimmunoassay (Seralute T_3, Bayropharm), normal range 80 – 120 ng/dl. As a measure of free T_4 and free T_3-SC, the ratio of SC of T_4 or T_3 to their serum uptakes was calculated and named free T_4 equivalent (FT_4E, normal range: 0.4 – 1.1) and free T_3 equivalent (FT_3E, normal range: 0.4 – 0.8) [3]. TSH was measured by the IRMA-assay hTSH-RIAgnost, Behring, using spline function for calculation of

Thyrotropin

values. After blood withdrawal, TRH-Tests were performed by rapidly injecting 200 μg TRH (Antepan®) i. v. and collecting blood again after 20 minutes. The maximal TRH-stimulated TSH value minus the basal TSH (bTSH) value was called delta TSH (dTSH). Pearson's r was used for calculating the correlation coefficients.

Results

The lower limit of detection for the TSH assay was 0.02 μU/ml in our laboratory. The inter-assay variance was 5.2% in the euthyroid range. The mean value of bTSH in the euthyroid patients was 1.36 ± 0.36 (mean ± SEM). The distribution of values was assymetric. Normal range was 0.5 to 4.5 μU/ml. In the 99 euthyroids, bTSH correlated closely with dTSH (6.5 ± 0.8 μU/ml, mean ± SEM) as shown by an r-value of 0.75 and a p-value of < 0.001 (fig. 1). When looking at the borderline hyperthyroids alone, bTSH (range: 0.02 – 0.5 μU/ml, 0.16 ± 0.02 μU/ml, mean ± SEM) demonstrated an even stronger correlation with dTSH (1.6 ± 0.77 μU/ml, mean ± SEM) with an r-value of 0.8 and a p-value less than 0.001 (fig. 2). T_4-SC (8.4 ± 0.27 μU/ml, mean ± SEM, n = 63) correlated with

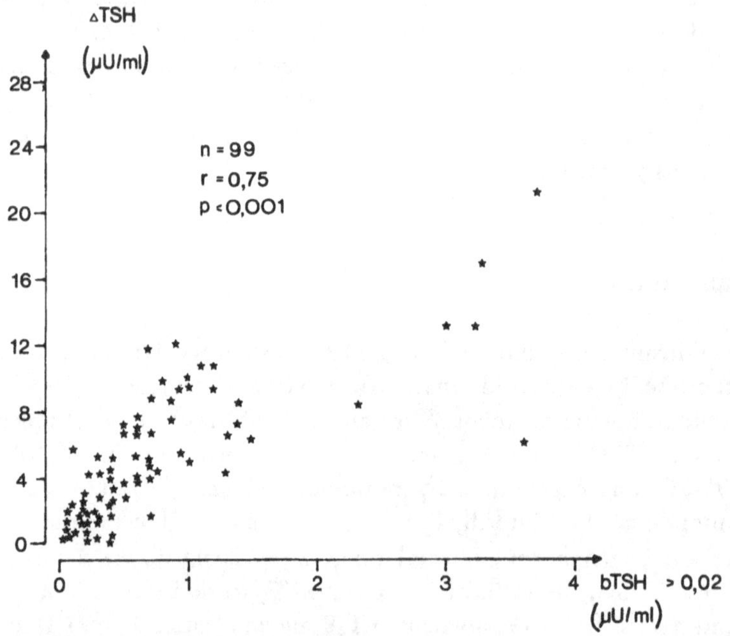

Fig. 1 Serum concentrations (SC) of TRH-stimulated TSH minus basal TSH (= *ΔTSH*) plotted against SC of basal TSH (= *bTSH*) in clinically euthyroids.

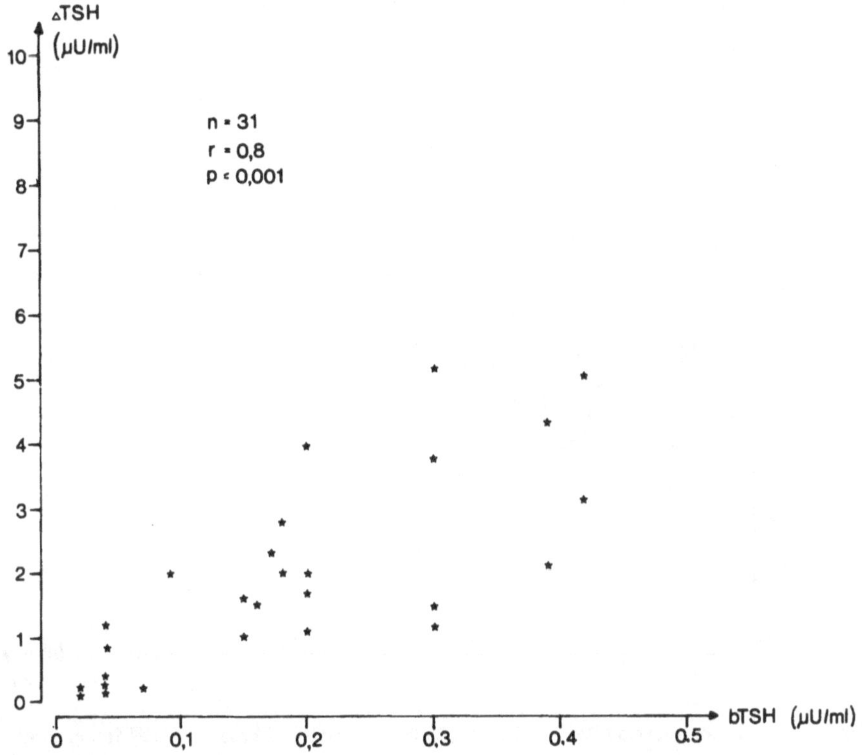

Fig. 2 Serum concentrations (SC) of TRH-stimulated TSH minus basal TSH (= *ΔTSH*) plotted against SC of basal TSH (= *bTSH*) in borderline hyperthyroids (bTSH 0.05 – 0.5 μU/ml).

Table 1 Correlations between serum concentrations (SC) of basal TSH *(bTSH)* and TRH-stimulated minus bTSH *(ΔTSH)* and SC of T_4 and T_3 as well as equivalents of free T_4SC *(FT_4E)* and of free T_3SC *(FT_3E)* in euthyroidism (bTSH 0.5 – 4.0 μU/ml) and in borderline hyperthyroidism (bTSH 0.02 – 0.5 μU/ml)

	T_4	FTE	T_3	FT_3E
bTSH (when bTSH < 0.5)	r = −0.49 $p < 0.001$	r = −0.28 $p < 0.05$	r = −0.17 n.s.	r = −0.04 n.s.
ΔTSH (n = 63)	r = −0.32 $p < 0.05$	r = −0.33 $p < 0.01$	r = −0.06 n.s.	r = −0.04 n.s.
bTSH (when bTSH 0.02 – 0.5)	r = −0.07 n.s.	r = −0.23 n.s.	r = 0.23 n.s.	r = −0.1 n.s.
ΔTSH (n = 31)	r = −0.03 n.s.	r = −0.23 n.s.	r = 0.23 n.s.	r = −0.32 n.s.

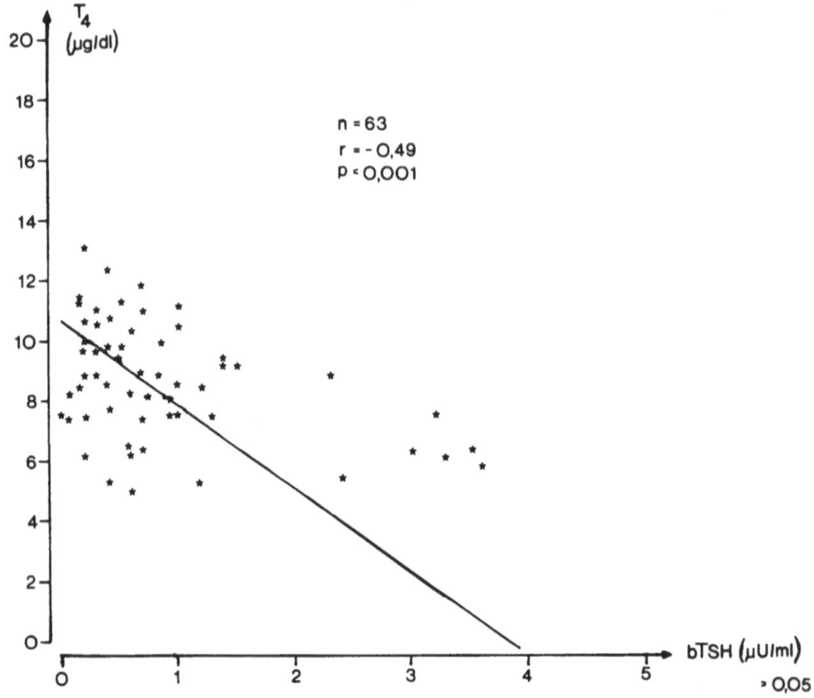

Fig. 3 Serum concentrations (SC) of T_4 (T_4) plotted against SC of basal TSH (*bTSH*) in euthyroidism.

bTSH significantly ($p < 0.001$) with the r-value of -0.49 demonstrating a negative feedback control of T_4-SC on bTSH-SC (fig. 3). The correlation of T_4-SC with dTSH was less pronounced (tab. 1). To a minor extent the FT_4E correlated with bTSH-SC as well as dTSH. However, the T_3-SC, and FT_3E did not show any correlation with bTSH or dTSH-SC. The borderline hyperthyroid cases did not show any correlation between the parameters of peripheral thyroid status and bTSH or dTSH.

Discussion and conclusions

The data obtained in this study demonstrate the clinical use of this supersensitive TSH-IRMA in the diagnosis of euthyroidism and borderline hyperthyroidism. Until recently it was postulated that the TRH-test is the most sensitive discriminator of hyperthyroidism. In this study it was found that bTSH-SC correlates closely with dTSH-SC, which is particulary pronounced in the borderline hyperthyroid patients. From these data, it is concluded, that in most cases, in this range of TSH, the TRH-test does not provide any additional information than use of basal TSH alone. However, the TRH-test can be of diagnostic importance in selected cases with borderline results. It is speculated that factors such as TSH autoantibodies might be responsible for low values of bTSH-SC, which can not be attributed to hyperthyroidism. In these cases TRH-test might be useful showing a response in case of autoantibody presence in euthyroidism [6]. – T_4-SC, and to a minor extent FT_4E, but not T_3-SC or FT_3E, correlate with both bTSH and dTSH. Therefore, it is suggested that the negative feedback control of the pituitary is mainly brought about by total T_4SC. Former studies in thyroidectomised patients under stepwise increasing substitution therapy demonstrated a highly significant correlation of T_3-SC with bTSH-SC was found to be mediated by serum T_4. Here again it is concluded that T_4 acts via intrapituitary conversion of T_4 to T_3. This is supported by the reports of Frumess et al. [1] and Larson [2]. The reason for the weaker correlation between FT_4E and bTSH-SC or dTSH-SC, when compaired with that of T_4, is not clear. A simple explanation would be a methodological problem in the FT_4E estimation in this range. Another explanation would be that an active uptake transport of proteinbound-T_4 into the pituitary is responsible for the feedback control. Interestingly the correlation between T_4-SC and bTSH-SC and that between T_4-SC and dTSH-SC are slightly different, which might be explained by differential effects of T_4-SC feedback control on TSH biosynthesis and secretion. The TRH-test from the theoretical point of view is just a test of pituitary reserve or secretory capacity, whereas bTSH-SC is an indirect measure of TSH-secretion. Further studies are in progresss to elucidate these findings.

Summary

In this study a supersensitive TSH-IRMA has been evaluated with respect to serum concentrations (SC) of thyroid hormones in 99 clinically euthyroids including 31 patients with laboratory evidence of borderline hyperthyroidism. In euthyroids basal TSH (bTSH)-SC correlated with delta TSH (dTSH) (maximal TRH stimulated TSH minus bTSH) ($r = 0.75$; $p < 0.001$). In borderline hyperthyroids bTSH (range: 0.02–0.5 μU/ml) correlated with dTSH ($r = 0.80$, $p < 0.001$). Thus, in most cases the TRH-test does not provide any additional diagnostic information than that provieded by bTSH alone. – bTSH also correlated with T_4-SC ($r = 0.44$, $p < 0.001$), but not with T_3 and Free Equivalent of T_3 (FT_3E). dTSH showed slight correlation with SC-T_4 and FT_4E only (in both $r = -0.33$, $p < 0.01$). This suggests that negative feedback control of the pituitary is mainly brought about by serum T_4.

References

[1] Frumess, R. D., P. R. Larsen: Correlation of serum triiodothyronine (T_3) and thyroxine (T_4) with the biologic effects of thyroid hormone replacement in propylthiouracil-treated rats. Metab. Clin. Exp. **24** (1975) 437–554.

[2] Larsen, P. R.: Regulation of Thyrotropin Secretion by 3,5,3'-Triiodothyronine and Thyroxine. Physiopathology of Endocrine Diseases and Mechanisms of Hormone Action, pp. 81–93, A. R. Liss, Inc., 150 Fifth Avenue, New York, NY 10011 (1981).

[3] Loos, U., R. Grau, E. F. Pfeiffer: Regulation der Schilddrüsen-Stoffwechsellage in der Peripherie (Beeinflussung der T_4-Konversion) Schwerpunkt Medizin **4**, Suppl. (1981).

[4] Loos, U., F. S. Keck, R. Müller: The interrelation of T_4 and its peripheral conversion products T_3 and rT_3 with basal and TRH-stimulated TSH in athyrotic patients. Acta Endocrinol. **105**, Suppl. 264 (1984) 88.

[5] Mahlstedt, J., A. Hotze: Erste Erfahrungen mit einem ultrasensitiven immunradiometrischen TSH-Assay. Nuc. Compact **16** (1985) 72–76.

[6] Moncayo, R., W. Scherbaum, G. Kratzsch, et al.: TSH-Antikörper bei verschiedenen Funktionszuständen der Schilddrüse. Klin. Wochenschr. **63** (Suppl. IV) (1985) 70.

[7] Reichlin, S.: Neuroendocrinology. In: R. H. Williams, ed.) Textbook of endocrinology, pp. 589–645. W. B. Saunders, Philadelphia 1981.

[8] Rothenbuchner, G., J. Birk, U. Loos, et al.: Die TSH-Bestimmung: der empfindlichste Parameter in der Diagnose und Therapie der Schilddrüsenerkrankungen. Therapiewoche **26** (1976) 2105.

[9] Seidel, C. H., D. Ziegelitz, A. Weber, et al.: Zum klinischen Stellenwert eines empfindlichen TSH-RIA. Endokrinologie, 80, 2 (1982) 181–193.

[10] Spencer, C. A., J. T. Nicoloff: Improved radioimmunoassay for human TSH. Clin. Chim. Acta **108** (1980) 415–424.

The effect of Metoclopramide on the TSH and PRL response to TRH in patients treated for depression

B. Varl, V. Žvan, D. Lesjak, B. Salobir

Introduction

Monoamine neurotransmitters are involved in regulation of secretion of hypothalamic and pituitary hormones. Changes in the functional activity of one or more neurotransmitter systems may be expected to produce changes in a number of endocrine systems. Neuroendocrine changes during treatment with tricyclic antidepressants (TCAs) and neuroleptic drugs (NL) have been the subject of numerous studies, and the results have often been contradictory [5].

Last year we reported two cases of inadequate TSH secretion and reversible enlargement of the pituitary gland after several months of treatment with TCAs and NL [7]. In our present study we have tried to identify the factors which may contribute to the observed clinical phenomenon. In particular we were interested in antidepressant treatment influence on TSH, PRL and GH release.

Subjects and methods

The study included six female patients with involutional depression and one with puerperal depression. The diagnoses were made on the basis of DSM III. All the subjects received TCAs and NL. In addition, four of them (K. M., P. K., T. D., S. B.) were treated with benzodiazepines, and patient T. D. also received electroconvulsive treatment (ECT). The standard TRH stimulation test and the combined metoclopramide (MCL)TRH test were performed in the first days of treatment. Six patients (all except M. H.) were rested upon clinical recovery.

Test procedures

The patients were kept in bed and were fasted overnight. The first blood samples were taken at 8 a. m. and 30 minutes later for estimation of T_3, T_4, TSH, PRL and GH. Further blood samples for measurement of TSH, PRL and GH were

Thyrotropin

obtained 30 and 60 minutes after i. v. administration of 200 µg TRH. Two days later a 10 mg dose of MCL was given orally at 8 a. m., and 90 minutes later an i. v. TRH stimulation test was performed. In each case blood was taken two times before MCL administration (0 and 30 min.) for estimation of T_3, T_4, TSH, PRL and GH, and at 60, 90, 120, 150, 180 min. for estimation of TSH, PRL and GH.

Analyses

The serum levels of T_3 and T_4 were measured by the RIA methods SPAC T_3 and SPAC T_4 (Mallinckrodt). TSH and PRL were determined by the RIA methods TSH MAIA and PRL MAIA (Biodata). For GH the RIA method GH-TER (Biodata) was employed.

The reference ranges were:
T_3: 1.40 – 3.25 nmol/l; T_4: 59 – 163 nmol/l; TSH: 0.9 – 3.7 mU/l; GH: 0 – 5.6 µg/l; PRL < 20 µg/l, in menopause < 12 µg/l.

Results

Mean serum T_4 level were 130 (92 – 139) nmol/l during the acute depressive episode, and decreased to 100 (90 – 107) nmol/l after antidepressant treatment. The decrease was significant ($p < 0.01$) in patients with involutional depression (5 patients).

Means serum T_3 levels were 1.8 (1.7 – 1.9) nmol/l initially, and there were no changes on clinical recovery.

The TSH responses to TRH during acute depression varied from subject to subject: there was one non-responder (M. B.), one patient showed a blunted response (K. M.), four were normal responders, and one was a hyperresponder (S. B.) (tab. 1). Basal TSH was elevated in two patients (S. B., M. M.).

The degree of TSH response to TRH was significantly greater ($p < 0.05$) after treatment with TCAs and NL (2 hyperresponders).

During acute depression, four patients (T. D., S. M., M. B., M. M.) showed increased TSH responses to TRH following administration of MCL, compared to the standard TRH stimulation (tab. 2). In one subject (K. M.) MCL had no effect on the TSH response to TRH. In patient S. B., who was TSH hyperresponsive to TRH in the standard test, the response normalized after MCL. It should be pointed out, however, that this patient's basal TSH level at the time of combined test had been normal, too.

Table 1 Serum levels of TSH before (0,30 min) and after i.v. TRH (60, 90 min)

Patients		Times (minutes)			
		0	30	60	90
K.M.	1	2.2	3.0	5.0	3.9
	2	0.8	0.8	5.8	3.7
S.M.	1	2.4	2.3	9.7	10.4
	2	4.7	5.6	24.6	18.4
T.D.	1	2.9	2.7	11.2	9.6
	2	3.3	3.0	19.9	13.4
S.B.	1	8.5	6.8	42.4	37.6
	2	12.7	10.7	55.4	64.8
P.K.	1	3.1	2.8	8.4	6.0
	2	3.0	2.8	16.7	10.8
M.B.	1	1.1	1.2	1.4	1.4
	2	1.6	2.2	7.9	5.9
M.M.	1	4.8	3.1	17.3	18.2
	2	–	–	–	–

1 = in acute depressive episode 2 = on clinical recovery

Table 2 Basal serum levels of TSH (0,30 min) after oral administration of 10 mg metoclopramide (90, 120 min) and after i.v. 150, 180 min) MCL administration at 30 min, i.v. TRH at 120 min

Patients		Times (minutes)					
		0	30	90	120	150	180
K.M.	1	1.5	2.4	2.1	1.5	3.5	2.5
	2	1.3	1.3	1.1	1.3	6.8	4.3
S.M.	1	2.4	3.4	3.8	3.3	14.7	10.2
	2	4.6	4.5	4.7	4.2	23.4	16.7
T.D.	1	7.7	6.5	6.7	5.7	45.1	45.2
	2	2.7	1.8	2.1	2.4	17.6	13.8
S.B.	1	2.9	2.1	2.6	2.4	14.6	10.3
	2	8.5	6.6	7.2	6.2	49.5	53.4
P.K.	1	3.3	2.4	2.7	2.4	14.6	10.1
	2	4.0	4.2	2.3	2.4	20.7	14.2
M.B.	1	1.1	1.4	1.5	0.9	7.5	6.9
	2	1.2	0.9	1.0	1.1	7.4	5.8
M.M.	1	3.2	7.8	2.5	2.4	24.7	20.4
	2	–	–	–	–	–	–

Table 3 Serum levels of PRL before (0,30 min) and after i.v. TRH (60, 90 min)

Patients		Times (minutes)			
		0	30	60	90
K.M.	1	4.8	5.2	40.4	12.4
	2	53.0	51.7	193.0	145.0
S.M.	1	14.6	14.8	126.2	54.1
	2	13.7	10.9	94.7	59.2
T.D.	1	7.7	6.6	23.4	16.2
	2	10.6	5.6	27.7	10.3
S.B.	1	79.7	71.5	140.0	137.6
	2	128.0	183.0	331.0	349.0
P.K.	1	8.5	6.2	33.1	34.8
	2	6.5	7.0	37.3	30.2
M.B.	1	94.9	164.0	172.0	315.0
	2	562.0	> 800.0	> 800.0	528.0
M.M.	1	8.1	7.5	43.3	22.5
	2	–	–	–	–

1 = in acute depressive episode 2 = on clinical recovery

Table 4 Basal serum levels of PRL (0,30 min) after oral administration of 10 mg metoclopramide (90, 120 min) and after i.v. TRH (150, 180 min) MCL administration at 30 min i.v. TRH at 120 min

Patients		Times (minutes)					
		0	30	90	120	150	180
K.M.	1	7.2	11.2	12.4	18.1	120	150
	2	47.4	57.8	143	153	203	200
S.M.	1	13.5	12.2	110	113	125	162
	2	13.2	11.8	86	140	183	156
T.D.	1	7.2	5.3	4.9	6.3	108	61.7
	2	6.8	5.6	17.2	94.3	128	97.8
S.B.	1	76.4	82.3	140.2	127	169	146
	2	114	117	159	302	663	452
P.K.	1	9.9	9.4	15.3	45.4	42.2	47.7
	2	9.8	7.2	9.3	31.9	110	67.0
M.B.	1	331	315	505	435	523	430
	2	511	484	> 800	638	542	791
M.M.	1	8.8	9.6	11.0	35.3	76.6	65.2
	2	–	–	–	–	–	–

On clinical recovery, the TSH responses to the standard TRH stimulation and to MCL/TRH stimulation were equivalent.

Neither during acute depression nor in the recovery period did MCL alone produce a significant change in the TSH levels within 90 minutes of administration.

Patients M.B. and S.B. were hyperprolactinaemic both during acute depression and upon clinical recovery, whereas K.M. grew hyperprolactinaemic on recovery (tab. 3). In the recovery period, all the three patients showed greater PRL responses to MCL (946%, max: 203, 542, 663 μg/l) and a faster rise in the PRL levels, compared to their normoprolactinaemic counterparts (236%, max: 183, 128, 110 μg/l) (tab. 4). Only one patient (M.B.) had a paradoxical GH rise both in the standard TRH test and in the MCL/TRH test. On clinical recovery TRH failed to elicit a rise in GH levels.

Discussion

In six depressive patients treatment with TCAs, NL and anxiolytic drugs led to a significant decrease in the mean serum T_4 level, converted the blunted TSH responses to TRH into normal responses, and enhanced the normal as well as the exaggerated TSH responses to TRH (figs. 1a, 1b).

Of the two patients who had blunted TSH responses to TRH during acute depression, one was hyperprolactinaemic throughout the study and the other grew hyperprolactinaemic on clinical recovery.

The patients who were normal TSH responders (S.M., T.D., P.K.) were mildly hyperprolactinaemic (S.M.) or normoprolactinaemic, and their PRL responses to MCL/TRH increased on recovery.

TSH hyperresponders to TRH were hyperprolactinaemic, and their basal TSH levels were elevated. These patients did not differ biochemically from manifest primary hypothyroidism in respect of their TSH responsiveness to TRH (figs. 2a, 2b). They were TSH non-responders to MCL, and MCL did not influence their TSH response to TRH. On recovery all our patients were TSH non-responders to MCL and they had blunted PRL responses to MCL, but pretreatment with MCL enchanced the PRL response induced by TRH (figs. 3a, 3b). This mode of TSH and PRL responsiveness to MCL differentiates our patients with an exaggerated TSH response to TRH from hypothyroid patients. In a study of primary hypothyroid patients Frey and Hang [4] have demonstrated an increased PRL response to MCL (1460%) and a reduced PRL response to iv. TRH in more than 50% of their subjects if pretreated by MCL (figs. 4a, 4b). The impairment of PRL stimulation by MCL is evidence of a defective pituitary

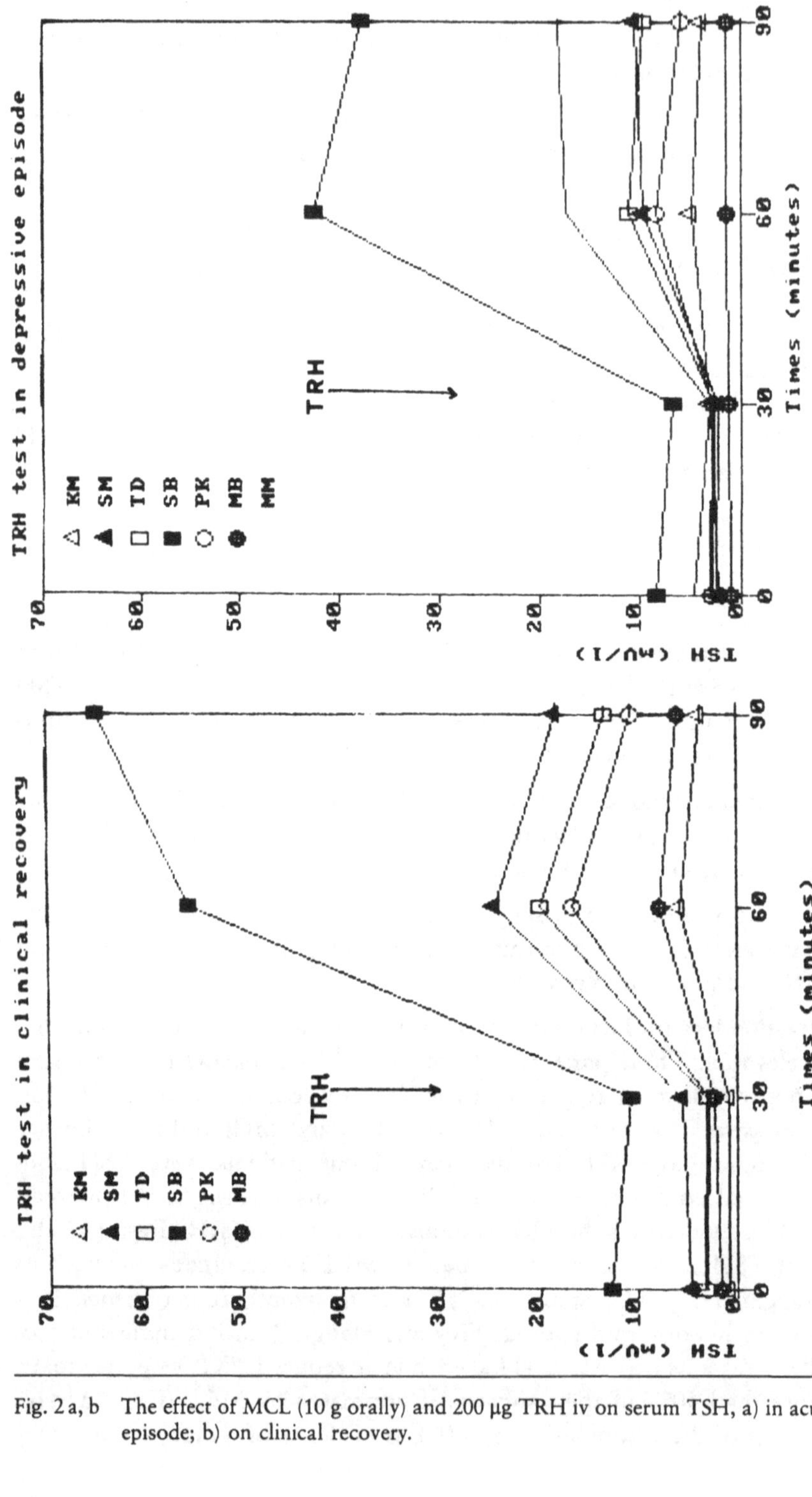

Fig. 1 a, b The effect of iv administration of thyrotropin releasing hormone on serum TSH, a) in acute depressive apisode; b) on clinical recovery.

Fig. 2 a, b The effect of MCL (10 g orally) and 200 μg TRH iv on serum TSH, a) in acute depressive episode; b) on clinical recovery.

MCL + TRH test in depressive episode

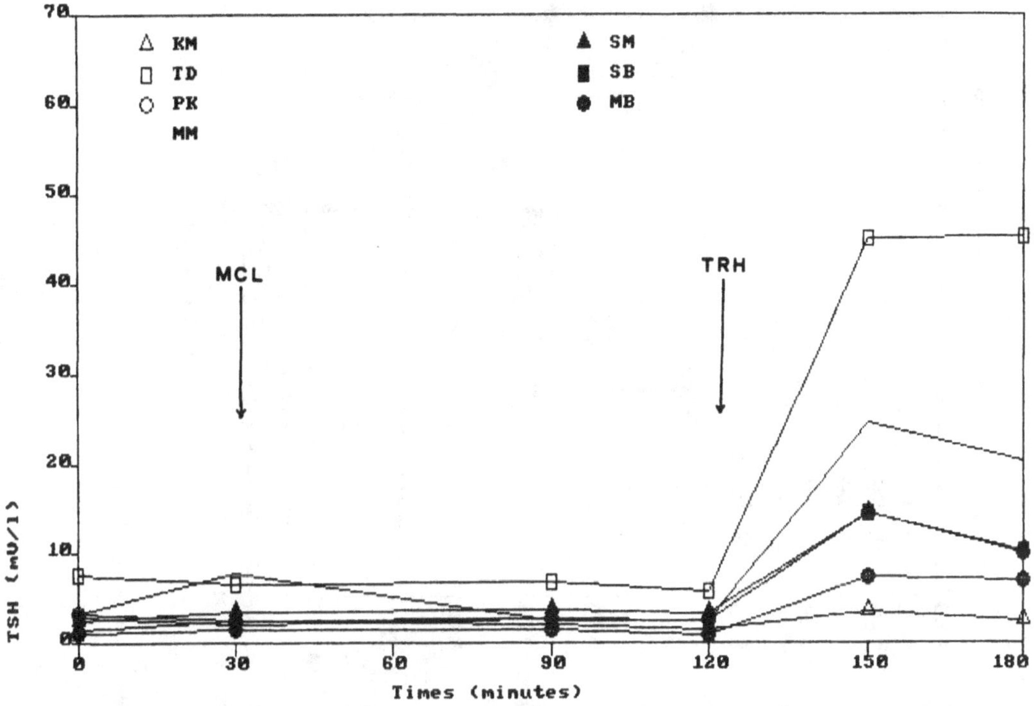

MCL + TRH test in clinical recovery

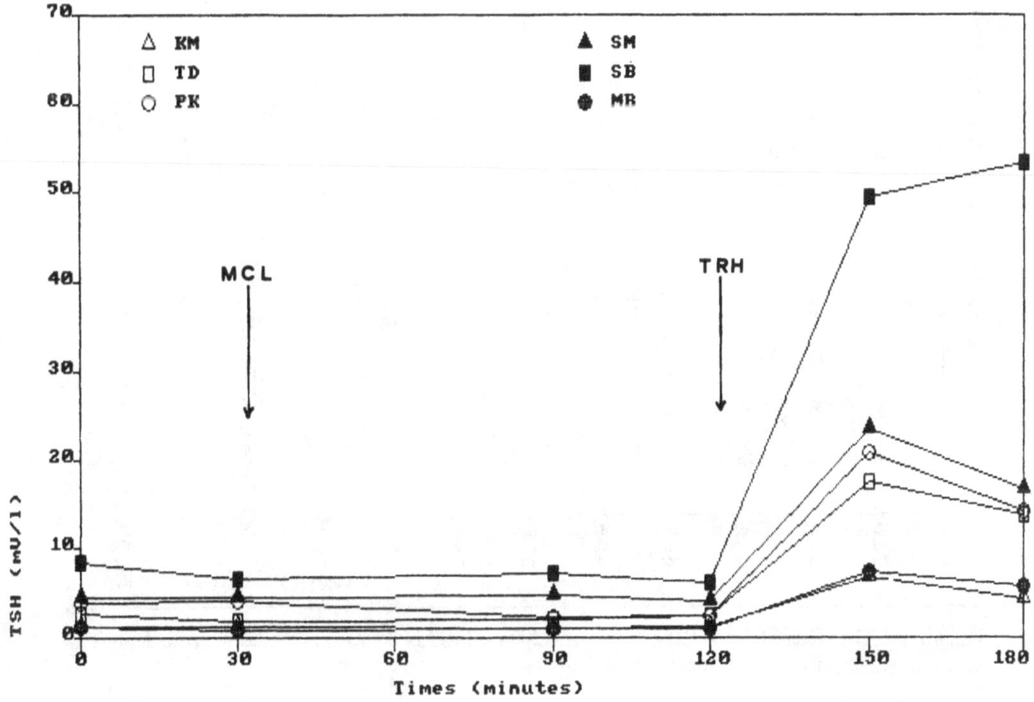

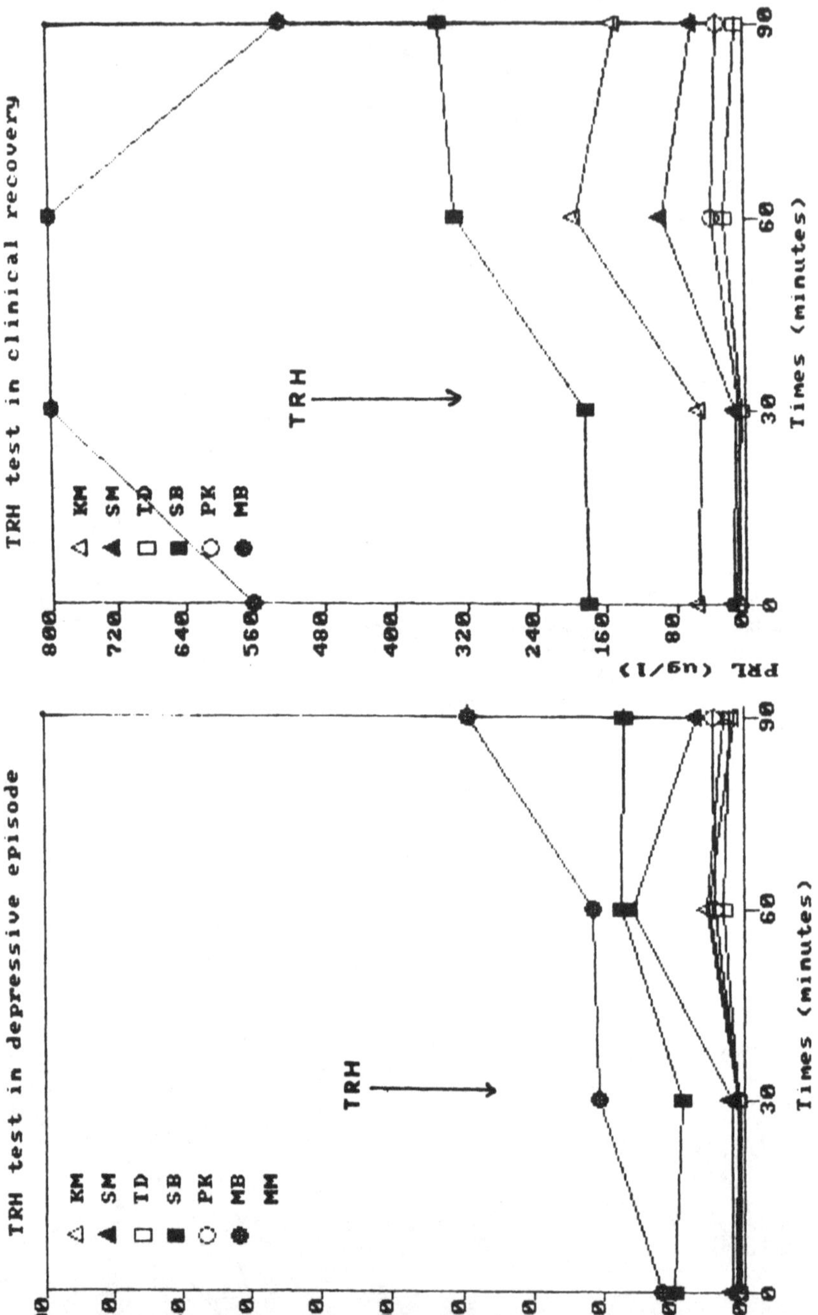

Fig. 3 a, b The effect of 200 µg TRH on serum PRL, a) in acute depressive episode; b) on clinical recovery.

Fig. 4 a, b The effect of MCL (10 g orally) and 200 µg TRH iv on serum PRL, a) in acute depresssive episode; b) on clinical recovery.

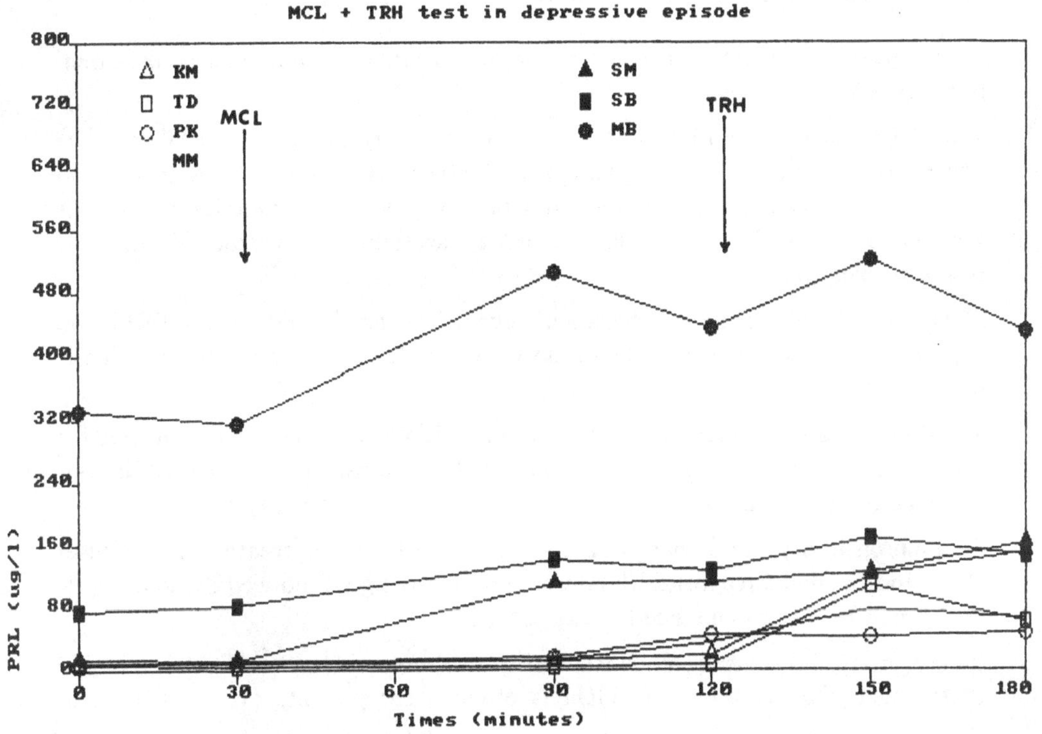
MCL + TRH test in depressive episode
KM
TD
PK
MM
SM
SB
MB
MCL
TRH
800
720
640
560
480
400
320
240
160
80
0
0
30
60
90
120
150
180
PRL (ug/l)
Times (minutes)

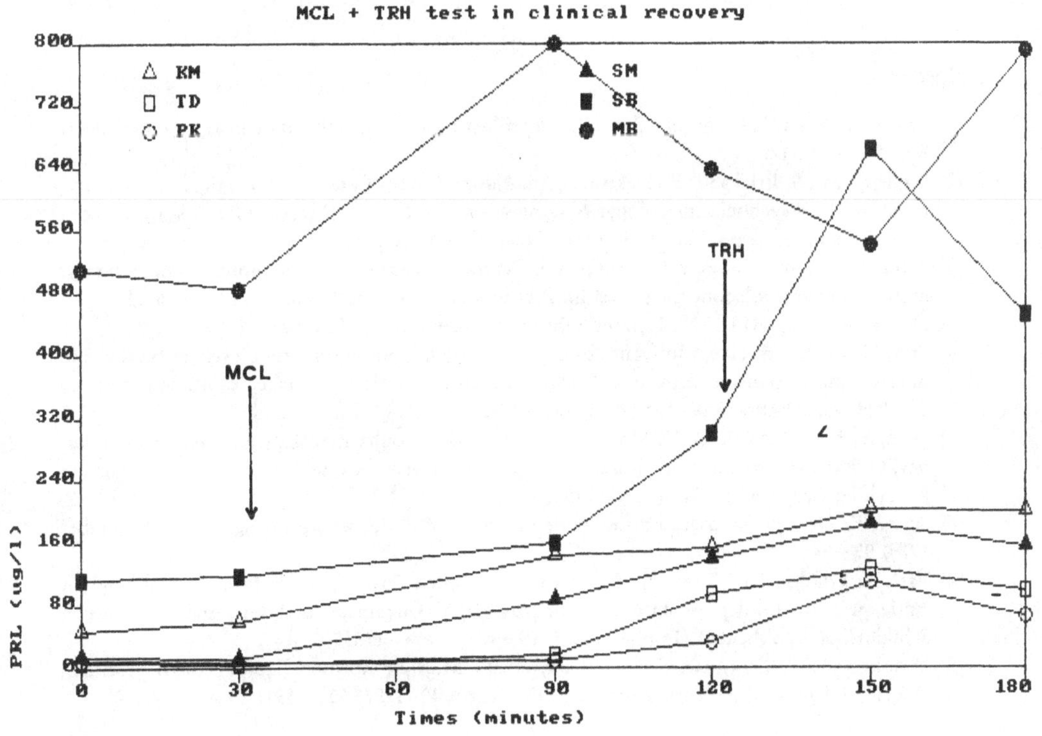
MCL + TRH test in clinical recovery
KM
TD
PK
SM
SB
MB
TRH
MCL
800
720
640
560
480
400
320
240
160
80
0
0
30
60
90
120
150
180
PRL (ug/l)
Times (minutes)

dopamine concentration [3] or a defective intracellular conductance of the dopaminergic signal.

The heightened variability of pituitary hormone response to TRH in acute depressive episode might be explained on the basis of a clinical heterogenity and these findings relate to a fundamental aspect of physiologic function in patients with endogenous depression, ie, increased variability of neuroendocrinologic responsiveness [8].

There is a high correlation between neuroleptic levels and serum PRL, and individuals on the same neuroleptic dose vary widely in their serum neuroleptic levels [1, 2].

Thus we can assume that different neuroleptic levels also may be responsible for the day-to-day variations of TSH and PRL responsiveness observed in our patients, notably S. B. and T. Dž. during the acute depressive episode.

The subsensitivity of adrenergic receptor induced by TCAs treatment [6] (Sulser 1979) and the defective intracellulare dopaminergic signal induced by neuroleptic drugs may be due to enhanced release of TSH.

In our study, however a tendency to the increment of serum TSH levels and to stronger TSH response to TRH is obvious for patients on antidepressant treatment.

References

[1] Brown, W. A., T. P. Laughren: Tolerance to prolactin elevating effect of neuroleptics. Psychiatry Res. 5 (1981) 317.

[2] Davis, J. M., S. Erickson, H. Dekirmenjian: Plasma levels of anti-psychotic drugs and clinical response. In: Psychopharmacology: A Generation of Progress (M. A. Lipton, A. D. Mascio, K. F. Killman, eds.) pp. 905–915, Raven Press New York 1972.

[3] Ferrari, C., A. M. Mattei, P. G. Crosignani: Central nervous system and pituitary dopaminergic defects in hyperprolactinemic states. In: Psychoneuroendocrine dysfunction (N. S. Shah, A. G. Donald, eds.) pp. 613–629. Plenum Publishing Corporation, New York. 1984.

[4] Frey, H. M. M., E. Haug: Influence of dopaminergic inhibition on serum levels of thyrotropin on prolactin in patients with hypothyroidism before and after prolonged oral administration of TRH. Acta Endocrinol. **104** (1983) 183–188.

[5] Shah, A. B., N. S. Shah, D. W. Morgan, et al.: Psychoneuropharmacology and neuroendocrinology, in Psychoneuroendocrine dysfunction (N. S. Shah, A. G. Donald, eds.), pp. 1–44. Plenum Publishing Corporation, New York 1984.

[6] Sulser, F.: New perspectives on the mode of action of antidepressant drugs. TIPS (December 1979) 92–94.

[7] Varl, B.: Erhöhte TSH-Werte bei Patienten mit erhöhten Thyroxin unter Dauerbehandlung mit Antidepressiva. Oral presentation: Schilddrüse 1985. Diagnostik und Therapiekontrolle von Schilddrüsenkrankheiten. Homburg/Saar, 10–12 October 1985.

[8] Winokur, A., J. D. Amsterdam, J. Oler, et al.: Multiple hormonal responses to protirelin (TRH) in depressed patients. Arch. Gen. Psychiatry **40** (1983) 525–531.

Secondary hyperthyroidism associated with pituitary chromophobe adenoma: Study of TSH chemistry and release

W. Waldhäusl, P. R. Bratusch-Marrain, P. Nowotny, W. G. Forssman, H. Schuster

Introduction

Hyperthyroidism commonly is a consequence of a primary defect of the thyroid gland associated with suppression of TSH release due to excessive production of thyroid hormones. Hypersecretion of thyroid hormones as a result of increased TSH secretion with TSH levels being 10 – 20-fold above normal, however, is a rare disorder [1 – 5]. Associated pituitary adenoma secreting excessive amounts of TSH are considered to arise either autonomously, but have also been seen in response to long lasting hypothyroidism [6].

This case report describes a male patient, 56 years of age, suffering from severe secondary hyperthyroidism, chromophobe adenoma and an excessive overproduction of TSH and TSH-like polypeptides and provides a workup of biochemical and functional characteristics of the tumour [7].

Case report

Clinical data

The patient presented the first time with an enlarged thyroid gland and hyperthyroidism two years prior to his admission to this endocrine unit. At that time a subtotal thyroidectomy was performed without being clinically successful. One year later he was again hospitalized, this time with psychotic behaviour and sellar enlargement. X-ray examination now revealed an intrasellar tumour with a sand-glass like suprasellar extension which was demonstrated angiographically.

Plasma concentrations of TSH were 480 μU/ml in the presence of normal total thyroxine concentration (T 4) and during treatment with methimazole. When methimazole was removed T 4 rose to 18 μU/ml and T 3 to 230 ng/ml, while immunoreactive TSH still remained extremely elevated (350 μU/ml).

Thyrotropin

Craniotomy and transcerebral removal of a large tumour weighing 8.4 g caused a fall in plasma TSH to 81 μU/ml. This concentration was still sufficient to induce a relapse of hyperthyroidism after stopping antithyroidal drugs. Finally, a second craniotomy became necessary to normalize TSH levels to 1.2 μU/ml and to cure hyperthyroidism. The patient was doing well thereafter and lived without relapse of this TSH producing tumour for more than 6 years, when he died from myocardial infarction at age 61 years.

Hormone determinations

Analyzing plasma hormone concentrations in detail (fig. 1) it is apparent that serum TSH was 250-fold above normal preoperatively. Postoperatively, it fell by 80% to concentrations 50-fold above the 2 μU/ml commonly seen in control subjects. Simultaneously, alpha-TSH was elevated to 66 ± 4 (SD) ng/ml. It fell to 10.3 ± 1.6 ng/ml (n = 9) upon operation. In contrast, βTSH which was preoperatively in the normal range (0.84 ± 0.7 ng/ml; n = 5), rose postoperatively 8-fold to 6.3 ± 1.5 ng/ml. βTSH decreased consecutively again thereby indicating that its rise was induced by surgery.

Administration of TRH (thyrotropin releasing hormone), which induces in healthy controls a 4–5-fold rise in serum TSH was without any effect upon TSH-release in the propositus. Response of plasma TSH upon TRH remained also uninfluenced by the administration of methimazole, or triiodothyronine or

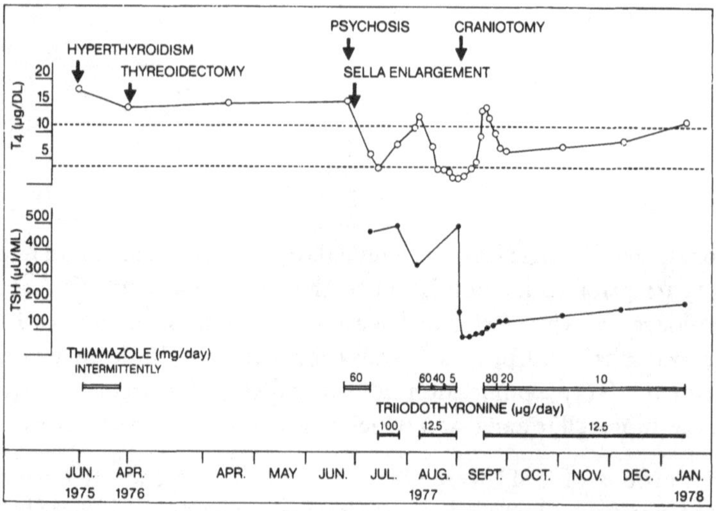

Fig. 1 Case history of a patient with chromophobe pituitary adenoma and secondary hyperthyroidism.

somatostatin. A normal response to TRH was, however, seen as far as serum prolactin (PRL) was concerned.

Stimulation of dopamine receptors by 2-Br-ergocryptine was without any effect on TSH-levels even when doses up to 10 mg were administered per day, while PRL release was suppressed in parallel.

Administration of metoclopramide (10 mg) which blocks dopamine receptors [8] did not induce the expected rise in either TSH, or alpha-TSH or β-TSH, but caused a rise in serum prolactin.

A normal release of pituitary hormones upon an adequate stimulus was observed in the propositus for LH after LH-RH, and for PRL upon intravenous arginine. In contrast, growth hormone and FSH release were not increased by arginine infusion.

Histological workup

The tissue removed by surgery was studied with differential staining, immunocytochemistry and electron microscopy. The chromophobe adenoma showed considerable pleiomorphism. Most cells were fairly large and spindle shaped, but others were round and ovoid and often contained several nuclei. Immunostained thyrotrophs (fig. 2) constituted the majority of cells, which displayed considerable variability in staining with TSH-antibodies using the peroxydase-antiperoxydase

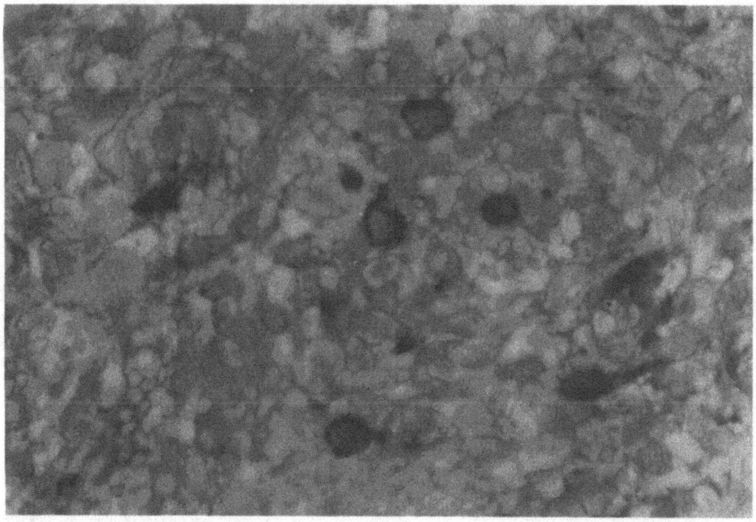

Fig. 2 Immunostained TSH-positive pituitary tissue (chromophobe adenoma) of a patient with secondary hyperthyroidism.

method, which indicated variable hormone content of the thyrotrophs. Specificity of immunostaining was proven by supression by prior antibody adsorption with TSH.

Some cells were also stained by antisomatostatin, but in this case antibody adsorption with somatostatin was without any effect. Antibodies vs. neurotensin, glucagon, gastrin, cholecystkinin, β-endorphin, met-enkephaline. substance-P and motilin did not react with the tumour tissue.

Electron microscopy revealed endocrine cells with secretory granules of 100, 200 and 300 nm diameter. Both TSH positive cells with small granula and a great number of mitochondria were seen as well as cells with larger granula.

Chemical workup

The supernatant of the tumour extract contained after its centrifugation at 30 000 g 1.65 U TSH, 6 μU alpha-TSH and 1 μU β-TSH per gram tissue, respectively. Radioimmunological identity of TSH-MRC 68/38 and tumour TSH was shown by parallel dilution curves.

Electrofocussing of the tumour extract revealed multiple fractions of tumour TSH (TSH.T) with isoelectric points at pH 4.8, 6.1, 6.8, 7.5, 8.2 and 8.9. The relative content of TSH.T with an isoelectric point at pH 6.1 corresponding with that of TSH-MRC 68/38 was 16.3%. The relative share of the other individual fractions ranged from 3.6 – 27.6%. In addition, two fractions containing alpha-TSH and one fraction containing β-TSH were observed.

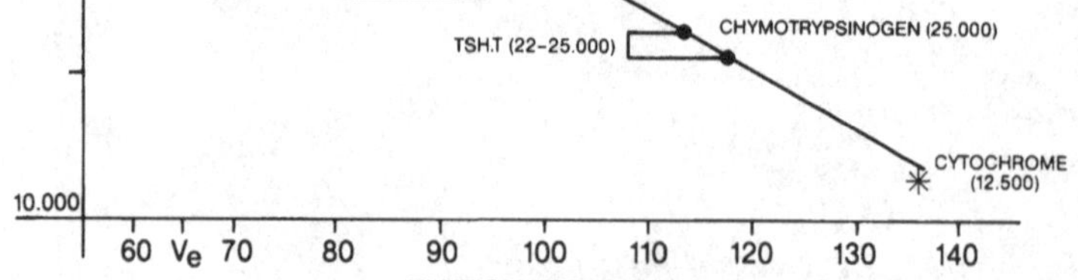

Fig. 3 Estimation of molecular weight by gel filtration on Sephadex G100 of different fractions of TSH.T obtained from pituitary tissue of a patient with secondary hyperthyroidism. TSH.T was prepurified by electrofocussing.

Estimation of the molecular weight by gel filtration on Sephadex G-100 of the various fractions of tumour TSH obtained after electrofocussing demonstrated three groups of the following apparent molecular size (fig. 3): F I – V: 38.000 – 44.000; F VI: 34.000; and F I, II, VI: 22.000 – 25.000 daltons. Thus, the majority of fractions contained TSH.T with a molecular weight in the range of TSH-MRC 68/38 (μ = 40.000) and of 125J-TSH (μ = 36.0000. There was no indication for a 'big TSH'.

Separation of TSH.T on concanavalin-A-sepharose showed that TSH.T behaved like a glycoprotein since it was bound like regular TSH and displaced by 0.1 M mannose (75%) and alpha-methyl-mannoside (25%).

Discussion and conclusion

The obtained data demonstrate in the propositus the presence of secondary hyperthyroidism associated with an excessive, autonomous overproduction of TSH.T by a chromophobe pituitary adenoma. On analysis TSH.T consisted of multiple fractions of different biochemical and biophysical properties, with only 16% coinciding with TSH-MRC 68/38, while the other fractions have to be regarded as paraneoplastic behaviour.

Since small amounts of methimazole were able to control the hyperthyroid state and TSH.T immunoreactivity corresponded only to 16% with that of TSH-MRC 68/38 only a small percentage of TSH.T appears to be biologically active, whereas TSH immunoreactivity was retained by all other molecules. From this it appears that the removed chromophobe adenoma, which also contained some immunoreactivity corresponding to somatostatin, synthesized primarily abnormal TSH molecules devoid of biological activity.

Studies of the common subunit of glycoprotein hormones and of the specific β-subunit of TSH in the patient showed markedly elevated plasma levels of alpha-TSH, which were not due to elevated levels of LH or FSH, but normal values for β-TSH. This situation was reversed after the first operation when alpha-TSH decreased, as has been shown by others [3], whereas β-TSH rose. Thus, it seems that high plasma levels of alpha-TSH indicate a pituitary tumour. In contrast, β-TSH is released only when the tumour tissue is disrupted by surgery. In this case, elevated values of β-TSH, possibly due to leakage from the tumour bed, permit monitoring of the recovery process. These findings that TSH subunits may serve as marker of a pituitary tumour are clinically important since release of subunits of human TSH is suppressed in patients with Graves disease, hyperfunctioning thyroid nodules, or secondary pituitary hypothyroidism, and do not respond to TRH [9].

Summary

Hyperthyroidism associated with pituitary adenoma is a rare disorder with TSH levels in the range from 1.7 – 34 μU/100 ml. This report describes a 57 yr old male suffering from hyperthyroidism (T4 14.3 μg/100 ml; ETI 1.3; T3 230 ng/100 ml) being primarily intractable by subtotal thyroidectomy. Secondary workup revealed elevated plasma TSH levels (480 μU/ml TSH-MRC 68/38/ml) and an enlarged sella due to a tumour (8.4 g) expanding into the suprasellar region. After two hypophysectomies plasma TSH fell to 20 μU/ml (T4 1.8 μg/100 ml; FTI 0.7).

The obtained biochemical data suggest 1. that TSH.T is released by the tumour almost completely independent from hypothalamic control; 2. that TSH.T is a glycoprotein which retained its immunological identity for all its components, and 3. that TSH.T exerts less biological activity than normal TSH.

References

[1] Jailer, J. W., D. A. Holub: Remission of Graves' disease following radiotherapy of a pituitary neoplasm. Am. J. Med. **28** (1960) 497.

[2] Lamberg, B. A., J. Ripatti, A. Gordin, et al.: Chromophobe pituitary adenoma with acromegaly and TSH-induced hyperthyroidism associated with parathyroid adenoma. Acta Endocrinol. (Copenh.) **60** (1969) 157.

[3] Kourides, I. A., E. C. Ridgway, B. D. Weintraub, et al.: Thyrotropin-induced hyperthyroidism: Use of alpha and beta subunit levels to identify patients with pituitary tumors. J. Clin. Endocrinol. Metab. **45** (1977) 534.

[4] Duello, T. M., N. S. Halmi: Pituitary adenoma producing thyrotropin and prolactin. Virchows Arch. (Pathol. Anat.) **376** (1977) 255.

[5] Tolis, G., C. Bird, G. Bertrand, et al.: Pituitary hyperthyroidism. Am. J. Med. **64** (1978) 177.

[6] Linquette, M., P. Fossati, M. Decoulx, et al.: Adénomes thyréotropes. In: Les Adénomes Hypophysaires Sécretants, p 155, Masson, Paris 1971.

[7] Waldhäusl, W., P. Bratusch-Marrain, P. Nowotny, et al.: Secondary hyperthyroidism due to thyrotropin hypersecretion: Study of pituitary tumor morphology and thyrotropin chemistry and release. J. Clin. Endocrinol. Metab. **49** (1979) 879.

[8] Healy, D. L., H. G. Burger: Increased prolactin and thyrotropin secretion following oral metoclopramide: Dose response relationships. Clin. Endocrinol. (Oxf.) **7** (1977) 195.

[9] Kourides, I. A., B. D. Weintraub, E. C. Ridgway, et al.: Pituitary secretion of free alpha and beta subunit of human thyrotropin in patients with thyroid disorders. J. Clin. Endocrinol. Metab. **40** (1975) 872.

Hyperthyroidism and thyroid hormone resistance

K.-J. Gräf, D. Witt, E. Kazner

Introduction

The syndrome of tissue resistance to the action of thyroid hormones together with the phenomenon of the inappropriately high thyrotropin (TSH) secretion was first described by Refetoff et al., 1967 [5]. Since then, various authors have published case reports of this very rare disorder, which together show that the clinical manifestation is rather variable [for review see 1, 4, 6]. In the present paper three case studies are added to this topic which underline the heterogeneity described in the literature.

Patients and methods

Case 1: a now 33-year-old female patient was first admitted to our clinic in 1974 with the only clinical symptom of a diffuse goiter (WHO II). There were no other pathological findings, in particular no signs of a thyroid dysfunction or endocrine ophthalmological symptoms. This was in clear contrast with the laboratory results which indicated a hyperthyroid dysfunction. Both total and free triiodothyronine (TT_3, FT_3) and thyroxine (TT_4, FT_4) levels were increased a finding which could be further substantiated by a distinct elevation of I-131 uptake (tab. 1). In consequence, the patient was treated with carbimazole, initially with 30 mg and later with lower dosages in combination with 50 – 100 µg levothyroxine (l-T_4). After 11 months of treatment, the I-131 uptake remained elevated as were the in vitro parameters for T_3 and T_4, while the enlargement of the thyroid gland had progressed. Therefore, the patient underwent a subtotal thyroidectomy followed by treatment with 100 – 150 µg l-T_4. Elevated basal TSH and normal TSH increase due to TRH stimulation (400 µg relefact (R) i. v.) were estimated for the first time in 1976 (here without any treatment and shortly before operation) and later in 1979 and 1981 (at these times most probably under the treatment with l-T_4) (fig. 1). However, the discrepancy between these results and the in vitro findings for T_3 and T_4 was ignored until 1982 when highly basal TSH levels (in 1982 the patient was without any l-T_4 treatment) with an only insignificant response to TRH were again measured several times (fig. 1 and tab. 1). Thus, with a latency of six years, the diagnoses of a secondary hyperthy-

Thyrotropin

Table 1 Synopsis of essential laboratory and clinical findings (case 1 – 3)

Patient (age)	Date (month/ year)	T_3 (%) (Hamolsky)	TT_3 (ng/ml)	FT_3 (ng/l)	TT_4 (ng/dl)	FT_4 (ng/dl)	TSH (µU/ml) basal/TRH stimulated	Varia (laboratory)	Clinical data (essentials)
R. C. (case 1) (*29. 06. 52)	7/1974	68			> 20				diff. goiter (WHO II); euthyroidism
	4/1975	68			16.8			I-131 uptake 2 h: 85% 24 h: 94% 48 h: 92%	treatment with carbimazole (4/75 – 5/76); euthyroidism
	5/1976	67	2.4		17		5.2 / 14.4	I-131 uptake (unchanged, see 1975) TAK ∅; MAK ∅	euthyroidism; goiter (WHO III) 5/76 thyroidectomy (subtotal) 5/76 1981: 100 – 150 µg l-T_4
	7/1982		3.1		18.4	4.7	21 / 22.8	PRL: 62 ng/ml GH: < 0.3 ng/ml	euthyroidism; goiter 12/82 adenomectomy (transnasal)
	5/1983		9.9	14	19.8	4.6	3.3	PRL: 15.2 ng/ml GH: < 0.3 ng/ml LH: 5.2 mlU/ml Cortisol: 258 mmol/l Progesteron: 0.3 ng/ml E_2: 8.5 pg/ml	2/83 2nd adenomectomy (transcranial); 4/83 irradiation; euthyroidism; no hypophyseal insufficiency; between 8/83 and 6/85 various treatment trials with bromocriptine, lisuride, terguride, TRIAC, d-T_4 and T_3
	1/1986		2.1	9.7	12.8	2.6	6.4		no treatment; euthyroidism; diffuse goiter
K.-S. G. (case 2) (*08. 09. 35)	9/1967	42						I-131 uptake 2 h: 63% 24 h: 84% 48 h: 78%	euthyroidism; diffuse goiter 2/68: (as 1952 and 1961) thyroidectomy (subtotal) 4/77: I-131 radiatio; euthyroidism; diff. goiter (WHO I); 12/77 – 4/86: 100 – 300 µg l-T_4

	11/1978	62	1.9		11		1.9 – 8	/ >50		euthyroidism
	11/1984		1.8	5.2	16	20	32.5	59.8		treatment with 100 µg l-T_4/daily
	6/1985		1.4	5.0	84	12	169	/ 15′ 182 30′ 187 90′ 184 120′ 206	PRL: 11.8 µg/ml	euthyroidism; goiter; no therapy with l-T_4 since 4 weeks; acute treatment trial with TRIAC (1 mg p.o.) given directly before the intranasal application of TRH
	4/1986		1.3	2.9	164	29	28			during treatment with 175 µg l-T_4; goiter clinically euthyroidism
S. A. (case 3) (*12. 01. 63)	8/1978		3.0 – 4.6		7.2 – 11.5		10 – 13		TAK ∅, MAK ∅	hyperthyroidism, diffuse and multinodular goiter (WHO II)
	12/1979	58	2.7		16		9.2	/ >50	PRL: 6.2 ng/ml	hyperthyroidism, unchanged goiter
	1/1981	66	2.3		15.8		2.3	/ 19		during treatment with 175 µg l-T_4; hyperthyroidism, unchanged goiter
	4/1986		2.5	6.5	10.9	17.8	61	/ 320	PRL: 2.7 ng/ml	hyperthyroidism, diffuse and multinodular goiter (WHO III) 10/85 thyroidectomy (subtotal)
	5/1986		1.8	6.2	17.8	78	21			during treatment with 150 µg l-T_4

Normal ranges: T_3 (Hamolsky): 40 – 67%; TT_3 (RIA): 1.2 – 1.9 ng/ml; FT_3 (RIA): 2.8 – 6.8 ng/l;
basal TSH (RIA): 0.6 – 3.9 µU/ml; TT_4 (RIA): 5 – 15 ng/dl; FT_4 (RIA): 1.1 – 2.5 ng/dl

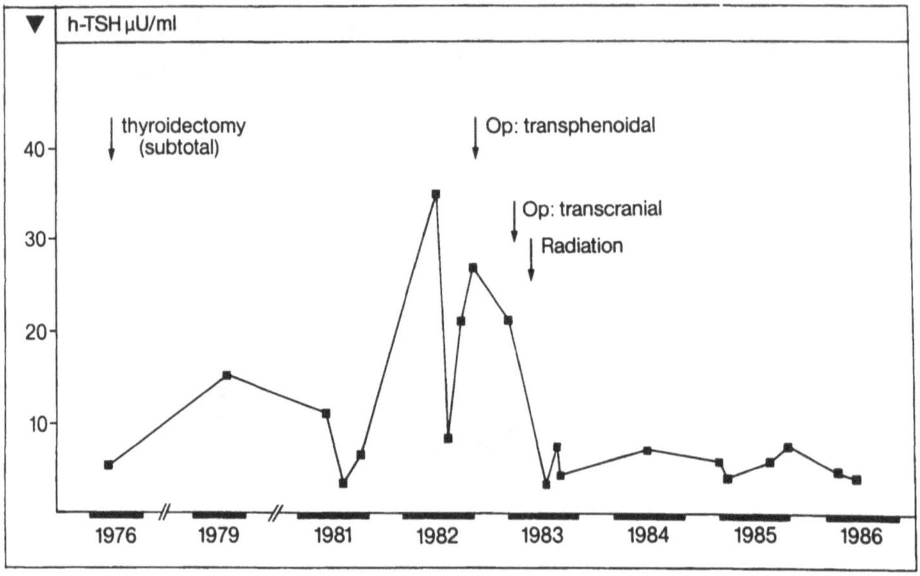

Fig. 1 TSH follow-up data from patient R. C. between 1976 and 1986.

roidism and a tissue resistance to thyroid hormones was first assumed in this year. The contrast enhanced CT scan of the sella region showed a large pituitary tumor with extensive suprasellar growth (fig. 2). Surgery was performed twice, at first by transphenoidal and 2 months later by transfrontal approach, followed by conventional irradiation with 50 GY because the tumor could not be excised in toto. The immunocytochemical studies on the excised tumor material showed that about 20% of the cells were positive for prolactin (PRL), 10% for growth hormone (GH). 5% for β-TSH and 50% for the α-subunit. After neurosurgery and irradiation, the TSH levels dropped significantly but did not return to normal (tab. 1, fig. 1). All the other endocrinological control studies performed repeatedly after operation and irradiation revealed no signs of a hypophyseal insufficiency, and the T_3 and T_4 levels remained essentially unchanged (tab. 1). However, the PRL levels – primarily found to be slightly elevated – felt from 62 ng/ml (preoperatively) to 7–10 ng/ml (postoperatively) within the normal range. Against this background, various drugs were given to suppress TSH secretion and thus to inhibit a further growth of the thyroid gland and regrowth of the pituitary adenoma residue. The treatment periods varied between 8 and 18 weeks, and the drugs used were the dopamine agonists Pravidel (R) (bromocriptine), Dopergin (R) (lisuride) and terguride (transdihydrolisurid); then Thybon (R) (triiodothyronine), Dynothel (R) (dextro-thyroxine), the biologically inactive T_4 derivative; and the T_3 analogue TRIAC (triiodo-l-thyroacetic acid). The dosages

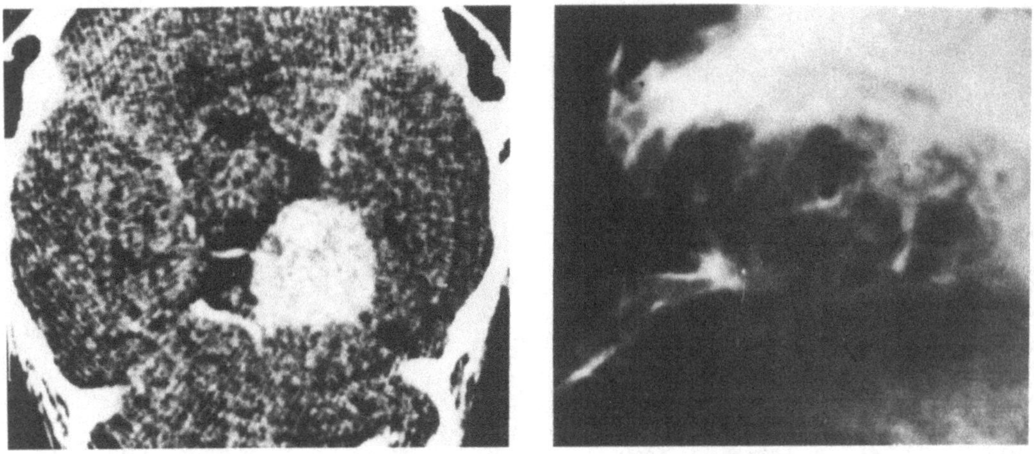

Fig. 2 Patient R. C. (case 1): TSH secreting pituitary adenoma. Left: Conventional X-ray of the sella region. Total destruction of the cavum sellae (dorsum and bottom). Right: CT scan (axial) of the supra sellar part of the macroadenoma near to the third ventricle.

given are listed in tab. 2. For terguride and TRIAC, two drugs in the clinical phase of development, written informed consent was obtained from the patient. According to the literature, bromocriptine, T_3, dextrothyroxine, and TRIAC effectively suppress TSH secretion – at least in some cases [3, 4]. No data have yet been attained with lisuride, a 'pure' dopamine agonist comparable to bromocriptine, and with terguride, a lisuride derivative which combines dopamine

Table 2 Influence of various drugs on thyroid hormones in patient R. C.

RIA / Substance	T_4	FT_4	T_3	FT_3	side effects
Pravidel® (2.5 mg t.i.d.)	=	=	↓	(↓)	tiredness
Dopergin® (0.1 mg t.i.d.)	=	=	↓	↓	none
Tergurid (0.25 mg t.i.d.)	=	=	(↓)	=	none
Dynothel® (1 mg t.i.d.)	↑*	↑*	↓	=	none
Thybon® (80 μg daily)	=	=	↑*	↑*	none
TRIAC (1 mg b.i.d.)	=	=	↑↑*	↑↑*	none

= unchanged ↓ lowered ↑ elevated ( ) uncertain change * due to cross reactivity

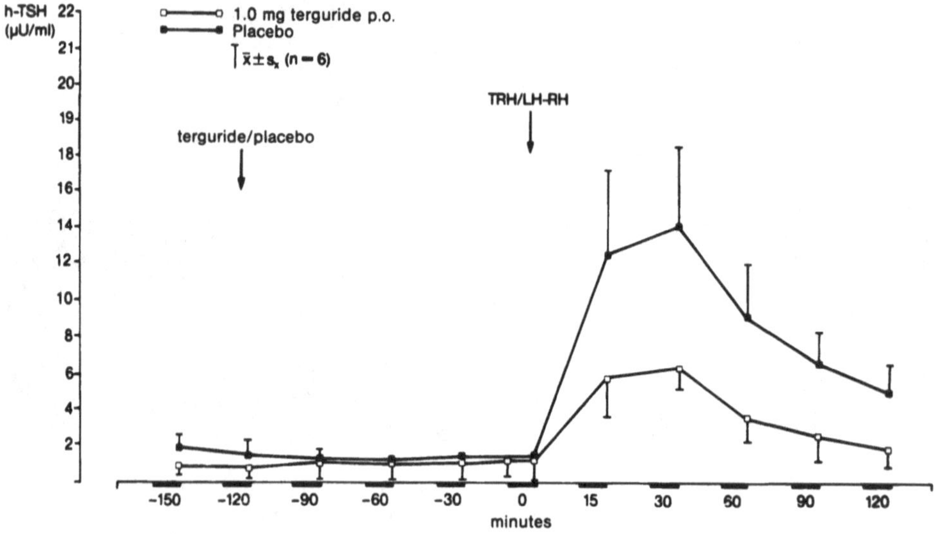

Fig. 3 TSH levels due to TRH/LH-RH stimulation in male volunteers pretreated with placebo or terguride. Dosages: TRH 200 µg i. v., LH-RH 100 µg i. v.

agonistic and antagonistic potencies [2,7]. The use of these drugs was of special interest since in human pharmacological studies especially terguride has been effective in lowering TRH-stimulated TSH levels (fig. 3). However, as regards TSH suppressive potency, none of the tested drugs proved to be effective (fig. 4). As regards the T_3 and T_4 levels and the clinical situation throughout the various treatment periods, the following characteristics are notable (tab. 2): the TT_3 and FT_3 levels were found to be slightly lowered throughout the use of Pravidel (R), Dopergin (R) and terguride. Thybon led to an increase of TT_3 and FT_3 levels, which is due to the expected cross-reactivity. In line with the assumption of a peripheral resistance to thyroid hormones is the fact that even relatively high in vitro levels (e. g. 5.8 ng/ml for TT_3 and 16.1 ng/l for FT_3) were tolerated without any clinical symptoms – especially with no signs of hyperthyroidism. Nor were any clinical correlates found during treatment with Dynothel (R), which led – also due to cross reactivity phenomenons – to an increase of TT_4 levels up to a maximum of 36 ng/dl and of 9.8 ng/dl for FT_4 levels. Finally, under the treatment with TRIAC high TT_3 (up to 8.2 µg/l) and FT_3 (up to 20 ng/l) levels were measured – even higher than during the treatment with Thybon (R) – and again the patient had no complaints. With the exception of Dynothel (R), the TT_4 and FT_4 levels remained more or less unchanged throughout the different treatments.

At present, the patient is receiving no drug treatment; the TSH levels have so far remained stable between 4 and 7.7 ng/l; the T_3 and T_4 levels are still (or even

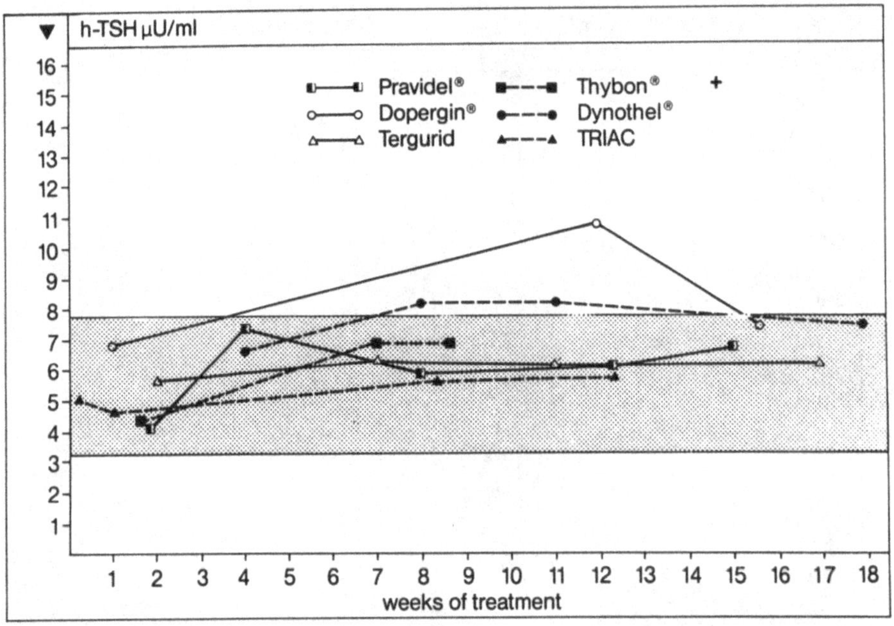

Fig. 4 TSH follow-up data from patient R. C. under various treatment regimes. + dosages see table 2.

more) elevated, while the patient has remained clinically euthyroid (see fig. 1 and tab. 1).

Case 2: Patient K.-S. G. a now 50-year-old female patient was first admitted to our clinic in 1967. At that time clinically the patient had a diffuse and bilateral nodular goiter (WHO II); otherwise she was clinically euthyroid and without any endocrine ophthalmological symptoms; the Hamoslky test was found to be within the normal range and the I-131 uptake was slightly elevated (see tab. 1). The in vitro results from 1976 – when most of the specific radioimmunoassays were introduced in the clinics – substantiated the clinical findings of euthyroidism in that the total and free T_3 and T_4 levels were all within the normal range. The antibodies TAK and MAK were both non detectable whereas the basal and the TRH-stimulated TSH levels were clearly elevated (see tab. 1).

Besides the laboratory findings which have essentially all remained unchanged since 1976 the patient had a peculiar clinical history with repeated subtotal thyroidectomies in the years 1952, 1961 and 1968. Since 1968 she has been treated with l-T_4 (in dosages between 50 and 300 μg daily); a treatment which could not prevent a further enlargement of the thyroid gland. In the years between 1977 and 1986 no major clinical changes in the thyroid growth was demonstrable. The TSH follow-up data are summarized in figure 5 which clearly demonstrates

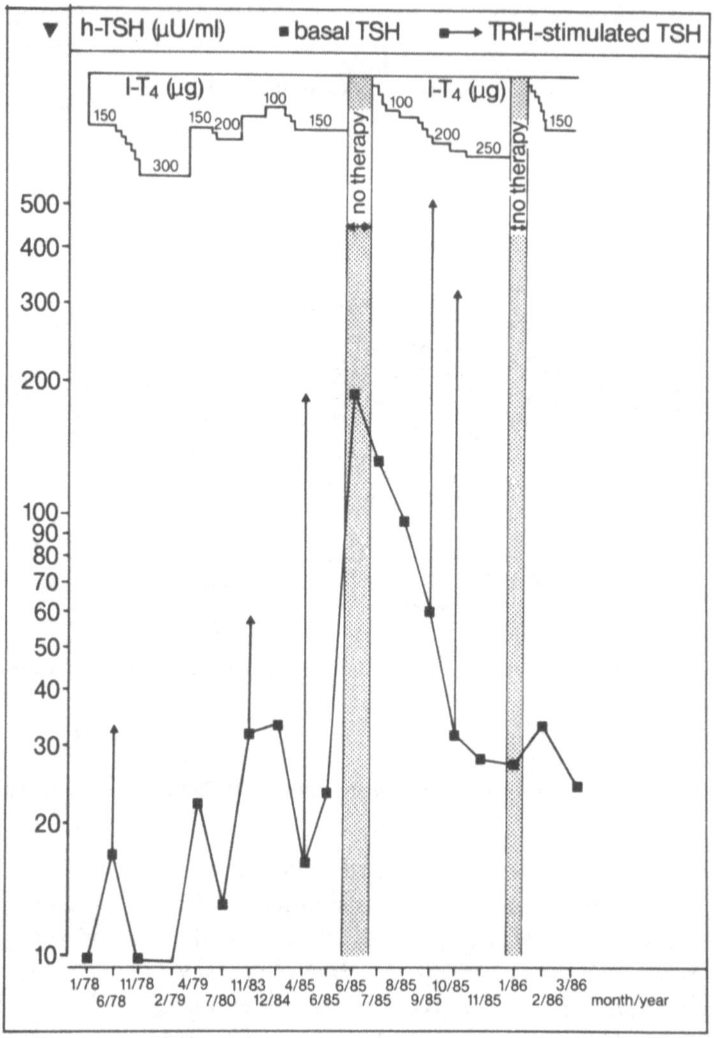

Fig. 5 TSH follow-up data from patient K.-S. G. with or without l-T_4 treatment.

a close negative correlationship between the height of the TSH levels and the dosages of the treatment with l-T_4. With regard to the diagnosis of a tissue resistance to thyroid hormones, it is of special interest in this patient that she always developed clinical signs of hyperthyroidism only when the dosages of l-T_4 was increased to more than 150 µg daily. However, in order to suppress basal TSH secretion to at least 5 mU/l, dosages of about 300 µg l-T_4 were necessary. These very high dosage were tolerated only if one increased the dosages very, very slowly over weeks and months in 12.5 µg steps so that the patient had time enough to adapt.

A treatment trial with TRIAC in the low dosage of 2 mg daily had to be stopped because of side effects, e.g. excessive sweating, headaches and severe emotional instability. However, TRIAC suppressed the highly elevated basal TSH levels within 7 days from 169 to 65 mU/l, whereas the TT_4 levels decreased from 84 to 20 µg/l, the FT_4 levels from 12 to 5 ng/L. The FT_3 levels were increased from 5 to 16 ng/l (again due to the expected cross reactivity). In an acute trial with a single oral dosage of TRIAC (1 mg) no TSH suppressive effect was found (tab. 1). In particular, the clinical symptoms described indicate that – in this case – there is no peripheral tissue resistance to thyroid hormones as is the case – at least in part – at the hypothalamohypophyseal level.

The intensitivity of TSH secretion to the feedback control mechanisms is most probably – in contrast to the first case presented – not attributable to an autonomous TSH secretion of a hypophyseal adenoma. This is substantiated to some extent by the fact that the TRH stimulation test has repeatedly been found to be highly positive (fig. 5). Moreover, the CT and NMR imaging studies have been entirely normal as were all the other endocrine functions of the pituitary.

Of further interest is especially the familial history of this patient. Although there are no definite details, it is notable that several members of the maternal side of the patient's family also had very large goiters. Furthermore, one of her two sons also has an enlargement of the thyroid gland due to an inappropriate TSH secretion (see case 3).

Case 3: Patient S. A., born in 1963, first received attention because of nervousness at the age of 2! He was treated in 1965 and 1966 at first with a sedative drug, thereafter with the thioamide derivative carbimazole. Details of endocrinological findings from this time are not available. The endocrinological findings can be followed back to 1978 when the patient was first examined in our clinic again because of nervousness and excessive sweating. His mother told us that he had been restless and nervous since early childhood. Furthermore, she had first noticed an enlargement of the thyroid gland several years earlier. In addition to the symptoms already mentioned clinically the patient had now a diffuse and multinodular goiter (WHO II), a tachycardia (124 per minute) and a labile hypertension with levels up to 160 (systolic) and to 100 mmHg (diastolic). The laboratory studies confirmed the clinical assumption of hyperthyroidism (tab. 1). From 1978 to 1986, repeatedly marginal or highly elevated in vitro levels were found for T_3 and T_4, whereas the basal and the TRH-stimulated TSH levels were found to be increased (fig. 6, tab. 1). The patient was temporarily treated in 1978 and 1979 with Nuran (R) (cyproheptadine, 4 mg t. i. d.), which lowered the TSH levels slightly. This treatment was stopped because of unwanted weight gain and irregular intake. In 1979 the patient was first treated with l-T_4 up to 200 µg daily, and the follow-up data indicate that in the dose range between 100 and 200 µg l-T_4 this treatment regime effectively suppressed the TSH secretion.

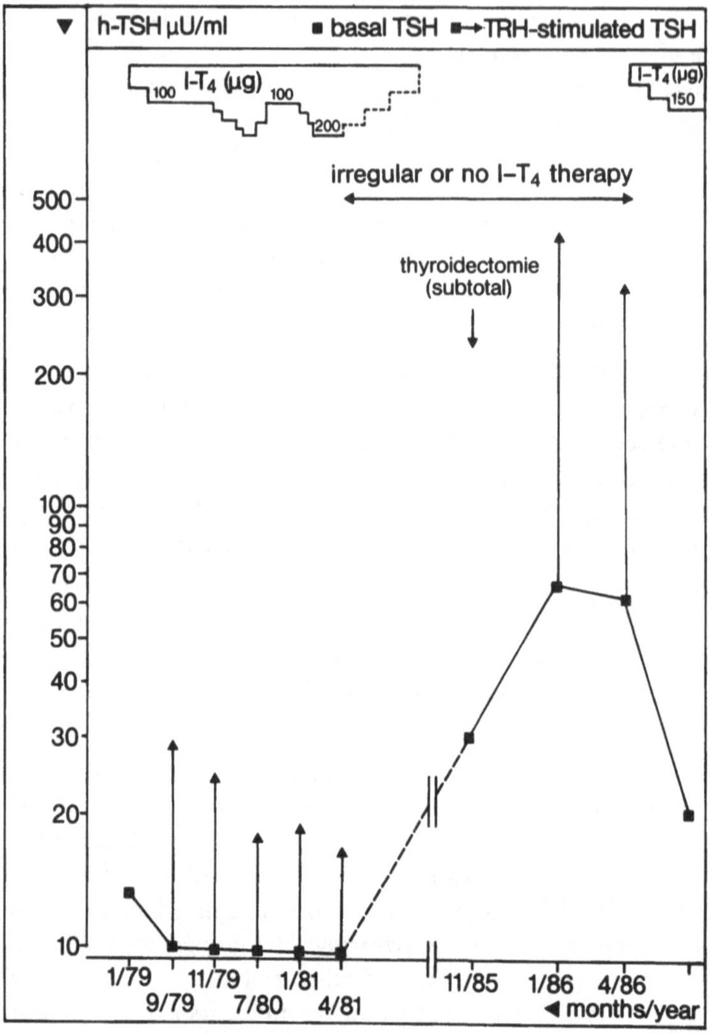

Fig. 6 TSH follow-up data from patient S. A. between 1979 and 1986.

When the l-T_4 therapy was stopped at the patient's request, the TSH secretion increased dramatically (fig. 6), and the enlargement of the thyroid progressed. In 1985 the patient underwent – due to a diffuse and nodular goiter (now WHO III) – subtotal thyroidectomy. Then the patient initially had refused the intake of l-T_4 and so again the TSH levels increased markedly (fig. 6). In consequence the patient has now agreed to take l-T_4. During the short treatment period (2 weeks) with 150 µg l-T_4 daily – which is well tolerated – the basal TSH levels were found to be lowered from the maximum of 61 µU/ml to 21 µU/ml, concomitantly the TT_4 and FT_4 levels increased whereas the TT_3 and FT_3 levels decreased (fig. 6 and tab. 1).

Summary

The three case reports substantiate earlier studies that the syndrome of the inappropriate TSH secretion and tissue resistance to thyroid hormone can occur in combination with and without a TSH secreting pituitary adenoma. Furthermore, the clinical symptoms described underline oncemore the heterogeneity of this syndrome. In principle one has to distinguish mainly between a central resistance to thyroid hormones, with the main clinical findings of euthyroidism and goiter – as this is the case in our first patient – and the global (central and peripheral) resistance, with clinical hyperthyroidism and goiter (see case reports 2 and 3). As regards the therapy and with respect to the data presented, a TSH-suppressive effect due to the treatment with l-T_4 cannot be excluded. This supports the assumption that at least in certain cases, the resistance to thyroid hormones is not complete, which in turn suggests that in these cases a treatment trial with l-T_4 is advisable. While this procedure led to positive results in two of our cases (both without a hypophyseal adenoma) this treatment regime failed to be effective in the third case – a patient with a TSH-secreting pituitary adenoma. Furthermore in this case no success has been had also with various other drugs, such as bromocriptine, lisuride, terguride, TRIAC, dextrothyroxine and high T_3 dosages. This is in some contrast to the literature, since in several cases dopamine agonists, TRIAC and dextrothyroxine suppressed TSH-secretion very effectively.

Acknowledgements

I wish to thank Dr. Jautzke (Klinikum Steglitz, Berlin) for the immunocytochemical studies. TRIAC was a gift from Henning, Berlin and terguride was kindly supplied by Schering AG, Berlin/Bergkamen. Neurosurgery was performed by Prof. Kazner (Klinikum Charlottenburg, Berlin). We are grateful to the staff of the Dept. of Radiology and Internal Medicine for laboratory assistance and for their care of the patients referred to in this paper.

References

[1] Bürgi, H.: Periphere Resistenz gegen Schilddrüsenhormon mit Hypothyreose oder Hyperthyreose bei TSH-Übersekretion – ein weites Spektrum von seltenen Funktionsstörungen mit TSH Übersekretion. Schweiz. Med. Wochenschr. **114** (1984) 16.

[2] Gräf, K.-J., D. Köhler, R. Horowski, et al.: Rapid regression of macroprolactinomas by the new dopamine partial agonist terguride. Acta Endocrinol. **111** (1986) 460–466.

[3] Hehrmann, R., J. Joost: Hyperthyreosen mit gesteigerter bzw. inappropriater Thyreotropin-Sekretion. In: Schilddrüse 1983 (C. R. Pickardt, H. Schleusener, eds.) pp. 256–265. Georg Thieme Verlag, Stuttgart – New York 1985.
[4] Refetoff, S.: Syndromes of thyroid hormone resistance. The American Physiological Society E 88 – E 98 (1982).
[5] Refetoff, S., T. Loren, L. T. DeWind, et al.: Familial syndrome combining deaf-mutism, stippled epiphysis, goiter and abnormally high PBI: Possible target organ refractoriness to thyroid hormone. J. Clin. Endocr. 27 (1967) 279.
[6] Seif, F. J.: Differentialdiagnostik der Gewerbsresistenz gegenüber Schilddrüsenhormonen. Act. Endocrinol. Stoffw. 3 (1982) 113 – 118.
[7] Wachtel, H., R. Dorow: Dual action on central dopamine function of transdihydrolisuride, a 9, 10 – dihydrogenated analogue of the dopamine agonist lisuride. Life Sciences 32 (1983) 421 – 432.

Comparison of TSH secretory response and plasma TRH levels after intravenous and nasal TRH administration*

D. Hadjidakis, S. Raptis, E. Katoulis, P. Portokalakis,
A. Souvatzoglou, U. Loos, L. Duntas, E. F. Pfeiffer

Introduction

Thyrotropin stimulation by synthetic TRH (thyrotropin releasing hormone) has gained great value in the investigation of thyroid as well as certain pituitary disorders [3, 5, 10].

The availability of thyrotropin releasing factor (TRH) in a form suitable for intranasal application led to the question regarding the effectiveness of this route. If this holds true then a more practical and simple way would be applied in the investigation of hypothalamic-pituitary-thyroid axis. In fact few studies so far have shown that the nasal route is equally effective to the intravenous one in eliciting the TSH as well as prolactin response [1, 2, 4, 7].

However nothing is known concerning the levels of plasma TRH obtained by either route. For this purpose besides studying the behavior of TSH response after the intravenous and intranasal TRH administration we extended our investigation on the pharmacokinetics of TRH in terms of time of peak levels and total circulating quantity during the observation period.

Material and methods

Ten healthy volunteers (7 males, 3 females aged 22 to 58 years, Group I) and 5 patients with hyperthyroidism participated to the study. After an overnight fasting and being recumbent for one hour they received in time 0′ either 200 μg of TRH (TRH Relefact, Hoechst A. G.) intravenously as a bolus or 2000 μg of TRH (HOE 011, kindly provided by Hoechst AG) in aerolized form by nasal

* This work was supported by grants from the Social Ministry, Athens, Greece; Department of Internal Medicine I, University of Ulm, FRG; Deutsche Forschungsgemeinschaft SFB 87 Endokrinologie Ulm, FRG; and the Alexander S. Onassis Foundation, Vaduz, Liechtenstein.

insuflation. Blood was sampled in 0, 15, 30, 45, 60. 90 and 120 minutes for radioimmunological determination of TSH and proclactin. Moreover in 0, 2, 5, 10 minutes and in the aforementioned time points serum TRH was measured by radioimmunoassay as well. An interval of at least 2 days intervened between the two tests which were performed in randomized order. Each time 6 ml of blood were drawn and at the time points mentioned 2 ml of them were placed into a glass tube containing 8 ml of 90% methanol which had been kept in deep freeze (−20 °C) for the previous 20 hours.

After gentle shaking the mixture was placed in 4 °C. Following this, it was shaken by vortex, transferred to plastic tube and centrifuged in 5000 g for 20 minutes. The supernatant was then aspirated placed in plastic tube and kept in −20 °C. After 24 hours it was centrifuged at 3200 g for 30 minutes and the supernatant was evaporized in dry atmosphere. The remaining material was subject to second evaporation after being extracted again with methanol, diluted in bidistilled water and lyophylized. In this product TRH RIA was performed.

Serum TSH was determined by radioimmunoassay using double antibody modified in our laboratory [8]. The intraassay variation in the region of 3 μU/ml was 9% and between 6 μU/ml and 12 μU/ml it was 5%. The interassay variation was 13% for the low values decreasing to 6% for the higher ones. Sensitivity was 0.39 μU/ml.

Serum TRH was determined by radioimmunoassay according to method Duntas after the appropriate extraction described above. The antiserum selected was the K.2B7 (final dilution 1 : 120 000) that gave the most sensitive displacement curve. The intraassay variation was 4.6%. The interassay variation in the region of 85%, 50% and 15% binding was 5.6%, 7.6% and 10% respectively. The sensitivity of the assay was 20 fmol/ml. Arterial blood pressure and pulse rate were recorded every 15 minutes. Values are expressed as mean ± SEM.

Statistical analysis was performed using the Student-t-test with the limit of statistical significant at 0.05.

Integrated TSH responses and total TRH concentrations over basal values during the observation time period were calculated according to Thompson's method ([9].

Results

After the intranasal as well as the intravenous administration of 2 mg and 200 μg TRH respectively a significant increase of basal TSH levels which peaked at 30 minutes occurred. In the case of intranasal administration there was at least a 4-fold increase (7.8 ± 0.6 μU/ml) while after the intravenous route 5-fold (9.3

± 1.2 μU/ml) (fig. 1). On the other hand TRH levels peaked at the 2nd minute after the intravenous administration (7360 ± 543 fmol/ml) while at the 5th minute when the intranasal route was used (3809.2 ± 760.7 fmol/ml) (fig. 2).

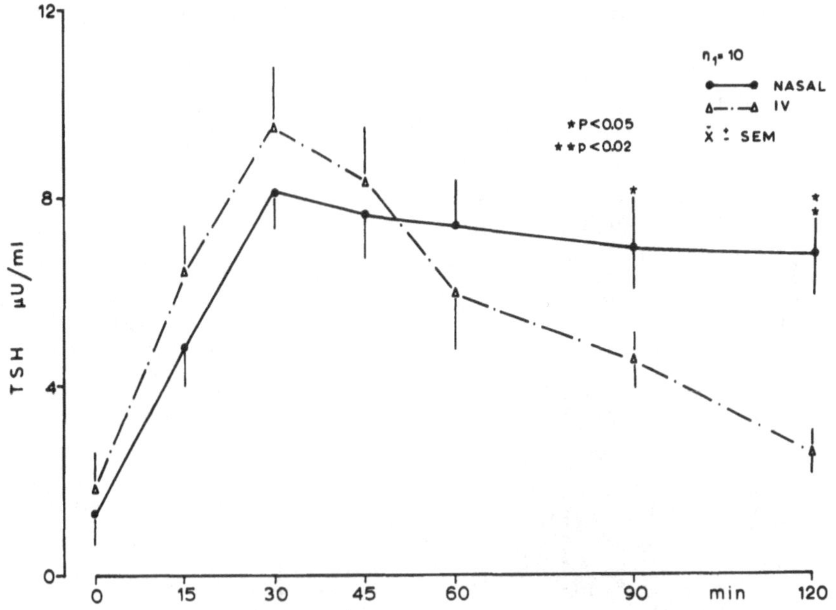

Fig. 1 Plasma TSH levels after intravenous △ –·–·– △ and intranasal ●——● administration of TRH.

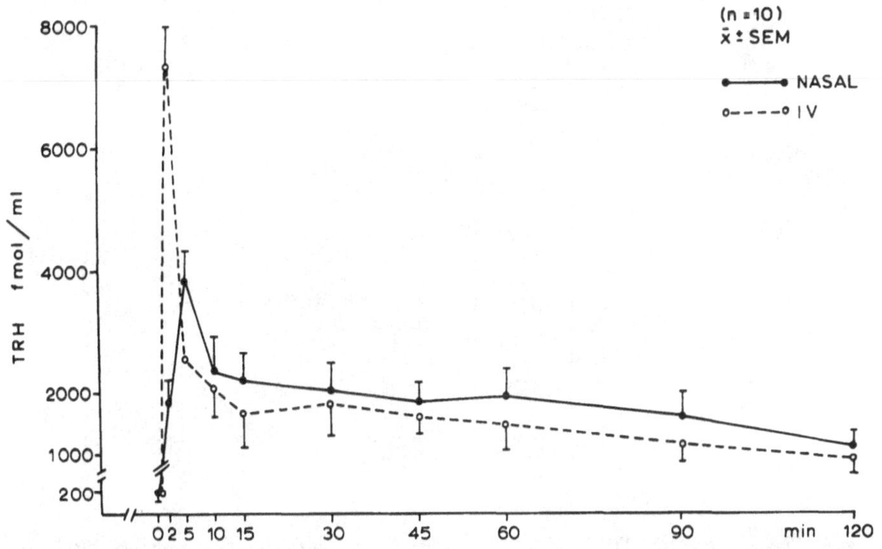

Fig. 2 Plasma TRH levels after intravenous and intranasal administration of TRH.

Thereafter the pattern of TSH curves was different in the descent, namely the trend of TSH decrease was slower under the intranasal form of TRH (TSH level at 90th minute 6.8 ± 1.1 μU/ml after nasal and 4.4 ± 0.5 μU/ml after intravenous administration, $p < 0.05$ and TSH level at the 120th minute 7 ± 0.8 μU/ml after nasal and 2.8 ± 0.4 μU/ml after intravenous administration, $p < 0.02$) (fig. 1).

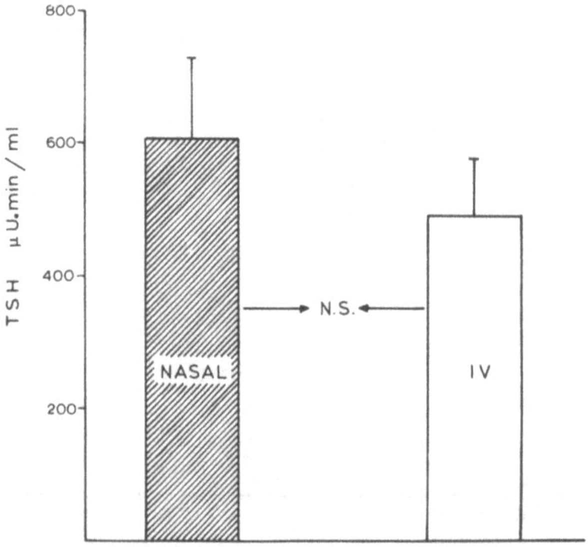

Fig. 3 Plasma integrated TSH responses over 120 minutes after administration of either intravenous or nasal form of TRH.

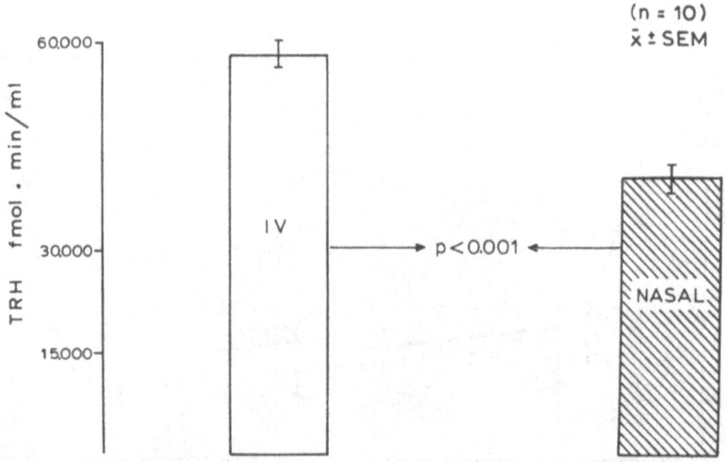

Fig. 4 Plasma integrated TRH concentrations over basal values after both routes of TRH administration.

For this reason the integrated TSH response over the basal value was calculated according to Thompson's method and no statistically significant difference was found between the two routes (610 ± 125 μU.min/ml nasal vs 494 ± 90 μU.min/ml intravenous, N. S.) (fig. 3).

As far as hyperthyroid subjects were concerned no increase of TSH was observed.

In contrast to what happened with the integrated TSH secretory responses between the two routes of administration, the integrated circulating quantities of TRH during the same period of observation exhibited statistically significant difference (58500 ± 1300 fmol.min/ml intravenous vs 40400 ± 1190 fmol.min/ml nasal, $p < 0.001$) (fig. 4).

Discussion

So far TRH tests using the intravenous, oral and intramuscular routes have been performed [2, 4, 6]. As it was shown the intranasal route of TRH administration is not only feasible and effective but it offers certain advantages over the intravenous and oral ones as well. In the case of our study we attempted to proceed to plasma TRH determination in addition to the estimation of TSH responses. As it can be demonstrated an appreciable increase of TSH levels occurred after both forms of TRH which peaked at 30 minutes in both occasions and did not differ significantly although the maximum was lower after the intranasal one. After the above time point the trend of TSH decrease was slower in the case of nasal administration and since the curves exhibited different patterns, the integrated TSH response over the period of observation was calculated. No statistically significant difference was observed between the intranasal and intravenous form. On the other hand regarding the achieved plasma TRH levels, despite the fact that the peak after the intranasal route was lower in comparison to that after the intravenous and occurred by 3 minutes later the obtained peak of stimulated TSH secretion did not differ statistically among the two forms of the administered peptide. Moreover the integrated circulating TRH quantity as expressed by Thompson's method was greater after the intravenous route. Since however the integrated TSH secondary response did not differ significantly between the two routes it can be assumed that the same effect in terms of total TSH secretion is achieved with less circulating quantity of TRH after the intranasal administration.

It is worthnoting that the stimulated TSH level decreases more slowly after the intranasal administration compared to the intravenous route, but faster than the oral route [2]. This can bear the practical importance that if a sample is taken at either the 90th or even the 120th minute, discrimination between low and non-responders can be achieved. Furthermore since no i. v. injection is necessary, the intranasal route offers the convenience that some member of the nursing staff may administer the substance and blood be drawn only for the determinations. As far as side effects are concerned facial flushing (2 persons), mild gastrointestinal disturbances (6 persons) and urgency for urination (1 person) were observed after the intravenous administration. Facial redenning was noted after the intranasal administration in only one occasion. No remarkable changes of either blood pressure or pulse rate were recorded.

In conclusion it can be said that the intranasal administration of TRH constitutes a safe, effective and convenient test in the investigation of thyroid disorders.

Summary

The availability of TRH in a form suitable for intranasal application led to the question about the effectiveness of this route and its possible superiority over the intravenous one. For this purpose, both TRH forms were administered to 10 healthy subjects and 5 patients with hyperthyroidism. 200 µg TRH Relefact® or 2 mg TRH in aerosol form were administered intravenously and intranasally respectively at 0 time. In 0, 2, 5, 10, 15, 30, 45, 60, 90, 120 TRH were determined radioimmunologically. After the administration of TRH to the normals and maximum of TSH secretion was observed in the 30th minute after both the intravenous (525% increase vs basal value) and intranasal (440% vs basal value) application. Since the course of both curves was different during the observation period, with the nasal one showing more prolonged action, the integrated response of TSH secretion was calculated. No statistically significant difference between the two routes of administration was noted (610 ± 125 µU.min/ml after nasal and 494 ± 90 µU.min/ml after intravenous). No increase in TSH was observed in any of the 5 hyperthyroid subjects after the administration of either TRH form. Regarding TRH levels, the peak occurred 2 minutes after iv. and 5 minutes after nasal administration. Integrated circulating TRH quantity during the period of 120 minutes is higher after iv. administration (58.500 ± 1.300 fmol.min/ml vs 40.400 ± 1.190 fmol.min/ml). However since the integrated TSH secretory response did not differ between the two routes it can be assumed that the same effect is obtained after intranasal TRH administration although the circulating TRH quantity in the latter case is less. It can be concluded that intranasal TRH administration is a safe, effective and well tolerated test in the evaluation of TSH secretion.

References

[1] Borkenstein, M.: TSH and PRL secretion after intranasal application of TRH. 18th Workshop for Paediatric Research. Eur. J. Pediatr. **138** (1982) 99.

[2] Jüngst, D., C. Sommerburg, S. Braun, et al.: Stimulation von TSH durch TRH – ein Vergleich von intravenöser, oraler and intranasaler Applikation. 5. Konferenz über die menschliche Schilddrüse, Homburg/Saar. In: Schilddrüse 1981, pp. 410–417. Georg Thieme Verlag, Stuttgart, New York 1982.

[3] Herschmann, J. M.: Clinical application of thyrotropin-releasing hormone. N. Engl. J. Med. **290** (1974) 886–890.

[4] Passath, A., G. Leb: Wirkungsvergleich von 2 mg TRH intransal and 200 µg TRH intravenös. Nuc. Compact. **12** (1981) 257–259.

[5] Rothenbuchner, G., L. Vanhaelst, J. Birk, et al.: Blood levels of TSH, HGH, Cortisol and ACTH after synthetic thyrotropin releasing factor (TRF). Horm. Metab. Res. **3** (1971) 139.

[6] Rothenbuchner, G., J. Birk, U. Loos, et al.: The dynamics of TSH-secretion after oral administration of synthetic Thyrotropin-Releasing Factor (TRF) in metabolically normal subjects. 18. Symp. Dtsch. Ges. Endokr., Hannover 1.–4. 3. 1972. Acta Endocrinol. (Copenh.), Suppl. **159** (1972) 2.

[7] Schäfgen, W., S. F. Grebe, J. Teuber, et al.: Personale TRH-Gabe: Verhalten von TSH, Prolaktin, Schilddrüsenhormon und Thyreglobulin in Vergleich zur intravenösen Injektion. 5. Konferenz über die menschliche Schilddrüse Homburg/Saar. In: Schilddrüse 1981, pp. 406–409. Georg Thieme Verlag Stuttgart, New York 1982.

[8] Souvatzoglou, A., G. Taliadouros, A. Kydonakis, et al.: The TRH stimulation test in endemic goitre in Greece. Klin. Wochenschr. **54** (1976) 25–29.

[9] Thompson, J. C., D. Reeder, H. Bunchman, et al.: Effect of secretin on circulating gastrin. Ann. Surg. **176** (1972) 384–390.

[10] Wilber, J. F.: Thyrotropin releasing hormone: secretion and actions. Ann. Rev. Med. **31** (1973) 137–145.

Thyrotropin serum concentration as a function of peripheral concentrations of thyroxine, triiodothyronine, reverse triiodothyronine, and thyroliberin

F. S. Keck, U. Loos, L. Duntas, S. Wieshammer, E. F. Pfeiffer

Introduction

This study was performed to evaluate the thyrotropic state of the human pituitary as reflected by thyrotropin (TSH) serum concentrations over a wide spectrum of peripheral thyroid hormone levels ranging from severe hypothyroidism to latent hyperthyroidism. An additional objective was to assess the relationship of TSH serum levels both with the levels of thyroxine (T4) and its degradation products triiodothyronine (T3) and reverse T3 (rT3) and with the blood concentration of thyroliberin (TRH).

Patients and methods

The study population consisted of 33 athyroid patients, who were assigned to two groups comprising 22 and 11 patients, resp. All patients had undergone thyroidectomy and radio-iodine therapy for thyroid cancer. They were found to be free of metastases at regular follow-up examinations. Substitution therapy with thyroxine was discontinued at least 4 weeks and triiodothyronine was withdrawn at least 10 days before the initial TRH-test was carried out (i. v. injection of 200 µg thyroliberin; serum thyrotropin determination before injection and after 20 min.). The substitution therapy with T4 was then restarted. The initial dose was 0.7 µg/kg body weight per day. In group I, this dose was increased by 0.7 µg/kg body weight every week, until the TRH-test became blunted (i. e. ΔTSH < 3 mU/l). The TRH-test was carried out at the last day of each level of substitution therapy. Blood samples were obtained at the time of the TRH-test. The specimens were frozen at $-20\,°C$; serum concentration of thyrotropin, thyroxine, triiodothyronine, and reverse triiodothyronine were determined by RIA and IRMA methods (thyroxine and triiodothyronine kit from Bayer-Diagnostic, sensitivity 0.5 µg/dl for thyroxine and 20 ng/dl for triiodothyronine, resp.; reverse triiodothyronine kit from Serono Diagnostics Inc., sensitivity 2 ng/dl;

Thyrotropin

TSH kit from Behring, sensitivity 0.02 mU/l). In order to detect any alterations in thyroid hormone binding, the T4-uptake was measured and the free thyroxine equivalent was determined (FTE [7]). In group II, the thyroxine dose was increased every 5 weeks as described above. In addition, the thyroliberin concentration in blood was determined at all levels of thyroxine substitution therapy, just before the dose was increased (sensitivity 20 fmols/ml [1]).

To analyze the interrelationship of the data, Pearson's simple correlation coefficient (r) was calculated. To detect the influence of any considered variable, the 1st and 2nd degree partial correlation coefficients (r_p) were derived from the data. The data are further analyzed by calculating the multiple correlation coefficient R and the multiple determination coefficient R^2.

Results

The thyroxine and triiodothyronine serum levels ranged from 0.5 to 15 µg/dl (normal range 4 – 12 µg/dl) and from 20 to 250 ng/dl (normal range 80 – 180 ng/dl), resp. The reverse triiodothyronine values were between 2 and 65 ng/dl (normal range < 40 ng/dl), and thyrotropin values ranged from 130 to 0.02 mU/l (basal, normal range 0.1 – 4 mU/l) and from 260 to 0.02 mU/l (stimulated, normal range 2 – 30 mU/l).

There was a close correlation between thyroxine serum concentration and FTE ($r = 0.89$), ruling out any alterations in thyroid hormone binding over the whole spectrum of thyroxine values. The data obtained from the two groups did not differ significantly from each other. Hence, as far as possible, the data were considered together for statistical analysis.

In the severe hypothyroid state, both basal TSH (bTSH) and stimulated TSH were elevated. The values increased with rising T4 levels and decreased steadily to zero, when tyhroxine serum concentration exceeded 2.5 µg/dl or 5.3 µg/dl, resp. In the low thyroxine concentration range (up to 2.5 µg/dl), there was a positive correlation between T4 and bTSH ($r[T4/bTSH] = 0.52$, $p < 0.001$, cf. fig. 1). With thyroxine levels exceeding 2.5 µg/dl, this correlation became negative: $r(T4/bTSH) = -0.79$ ($p < 0.001$).

In the low thyroxine range, the positive linear correlation between T4 and bTSH was confirmed by the partial correlation coefficient, which was calculated to eliminate any influence of triiodothyronine and reverse triiodothyronine on this association: $r_p(T4/bTSH\text{-}T3, rT3) = 0.84$, $p < 0.001$. For thyroxine levels exceeding 2.5 µg/dl, the negative correlation between T4 and bTSH was confirmed too: $r_p(T4/bTSH\text{-}T3, rT3) = -0.66$, $p < 0.001$. By contrast, the simple correlation between T3 and bTSH ($r[T3/bTSH] = -0.68$, cf. fig. 2) is disclosed

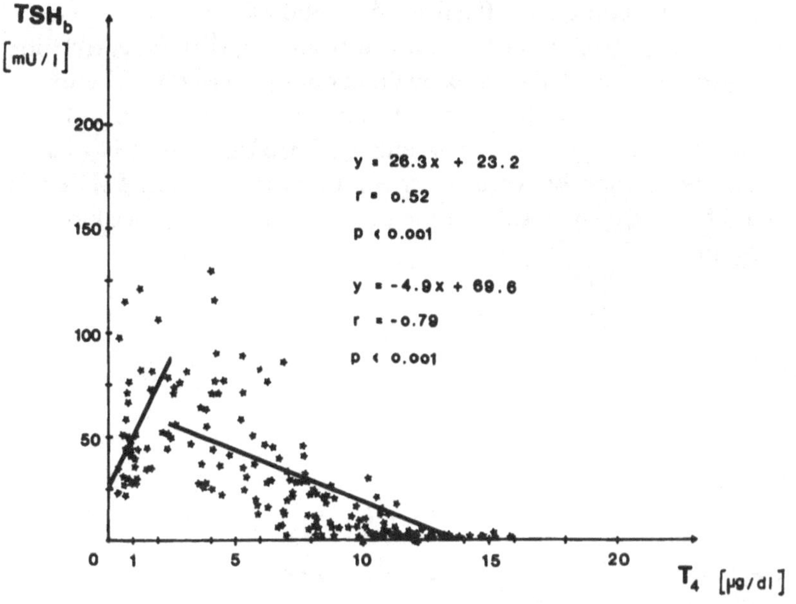

Fig. 1 Relation between basal TSH and thyroxine serum levels.

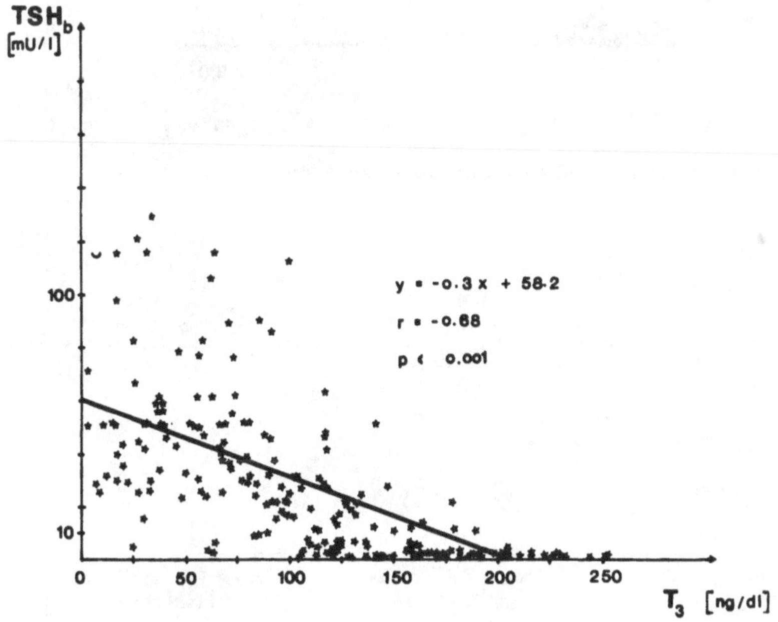

Fig. 2 Relation between basal TSH and triiodothyronine serum levels.

as being fictitious by eliminating the influences of T4 and rT3 on this association: r_p(T3/bTSH T4, rT3) = −0.05, n. s.). It is evident from this, that the correlation between triiodothyronine and bTSH was brought about by thyroxine. The simple correlation between rT3 and bTSH (r[rT3/bTSH] = −0.56, cf. fig. 3) was substantially lowered by the partial correlation: r_p(rT3/bTSH T4, T3) = 0.09, n. s. No significant association between the thyroliberin levels and bTSH could be demonstrated (cf. fig. 4). The results of the partial correlation procedures are summarized in figure 5.

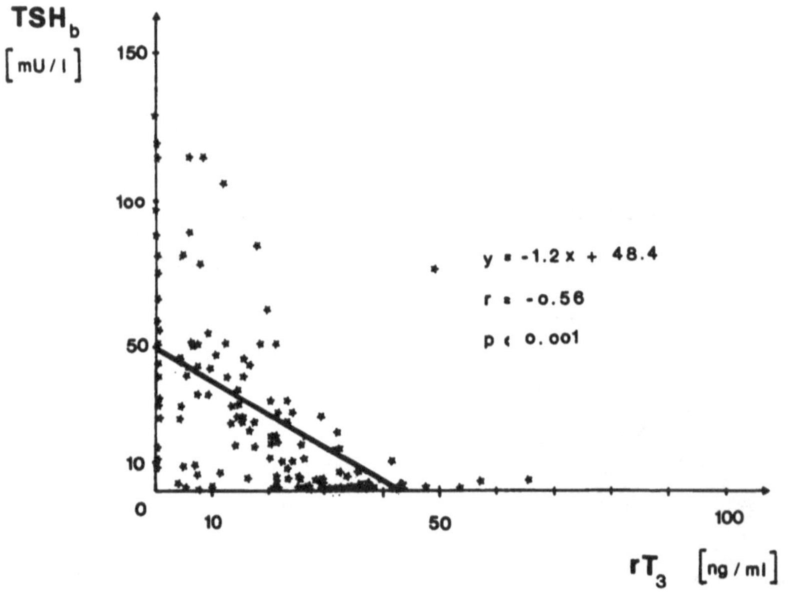

Fig. 3 Relation between basal TSH and reverse triiodothyronine serum levels.

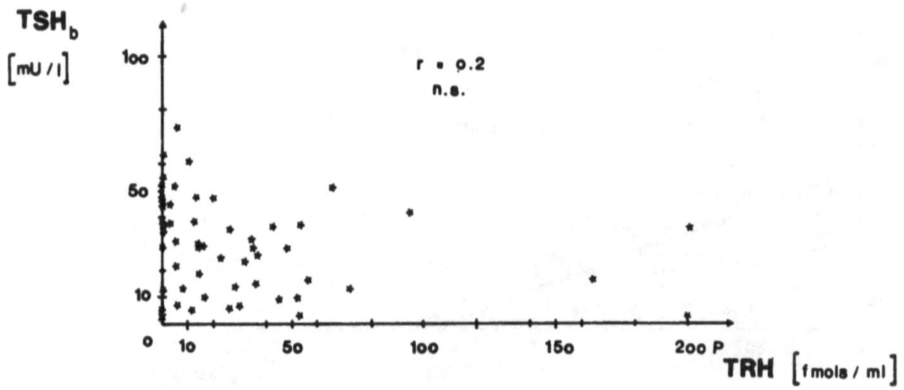

Fig. 4 Relation between basal TSH serum levels and thyroliberin blood levels.

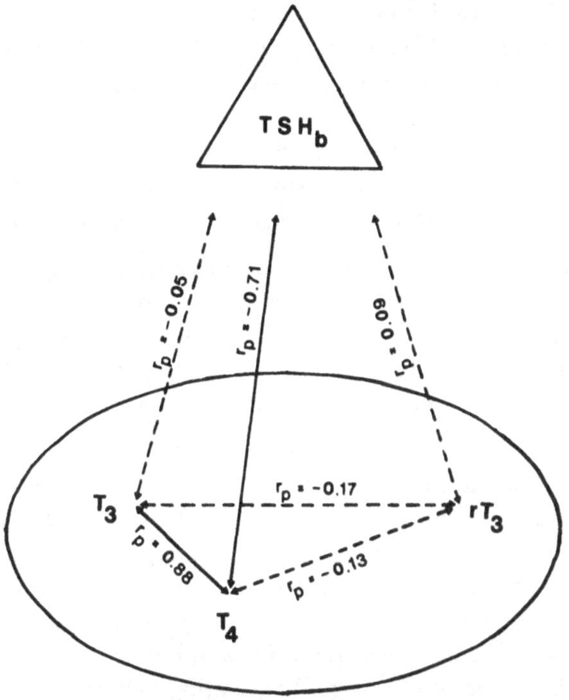

Fig. 5 Association between serum levels of thyroxine, triiodothyronine, and reverse triiodothyronine and basal TSH as assessed by partial correlation coefficients r_p (for T4 levels > 2.5 µg/dl).

As to stimulated TSH, the results were similar. All correlation coefficients were lower however. To determine the extent to which bTSH levels are influenced by T4, T3, and rT3 levels, the multiple correlation coefficient R was calculated. This parameter revealed a close association: $R = 0.91$, $p < 0.001$. It indicates, that 83 percent ($= R^2$) of the variance of the basal thyrotropin levels were determined by those peripheral parameters. If the TRH levels were included in the statistical analysis, this value remained essentially unchanged.

Discussion

The results of this study in man demonstrate, that the elevated thyrotropin levels in the severe hypothyroid state are further increased by small amounts of administered thyroxine for a short thyroxine serum concentration range (T4 levels < 2.5 µg/dl). A transient positive feedback regulation as previously described in rats [9] could account for this finding. As all patients were athyroid, T3 can only be produced by conversion of exogenously administered thyroxine. Studies in rats have shown, that the pituitary type II deiodinase activity is increased in the hypothyroid state [3, 4]. Therefore, it may be hypothesized, that the thyroxine serum concentration of 2.5 µg/dl indicates the point at which the dominant regulation of the thyrotropic function in the pituitary is switched from type II to type I deiodinase. With T4 levels exceeding 2.5 µg/dl, type I deiodinase appears to become predominant in pituitary T4 conversion. The close correlations of thyroxine levels with both T3 levels (positive correlation) and TSH levels (negative correlation) in that T4 serum concentration range supports this point of view.

As evidenced by the statistical analysis, thyroxine concentration is the most important variable in describing thyrotropic function. A peripheral mechanism of regulating serum T3 levels may account for the fact, that there is no causative association between serum T3 and TSH levels, as evidenced by the partial correlation procedures. This mechanism is not part of the pituitary-thyroid regulation system and is not dependent on TSH [2, 5, 6, 8].

Thyroliberin blood levels do not contribute to the variance of serum thyrotropin levels. The peripheral thyroid parameters T4, T3, and rT3, however, account for that variance nearly completely. Because of our findings it remains to be questionable, whether thyroliberin blood levels reflect hypothalamic function at all. As they do not correlate with any of the thyroid parameters measured, it may be presumed, that thyroliberin, as measured in peripheral blood, does not belong to and is produced outside of the thyroid regulating system.

References

[1] Duntas, L., D. Grouselle, F. S. Keck, et al.: Measurements of TRH-like immuno-reactivity in human blood in thyroid diseases. In: Frontiers in thyroid research (G. A. Medeiros-Neto, E. Gaitan, eds.). Plenum Press, New York (in press).

[2] Erickson, V. J., R. R. Cavalieri, L. L. Rosenberg: Thyroxine-5'-deiodinase of rat thyroid, but not that of liver, is dependent on thyrotropin. Endocrinology **111** (1982) 434–440.

[3] Kaplan, M. M.: Thyroxine 5'-monodeiodination in rat anterior pituitary homogenates. Endocrinology **106** (1980) 567–576.

[4] Kaplan, M. M.: The role of thyroid hormone deiodination in the regulation of hypothalamo-pituitary function. Neuroendocrinology **38** (1984) 254–260.

[5] Keck, F. S., R. Müller, L. Duntas, et al.: TSH has no effect on T4 conversion in man. Acta Endocrinol. Suppl. (Copenh.) **270** (1985) 76.

[6] Keck, F. S., U. Loos, L. Duntas, et al.: Evidence for peripheral autoregulation of thyroxine conversion. In: Frontiers in thyroid research (G. A. Medeiros-Neto, E. Gaitan, eds.). Plenum Press, New York (in press).

[7] Loos, U.: Die periphere T4-Konversion. Ihre Rolle für Klinik und Therapie der Schilddrüsenerkrankungen. Habilitationsschrift, Ulm 1981.

[8] Lum, S. M. C., J. T. Nocoloff, C. A. Spencer, et al.: Peripheral tissue mechanism for maintenance serum triiodothyronine values in a thyroxine-deficient state in man. J. Clin. Invest. **73** (1984) 570–575.

[9] Reichlin, S., J. B. Martin, M. Mitnick, et al.: The hypothalamus in pituitary-thyroid regulation. In: Recent progress in hormone research (E. B. Astwood, ed.). Academic Press, New York 1972.

II Sensitive methods for the measurements of TSH

Sensitive immunoassays for the determination of thyrotropin levels in serum

W. G. Wood

Introduction

Before discussing the merits of the second generation thyrotropin kits, which use solid-phase immunometric techniques, I would like to review the history of thyrotropin or TSH kits, and the improvements made in components and methodology over the past decade.

I shall not use the term "supersensitive" for the new kits, but rather the term "second generation", as sensitivity is a relative definition, and not an absolute term. It is better to say that the first generation radioimmunoassay or RIA kits were insensitive, as they were unable to differentiate between euthyroid and non-treated hyperthyroid patient sera without using a thyroliberin or TRH stimulation test.

The series of external quality assessment surveys carried out by the Munich group under Professor Scriba from 1974–1981 show the progress made, at least in Europe, in improving the performance of TSH kits of the first generation [1–3].

The recent spate of publications using second generation immunometric assays using a solid-phase sandwich principle, show that comparison between kits, in terms of correlation data, in the euthyroid range is usually good, although the results are different numerically, due to inadequate standardisation of calibrators or standards. This is reflected in the slope of the regression line, which deviates widely from unity in some cases, as we will later see.

The use of the new methods (tab. 1), whether labelled with ^{125}I or with fluorogens, luminogens or chromogens, in both diagnostic and experimental fields, will be discussed at length later, where it will be seen, that the antibody quality plays the more important role than the label, as far as sensitivity and specificity of the method are concerned.

Finally, I would like to discuss some new, and often still controversial uses, of the measurement of serum TSH in clinical diagnosis, using the new second generation TSH kits.

Thyrotropin

Table 1 Thyrotropin assays – first and second generation

First generation (polyclonal antibodies)	RIA – e.g. Henning IRMA – e.g. BIORAD
Second generation (monoclonal or polyclonal/monoclonal)	IRMA – e.g. Behring IEMA – e.g. Abbott/Boehringer IFMA – e.g. LKB ILMA – e.g. Henning/Corning/Amersham
Expected lower detection limits:	1st generation not under 0.5 mU/l 2nd generation down to 0.02 mU/l

History of the first generation (RIA) kits

I would now like to discuss the components and improvements in TSH-kits made over the past 10 years.

The external quality assessment scheme (EQAS) made by the Munich group in 1974 (fig. 1 a), showed that comparison between methods was abysmal, where coefficients of variation (c. v. s) over 100% were obtained! These results led to the work of Erhardt, Marschner and Scriba [4–5], which examined the reasons for such results. They found that for the RIA, standards of human TSH in human serum free of TSH improved the results, as did the introduction of a tracer-free pre-incubation step before addition of the radioactive TSH.

These results were accepted and implemented in kits produced in the Federal Republic of Germany by Henning and later by Byk-Mallinckrodt.

In the USA, the first firm to follow these suggestions was Diagnostic Products in 1980. Many firms in the US have until today kits which are antiquated, as far as optimisation is concerned.

Another finding was the need for a specific separation of bound and free TSH. This was possible using a second- or double-antibody separation. Charcoal, polymer or salt separation methods were unacceptable, as they were not specific enough.

The second EQAS (fig. 1 b), from 1977 showed an improvement of the situation. The c. vs were reduced, as we shall see in the comparison of the precision profiles of all three EQAS. The use of a unified algorithm, here the spline function described by Reinsch, and adapted for RIA by Marschner, for data reduction brought an improvement in comparison of results. The largest improvement, however, came from the incorporation of a hidden standard curve of human TSH in human TSH-free serum. This was used to construct the standard curve of each participant, from which his or her results were read off.

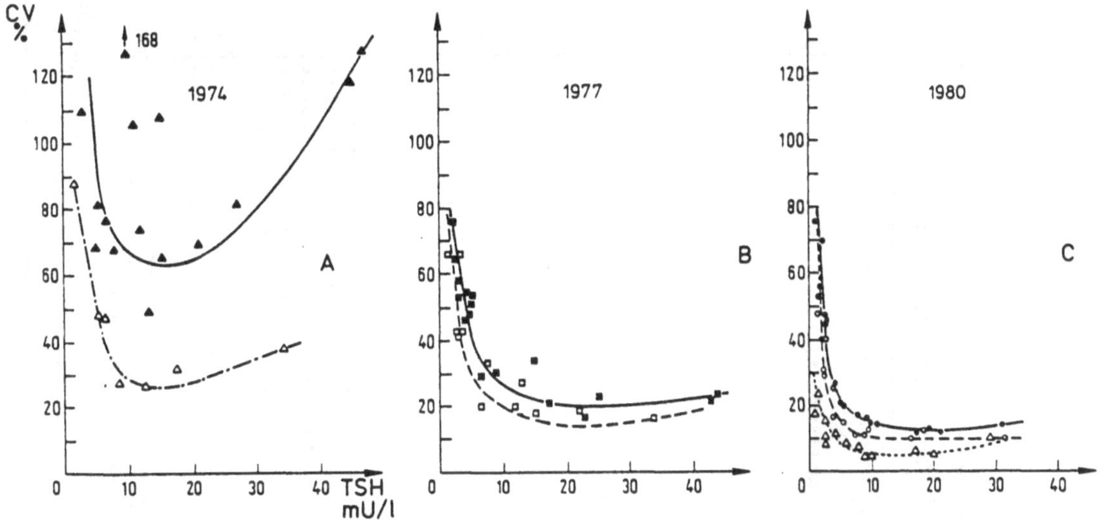

Fig. 1a–1c Compound precision profiles of the samples in the Munich-Model external quality assessment schemes, 1974 (A), 1977 (B) and 1980 (C).
Mean cv from participant's own data (———) and data reduction programme. Mean cv from hidden standard curve. (– – –) and spline function. Mean cv from "matched-reagents" group (---------) (1980) and spline function.

The third EQAS of the Munich group in 1981 (fig. 1c) showed the zenith of the RIA kits, with a further improvement of precision and comparison between kits. The results can only be seen as the progress on the West German Market. Results of similar studies from other countries will be presented here at this meeting, and it is interesting to see the state of the art in other countries.

What does the radioimmunoassay measure?

Does the radioimmunoassay measure TSH concentrations correctly? At low concentrations, most definitely not. One cannot believe the values from RIA, even so called sensitive assays with impractically long incubation times of up to 7 days! What happens in the assay tubes during this time? Not only antibody-antigen reactions, but also serum enzyme reactions, for example proteases, and one can play the devil's advocate and question whether the "sensitivity" of such assays is partially due to differential degradation in standards, which are composed of treated serum or plasma, and in patient samples, which are still "intact" so to say, with regards to proteolytic activity.

How can I back up claims, that the RIA is unreliable at low levels? One way is by comparing the results from hyperthyroid patients, who have not been treated,

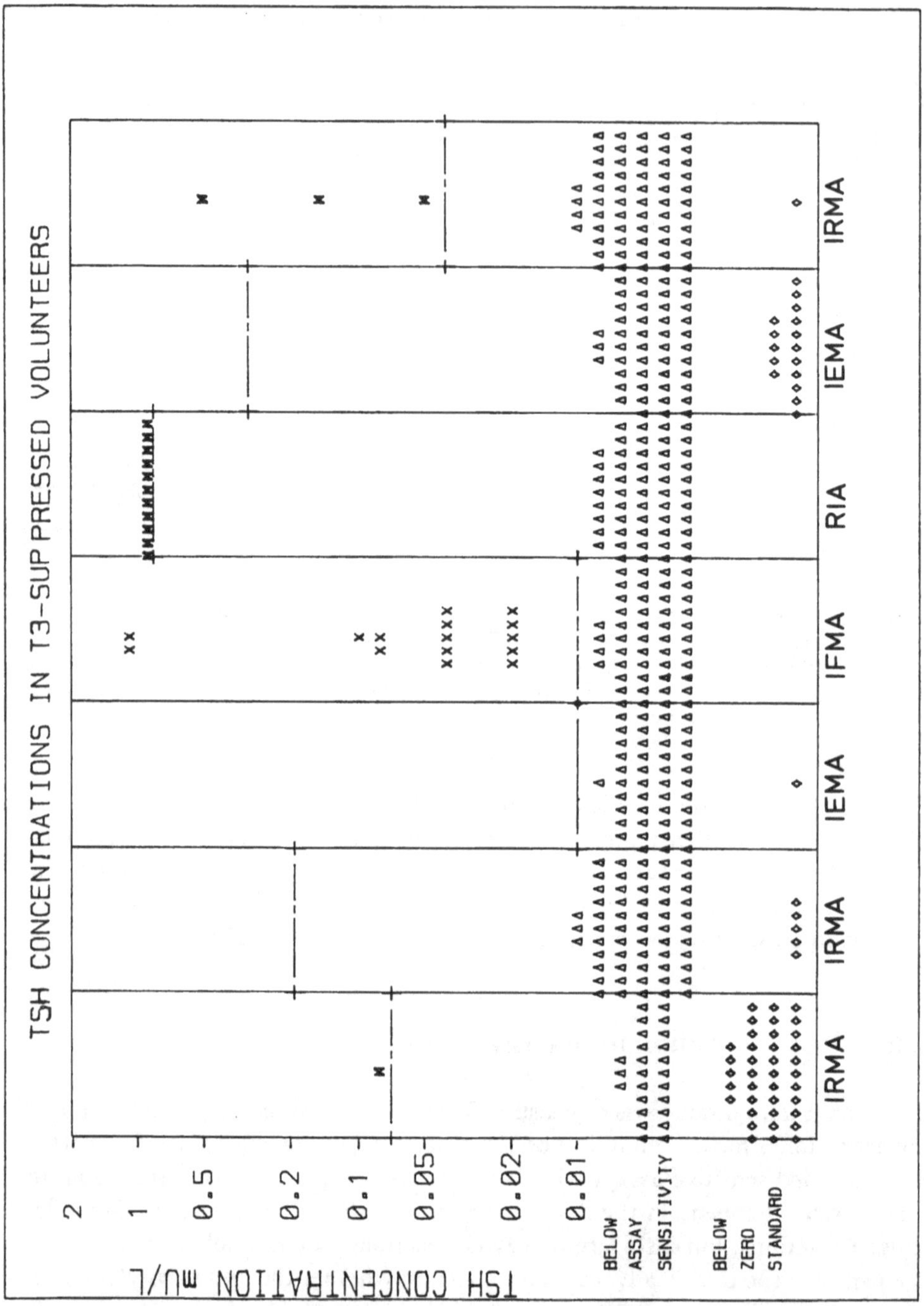

Fig. 2 TSH-levels in T_3-suppressed volunteers (5 days/80 μg/day) as measured in first (1) and second (2) generation kits.
Assay type: IRMA = immunoradiometric assay, IEMA = immunoenzymometric assay, IFMA = immunofluorimetric assay, RIA = Radioimmunoassay.
(The author wishes to thank Dr. Swift and Professor Ratcliffe of the University of Manchester for being able to use this figure.)

in RIA and IRMA, but this is not the only way. In 1974, we attempted to produce TSH-free serum for the first Munich group external quality assessment scheme, by subjecting volunteers to 100 µg T_3/day for a week. We obtained, to our surprise, only serum with immunoreactive TSH from these people. Ten years later, Professor Ratcliffe and Dr. Swift in Manchester performed similar experiments, and answered our question without knowing it. The serum was TSH-free, or nearly so in all cases when measured with the IRMA, but not with RIA kits. Figure 2, for which I must thank Dr. Swift, shows TSH levels in T_3-suppressed volunteers.

The implications of these results are wide reaching, inasmuch as all results for euthyroid and hyperthyroid patient sera, which were measured with a first-generation kit must be subject to re-examination. As is often the case, many unexplainable phenomena are due to technical problems rather than extremely complicated hormone regulation circuits. As one very distinguished scientist once said, "If a theory is exceedingly complicated, it is likely to be wrong!"

Second generation kits

Questions and a few answers

Now to the second generation kits using sandwich techniques, and to the question, "Is RIA dead, as far as TSH measurements are concerned?" The answer is yes, the days of the RIA are past. The sandwich assays constitute the methodology of the future, regardless of the label used. The use of selected monoclonal antibodies often make the choice of label secondary, as far as sensitivity and specificity are concerned. If we take the results of the Manchester group, as seen in figure 3, with suppression of human TSH over 5 days in serum from T_3-suppressed volunteers, it can be seen, that the sandwich methods suppressed as theoretically expected, whereas the conventional RIA did not suppress under ca. 1 mU/l.

What can we expect from second generation kits? Take two studies made in our laboratory, in which sera were assayed without the assayist knowing from which patient groups the sera came. The code was only broken, after the study had been completed. An established RIA, from Henning, Berlin, was used as a representative of the classical TSH kits, and was compared with five sandwich-type second generation kits with both radioactive and enzyme labelling [6].

The main groups of patients consisted of serum and citrated plasma from blood donors, serum from clinically euthyroid patients, from untreated hyperthyroid patients, from thyroliberin tests on euthyroid and hyperthyroid patients using 200 µg TRH i. v. together with a basal and 30 minute blood sample.

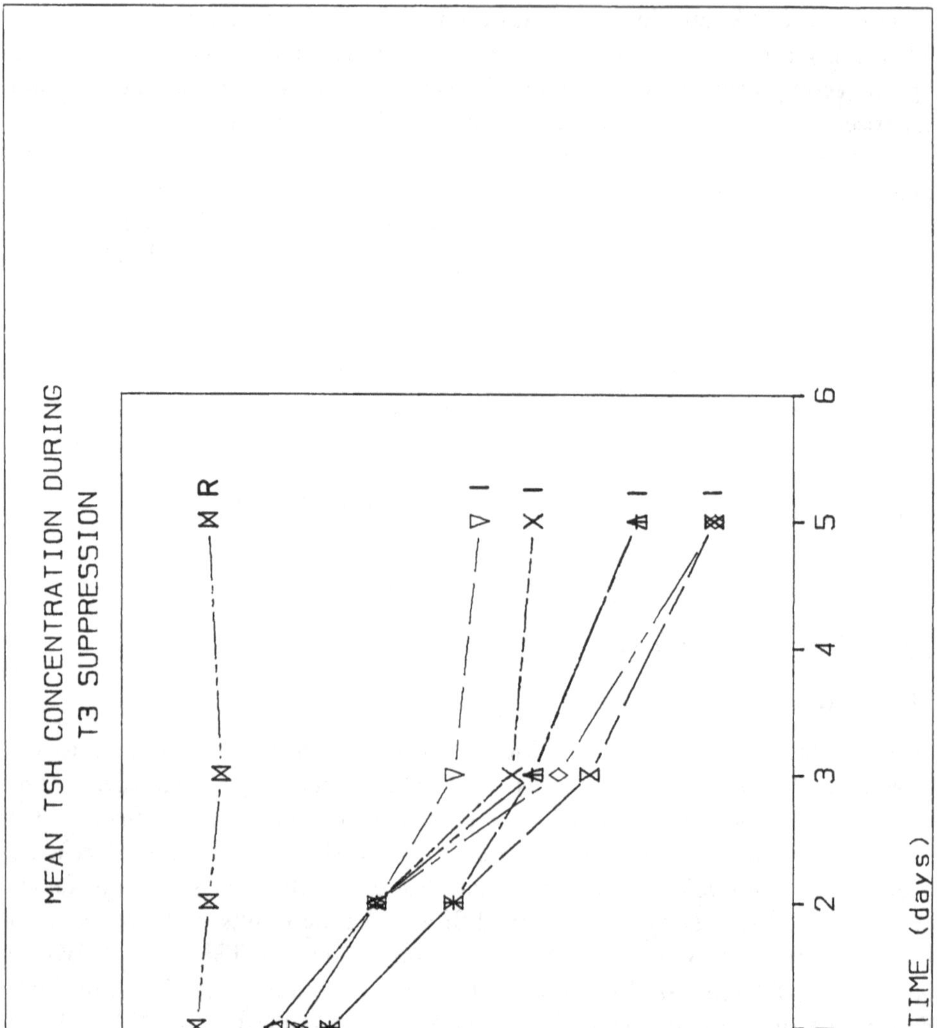

Fig. 3 Progressive suppression of serum TSH levels under T_3-dose of 80 μg/day. R = RIA, I = Immunometric method.
(The author wishes to thank Dr. Swift and Professor Ratcliffe of the University of Manchester for being able to use this figure.)

First, I would like to compare the results of citrated plasma and serum. There were no differences in the results obtained from all six kits tested.

How did the assays perform in measuring euthyroid and untreated hyperthyroid patient sera? The immunometric kits could distinguish statistically speaking, between euthyroid and non-treated hyperthyroid patients, although in two cases one hyperthyroid result lay within the euthyroid range. The conventional RIA, even in a "sensitive" overnight version, was unable to differentiate between euthyroid and hyperthyroid groups. The best performance was from an IRMA, (Behring), which gave results above the zero standard in 544 from 546 serum samples measured. For full results, see [6].

That not all second generation kits are without problems can be seen in the first version of one kit. A euthyroid patient serum was estimated to have over 50 mU/l TSH, before and after TRH. In all other kits, this patient showed a normal euthyroid response to TRH, with a basal level around 1 mU/l and a delta-TSH of around 12 mU/l. After addition of mouse immunoglobulin G to the assay buffer, this kit produced these results as well. Such anomalies have been noted by several groups, although it is still unclear as to what this or these factors are. It is unlikely that humans have a specific anti-mouse IgG antibody, and it is more likely, that these patients have anomalous proteins with the ability to bind to the monoclonal antibody and to the tracer. We have removed such anomalous binding in one case by the addition of an anti-rheumatoid factor antiserum, although the amount of rheumatoid factor in the patient serum was not elevated. As other groups have not found a correlation between anomalous binding in the immunometric assay and levels of rheumatoid factor, it is probable, that the interfering substances do not belong to a single class of serum proteins. Here is an interesting challenge to researchers in the thyroid field, who are looking for something to do!

What is to be seen in the TRH tests? Figure 4 shows the TSH serum levels in one patient, before and after TRH, as measured in all 7 kits. In this patient who had a total hypophyseotomy, four kits showed a normal response to TRH, the other three showed no response to TRH. The patient was clinically hypothyroid and needed thyroid hormone substitution. All one can say in such a case is that two kits represented the clinical situation, i. e. showed no response to TRH, the other two posed the question as to whether the hypophysectomy was complete, or whether tumour tissue was still present which was producing a non-biologically active form of the hormone? This is an awkward case which poses the question, "What do these kits really measure?". The answer at present seems to be, "Something like or near intact TSH, but not the same in each kit".

Table 2 shows the good correlation between the immunometric assays within the euthyroid range as seen by the correlation coefficients. The divergence of the slope, here the b-values, shows the non-optimised standardisation and calibration

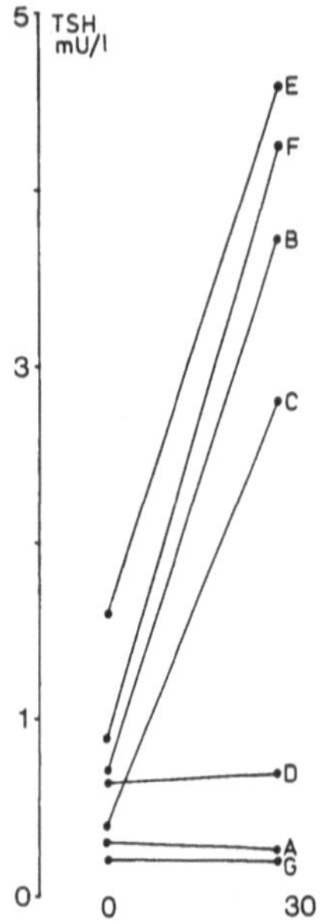

Fig. 4 TSH response to TRH in a patient who had undergone a total hypophysectomy. The kit identity is the same as in Table 2. The patient was clinically hypothyroid.

Table 2 Regression and correlation data for seven kits from sera in the euthyroid and hyperthyroid range (0–5 mU/l TSH)

Kit	Assay type	Solid phase	a_{yx}	b_{yx}	r
A	IRMA	Coated tubes	0.00	1.00	1.000
B	RIA	Microparticulate polymer	0.68	0.42	0.347
C	IRMA	Microparticulate polymer	0.55	0.72	0.851
D	IRMA	Magnetic particles	0.34	1.25	0.938
E	IEMA	Coated tubes	0.21	0.99	0.857
F	IRMA	Agarose	0.22	1.52	0.811
G	ILMA	Polystyrene ball	0.07	0.91	0.977

Regression line – $y = a + bx$

All kits were correlated with kit A, as this kit did not have any values lying below the zero standard.

of the kits. This data is in accordance with that from other groups, who have carried out recovery experiments in second generation kits, and have found values which diverge widely from 100% in some cases.

This emphasises the need for standardisation of kits. Even the best methods and components are useless without correct calibration, a fact true both for RIA as well as for the successors.

The precision of the new generation of TSH kits can be seen in precision profiles made in the euthyroid and hyperthyroid ranges, which are shown in figure 5a–5g.

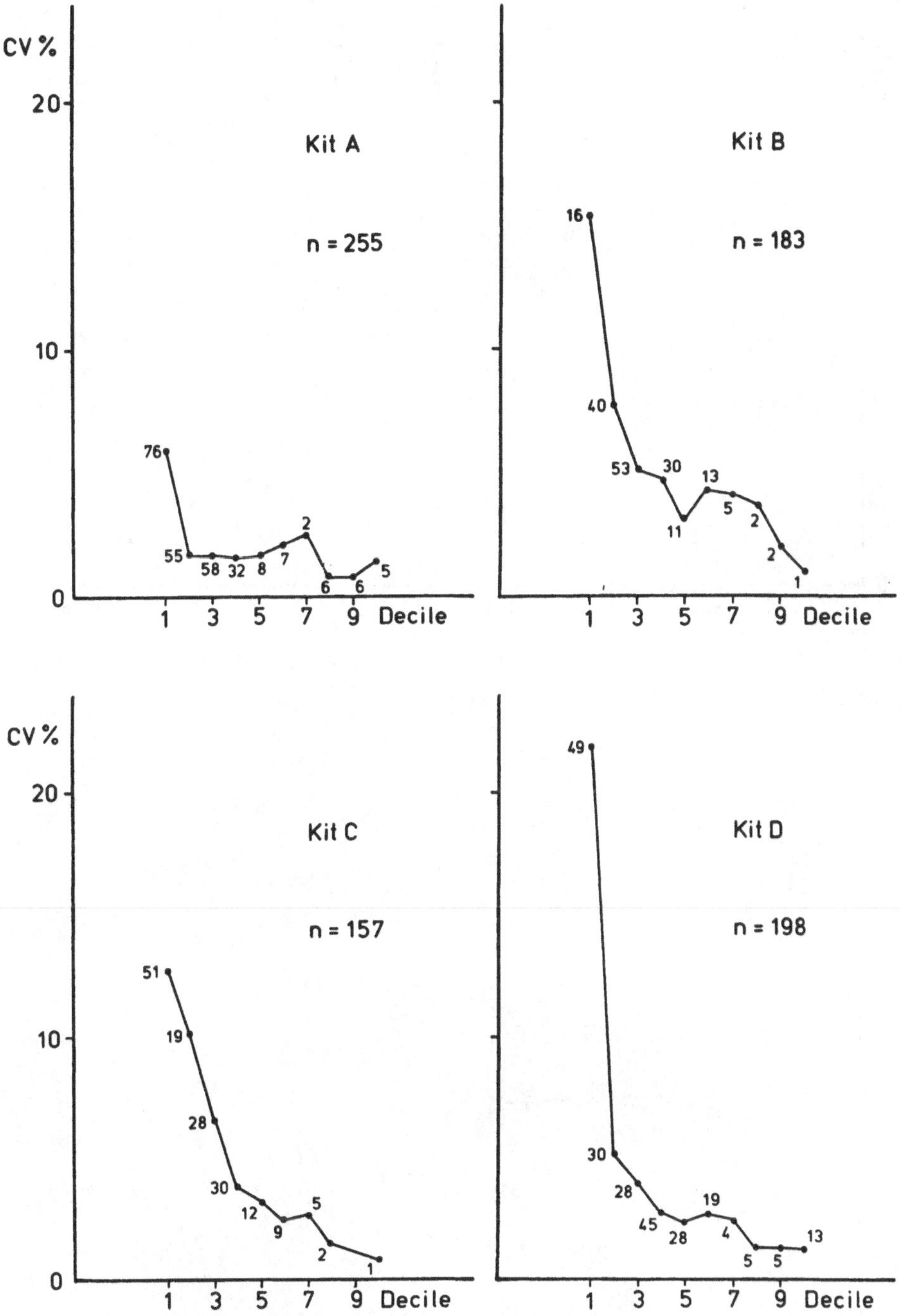

Fig. 5a–5d Compound precision profiles of the kits listed in table 2. The range covered in each case is 0–5 mU/l TSH, divied into deciles of 0.5 mU/l. The numbers at each point indicate the number of data pairs used to construct this point.

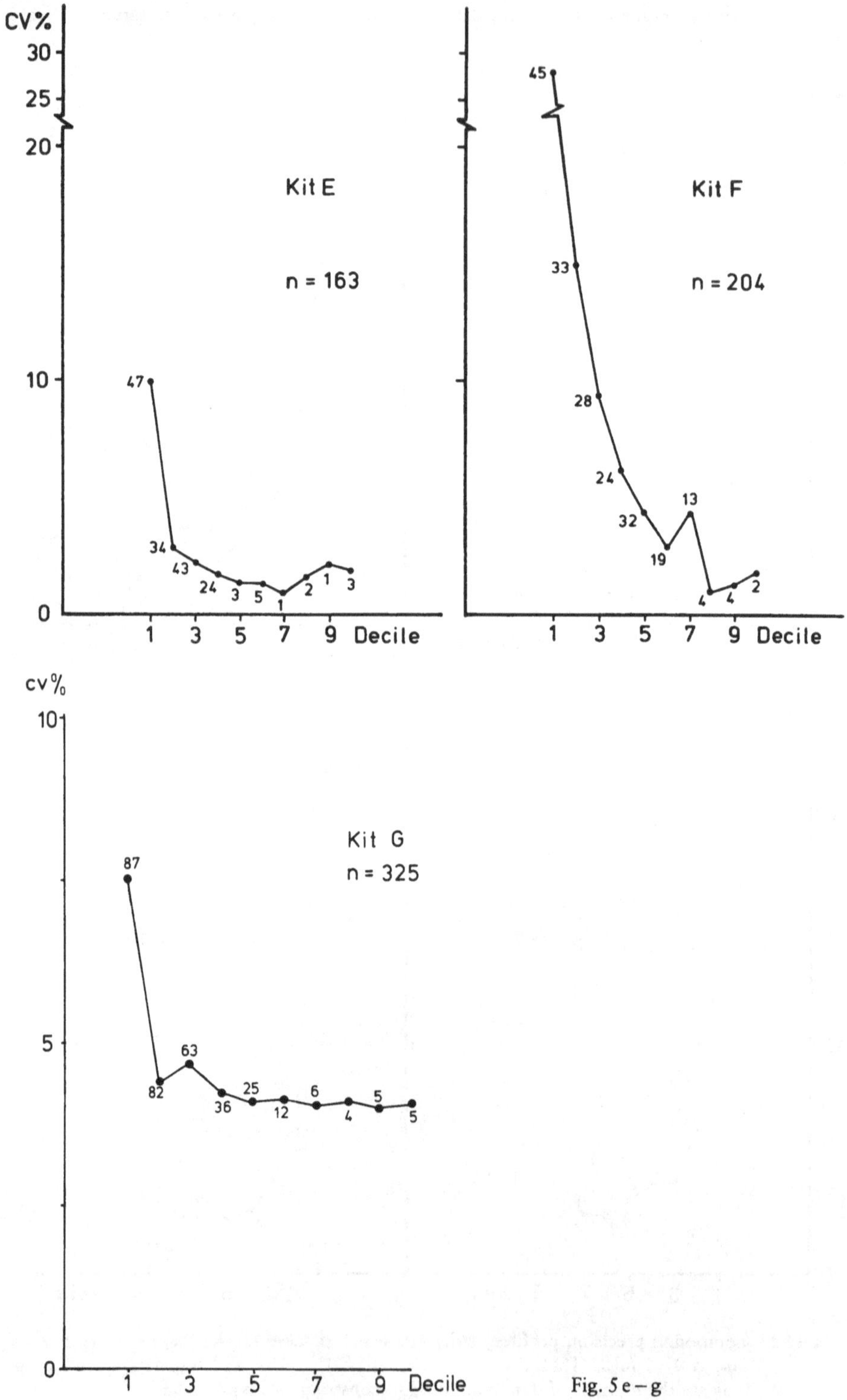
CV%
30
25
20
10
0
Kit E
n = 163
47
34
43
24
3
5
1
2
1
3
1 3 5 7 9 Decile
Kit F
n = 204
45
33
28
24
32
19
13
4
4
2
1 3 5 7 9 Decile
cv%
10
5
0
Kit G
n = 325
87
82
63
36
25
12
6
4
5
5
1 3 5 7 9 Decile

Fig. 5 e–g

Alternatives to radioactive labelling

What are the alternatives to RIA? Are they practical? Are they commercially available? These are shown in table 1.

Firstly, enzyme immunoassays. For example, the Abbott and Boeringer-Mannheim IEMA tests. These tests have good precision, and can be made to detect TSH levels under 0.2 mU/l. It is possible, that the measuring range of the assay is less than in other "alternative" methods due to the Beer-Lambert law governing photometric measurements. For example, in our study, [6], the Boehringer kit was able to measure in the range 0.05 to 6 mU/l.

Fluorescent labelled kits include the LKB DELFIA, which uses the fluorescent properties of europium. The theoretical sensitivity of this method is very low, although the methodology is somewhat complicated. The disadvantage of the LKB system, is that it is a closed system, the user being fully dependant upon the supplier. Conventional fluorescence immunoassays using, for example fluorescein or methyl umbelliferone as labels do not seem to be sensitive enough to measure TSH in normal serum samples.

A third alternative is the use of luminescent labels. The theoretical sensitivity of such assays is similar to those for the RIA and time-resolved fluorescence. Practically, the assays are similar in sensitivity to the IRMA. Commercial kits undergoing trials in our laboratories at present have shown that immunoluminometric assays are able to compete with immunometric assays in both simplicity and assay time, one step assays with a two-hour incubation at room temperature being possible. The availability of such kits and measuring equipment, i. e. clinically suitable luminometers, will to some extent determine whether ILMA will become a rival to IRMA. The advantage of luminescence systems available, is that they belong to the class of open systems, where the laboratory has the choice of reagents and tests, just as it has in RIA or IRMA.

An alternative, or better said, combination of enzyme and luminescence techniques can be seen in the Amerlite system, which is best described as a luminescence enhanced enzyme immunoassay. This system is closed, and preliminary results from our studies show that it is able to measure low TSH-levels.

An advantage of the Amerlite system is that one can measure the samples several times over a time period which varies from analyte to analyte, but which is at least 20 minutes. With conventional chemiluminescence, as employed in the kits from Ciba-Corning and Henning, the light initiation can only be made once.

Results from our laboratory using luminescent labels

I would now like to present a few results from our laboratory, using LIA as an example, as we have chosen this method as RIA-successor in our laboratory.

Table 3 shows the results from 16 consecutive assays, in which the signal for each standard has been averaged, together with the standard deviation of the signal, and the dynamic range, expressed as light signal from a given standard, compared with the light signal of the zero standard. Table 4 shows the "conventional" inter-assay variation determined in 6 commercially available control sera. Precision profiles and correlation data are given in figure 5 and table 2 respectively.

Table 3 Compound assay curve from 16 assays – Henning Lumitest ILMA

Standard mU/l TSH	Signal BLU/100 (+/– s.d.)	Dynamic range ($Signal_{std}/Signal_{zero}$)
0	90 (16)	1.00
0.31	249 (51)	2.77
1.25	573 (53)	6.37
5.00	1827 (145)	20.3
20.0	6792 (620)	77.0
80.0	21705 (195)	241

Key: RLU = Relative Light Units, proportional to the number of photons emitted.

Table 4 Inter-assay precision in 16 assays – Henning Lumitest ILMA

Serum	mean mU/l	ov %
HB 1	11.4	9.20
HB 2	2.98	6.24
HB 3	1.06	9.18
DPC IV	0.59	12.9
DPC V	3.45	5.39
DPC VI	16.9	7.37

Coefficients of variation determined from the means of duplicate determinations.

Results from other laboratories

I would like to summarise a few results from other groups who have investigated what can be done with the new sensitivity of the second generation kits. New questions such as "Can the new TSH kit generation replace the TRH test, and if so, when, or what are the limitations?" Table 5 shows a scheme for the initial diagnosis confirmation from the laboratory side of things, together with the tests needed for follow-up under treatment. I am grateful to Dr. R. Gutekunst, one of our endocrinologists for the scheme presented here. One must not forget, that the laboratory tests are subordinate to the clinical diagnosis formed from signs and symptoms. The full clinical picture can only be obtained by optimal cooperation between ward, clinic and laboratory, a point often overlooked by many medics and laboratory bosses.

Table 5

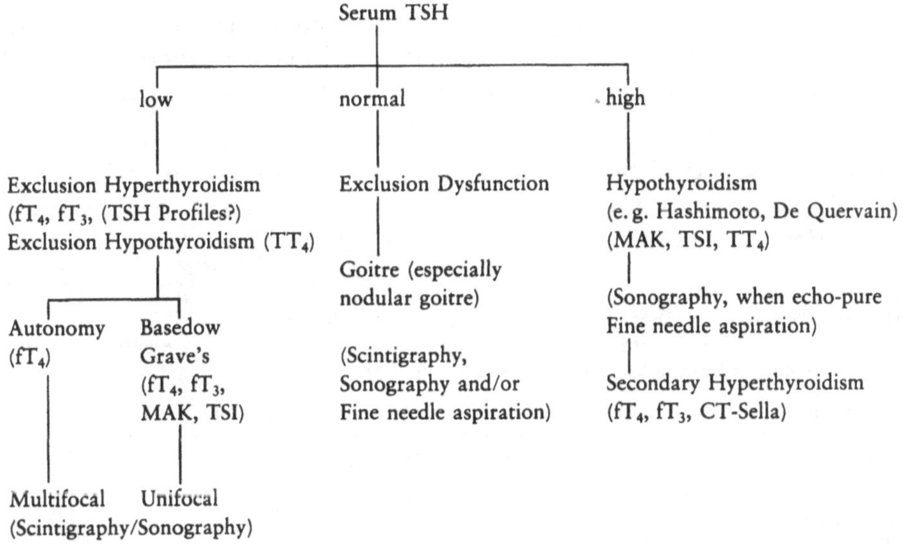

The TRH test may take on a new role in thyroid diagnosis. Delta TSH levels under 0.5 mU/l in the range 0.3 to 1 mU/l are easily detected by many second generation kits, and returning thyroid-pituitary interplay may be monitorable in hyperthyroid patients under treatment.

The Cardiff group, under Drs. Woodhead and Weeks have measured such returning interplay, not with TRH tests, but with returning episodal secretion of TSH, present in normal subjects, but absent in thyrotoxic patients. They were able to detect pulses of TSH secretion under 0.1 mU/l using a sensitive immunoluminometric assay.

Pulsatile release of TSH has been demonstrated recently by the Hannover group under Professors Hesch and von zur Mühlen. This episodal secretion of TSH in normal subjects shows that TSH behaves like many other pituitary hormones in this respect.

The Munich group under Professor Pickardt has shown that the new tests also have the same disadvantages as their first generation predecessors, i.e. they are not optimal for the diagnosis of early primary hypothyroidism.

For the clinician in his daily routine, the importance of the new tests may be reflected in the reduction of TRH tests needed, perhaps up to 90% of those at present carried out, provided that the clinical data is optimally used.

Neonatal screening is possible with the new methods, publications of fluorescence immunoassays from the Municipal Hospital [7] group in Munich, and luminescence and immunoradiometric assays from our group in Lübeck [8]. I will close with a couple of results (tab. 6) showing results for dry blood spot TSH test, with 2 or 4 hour incubation – a one-step method without centrifugation, to show what can be done in this field to allow a same-day reporting of results. This can be used for neonatal screening, or has been shown here, for samples obtained under difficult circumstances in Tanzania.

I have only scratched the surface of what is no doubt possible with the new second generation TSH kits in this short report, and await new and exciting applications in the coming months.

Table 6 TSH Neonatal IRMA (Behring) v ILMA (Lübeck-Henning)

Group I – non endemic goitre area (Tansania) – n = 188

Percentiles	Behring	Henning
2.5	n.d.	0.51 mU/l
16	n.d.	1.71
50 (median)	1.30	2.80
84	2.50	4.20
97.5	4.40	6.00
mean/median	1.06	1.06
z-value	– 10.8 (p < 0.001)	

Group II – endemic goitre area (Tansania) – n = 138

Percentiles	Behring	Henning
2.5	n.d.	n.d.
16	1.10	1.20
50 (median)	1.70	2.60
84	10.5	12.9
97.5	> 100	360
mean/median	6.74	7.98
z-value	– 1.48 (not significant)	

References

[1] Marschner, I., F. W. Erhardt, P. C. Scriba: Ringversuch zur radioimmunologischen Thyrotropin-bestimmung (hTSH). J. Clin. Chem. Clin. Biochem. **14** (1976) 345 – 351.

[2] Wood, W. G., J. Habermann, I. Marschner, et al.: The validity of serum TSH measurements by immunoassay. In: Radioimmunoassay of hormones, proteins and enzymes, (A. Albertini, ed.) pp. 39 – 47. International congress series no. 528, Exerpta Medica, Amsterdam, 1980.

[3] Marschner, I., W. G. Wood, P. C. Scriba: The Munich-model as external quality control educational programme. In: Radioimmunoassay and related procedures in medicine 1982, pp. 615 – 619, IAEA, Vienna, 1982.

[4] Erhardt, F. W., I. Marschner, C. R. Pickardt, et al.: Verbesserung und Qualitätskontrolle der radioimmunologischen Thyreotropin-Bestimmung. J. Clin. Chem. Clin. Biochem. **11** (1973) 381 – 387.

[5] Erhardt, F. W., P. C. Scriba: Probleme der radioimmunologischen hTSH Bestimmung. Ärztl. Lab. **20** (1974) 191 – 198.

[6] Wood, W. G., D. Waller, U. Hantke: A comparison of six sensitive TSH kits. J. Clin. Chem. Clin. Biochem. **23** (1985) 461 – 471.

[7] Von Reuss, K., K. D. Gerbitz: Fluoroimmunoassay for neonatal thyrotropin screening in dried blood spots. Fresenius' Z. Anal. Chem. (in Press).

[8] Rohde, C., M. Petrowski, Z. Huang, et al.: Same day neonatal screening for connatal hypothyroidism using dry blood spots and a one-step assay using either a radioactive or luminescent labelled immunometric assay. Fresenius' Z. Anal. Chem. (in press).

Studies on different hypersensitive TSH tests

S. F. Grebe, H. Müller, S. K. Grebe, I. Stute, G.-L. Fängewisch,
G. Kovaćs, B. W. Hoogendam

Introduction

Determination of serum TSH level normally enables only the identification of elevated values as seen in primary hypothyroidism [8]. By the use of ultrasensitive test methods it is possible to differentiate between normal values, which are found in euthyroid patients and depressed levels which can be seen in hyperthyroid patients [2, 5, 9–17].

Results of primary investigations

In a pilot study we saw significant overlap of values obtained in the various thyroid states (figs. 1–6).

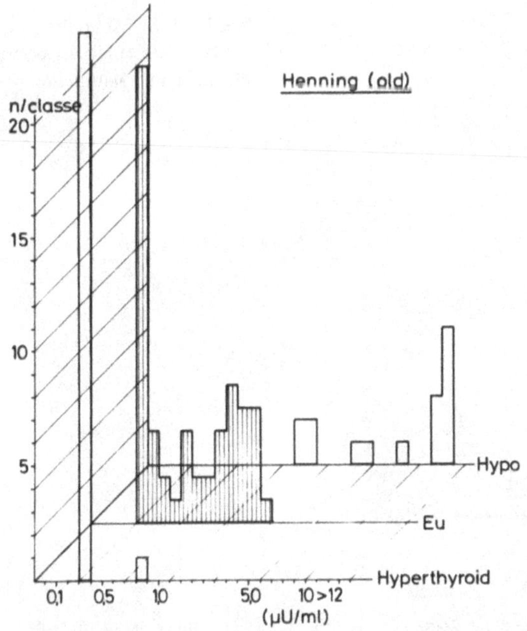

Fig. 1 TSH values using the RIA from Henning Berlin – old Henning –.

Thyrotropin

Figure 1 illustrates the results of the ordinary "old" TSH-RIA from Henning. Figure 2 shows the values found with the enzyme test from Boehringer-Mannheim using monoclonal antibodies. Both tests are unable to differentiate between normal and depressed values.

It is a different matter with the hypersensitive TSH RIA from Henning (fig. 3), the hypersensitive TSH-IRMA with monoclonal antibodies from Boots-Celltech.

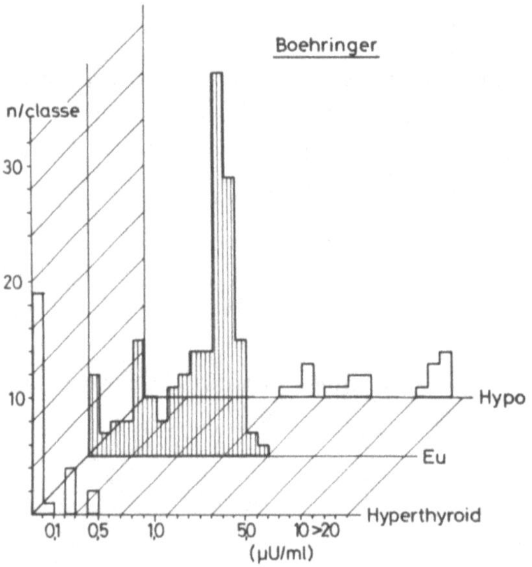

Fig. 2 TSH values using the enzymetest with monoclonal antibodies from Boehringer Mannheim.

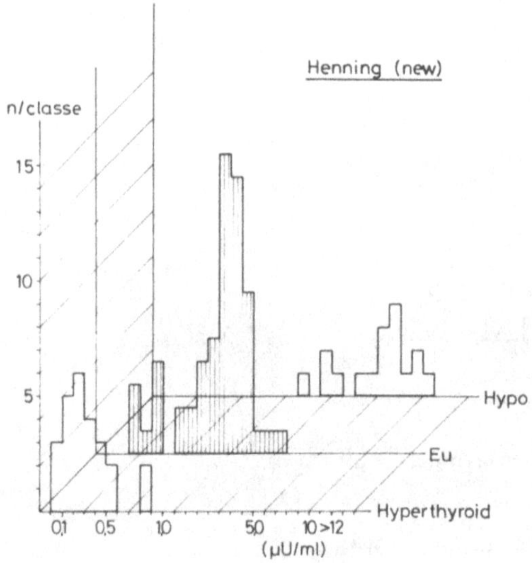

Fig. 3 TSH values using the ultrasensitive RIA from Henning Berlin.

Diagnostics (fig. 4) and the hypersensitive TSH-IRMA with monoclonal antibodies from Serono (fig. 5). These various test methods differ in the degree and size of overlap seen between the various patient states (fig. 6). The number of patients found to be hyper-, eu- or hypothyroid differs according to the test method used.

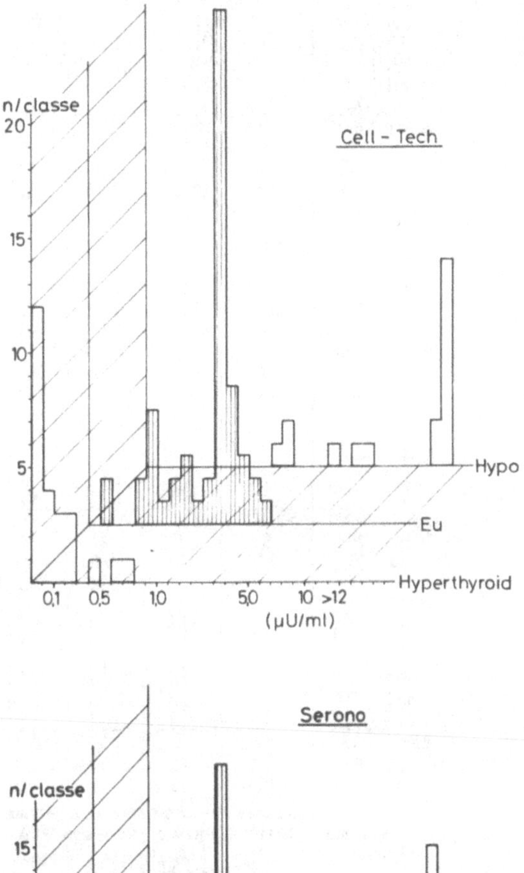

Fig. 4 TSH values using the hypersensitive IRMA from Boots Celltech.

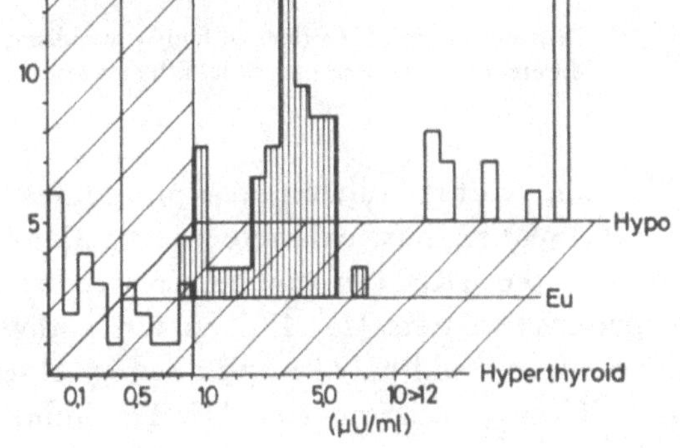

Fig. 5 TSH values using the supersensitive IRMA from Serono.

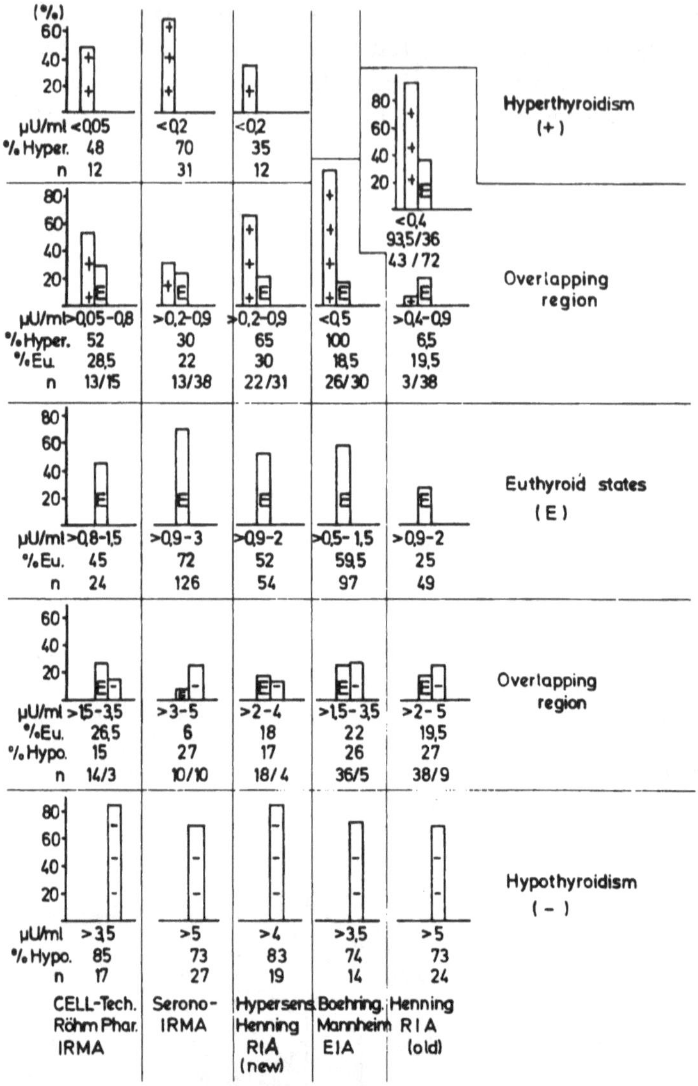

Fig. 6 Distribution of TSH values in hyperthyroidism, euthyroid state and hypothyroidism, in the different regions seen using the different tests.

The validity of the different test procedures varies along with the borderlines of the different regions, and more investigation is needed in this area. It is uncertain, whether the TRH test can be replaced by measuring the TSH value using a hypersensitive tests [15, 17]. So far, a thyroxine therapy for substitution or suppression could only be optimised by observing the changes of the TSH level after TRH application [1, 3, 11]. The influence of different thyroxine doses on the values measured by hypersensitive TSH tests is yet unknown. Moreover it is questionable whether measuring TSH values is a first step in screening diagnostics of the thyroid function [2, 13]. The aim of our investigations was to clear up these questions.

Material and methods

In more than 6000 sera the TSH value was measured in additon to other parameters (T3U-, T4-, T3-, FT4- and FT3-tests). A TRH test was carried out in most cases. The sera were taken from healthy individuals, hyper- or hypothyroid patients; patients who were treated with thyroid hormones, antithyroid drugs or other medicaments; patients who were contaminated or treated with iodide; patients having undergone a successful treatment of hyperthyroidism; patients with Graves' ophthalmopathy without hyperthyroidism, patients in intensive care; patients with kidney insufficiency, dialysis patients; patients with acute uremia and patients with T3 or T4 autoantibodies.

For most of the measurements two different hypersensitive tests were used, in many cases three to four and in some cases up to six different tests. At the beginning of our investigations, we used an "old" TSH RIA test in addition. These tests were:

1. IRMA methods with monoclonal antibodies
   SUCROSEP TSH-IRMA from Boots-Celltech
   TSH-MAIAclone from Serono
   RIAgnost h-TSH monoclonal from Behring
   TSH-IRMAclone from Henning
   TSH monoclonal from Ciba-Corning
   SPECTRIA-TSH from Organon Teknika
   TSH-NML-IRMA
   TSH-IRMA gammacoat from (Clinical Assays) Travenol
   ELSA-TSH from IDW-Cis
   TSH monoclonal from Hybritech
2. an RIA with special polyclonal antibodies
   TSH-RIA hypersensitive from Henning
3. EIA tests with monoclonal antibodies
   HTSH-EIA from Abbott
   ENZYMUN-TSH from Boehringer-Mannheim
4. an IRMA method
   QUANTIMUN-HTSH-IRMA from Bio-Rad
5. and for comparitive purposes an RIA test which has been used for many years in our laboratory
   TSH-RIA from Henning

Dilution studies were carried out with the new tests. For these studies we took numerous pooled sera from hypothyroid patients with high TSH levels and for dilution we used sera containing no TSH. Precision was established by analysing three panel samples (Lyphocheck Immunoassay Control Serum Bio-Rad) in replicates of five with the different assays; intra- and interassay coefficients of variation were calculated. For some test procedures the sera containing no TSH were measured in replicates of ten.

Results and discussion

The Quantimun HTSH IRMA test from Bio-Rad (fig. 7) is an IRMA method using iodine 125 labelled polyclonal antibodies. The advantage of the IRMA is its very good sensitivity [4]. This test differentiates between normal TSH values and depressed values. But the test shows a large overlap of normal TSH values with values for depressed levels.

The result of the dilution study (fig. 8) is a linear response for increasing dilution (decreasing TSH concentration) up to a value of 0.5 μIU/ml. Intra-assay CV was 3.75% (1.55 μIU/ml), 1.39% (10.88 μIU/ml) and 1.34% (28.8 μIU/ml), the corresponding interassay CVs were 7.01, 2.86 and 3.65%.

The RIAgnost h-TSH test from Behring (fig. 9) is a IRMA test using iodine 125 labelled monoclonal antibodies. This test shows a good classification of values for the different thyroid states, combined with a small degree of overlap. The dilution study (fig. 10) results in a nearly linear response for increasing dilution up to a value of 0.015 μIU/ml. The intraassay CVs were 3.15% (1.39 μIU/ml), 1.12% (9.63 μIU/ml) and 1.27% (23.8 μIU/ml), the corresponding interassay CVs were 2.09, 4.04 and 3.2%.

The HTSH-EIA from Abbott (fig. 11) is an IEMA using two different HRPO labelled monoclonal antibodies. This test differentiates as well as the most highly sensitive IRMA methods. The dilution study (fig. 12) shows a linear response with decreasing concentrations. The intraassay CVs were 4.46% (1.66 μIU/ml), 4.02% (12.2 μIU/ml) and 4.44% (36.29 μIU/ml). The corresponding interassay CVs were 4.33, 3.58 and 8.23%.

The other investigated IRMA tests with iodine 125 labelled monoclonal antibodies from different suppliers (fig. 13) show similar results to the tests from Abbott and Behring.

The results show that the borderlines between the different regions (unmeasurable TSH, overlapping normal, overlapping and elevated TSH values) vary for the individual tests from the various suppliers. This was also established by Wood [17].

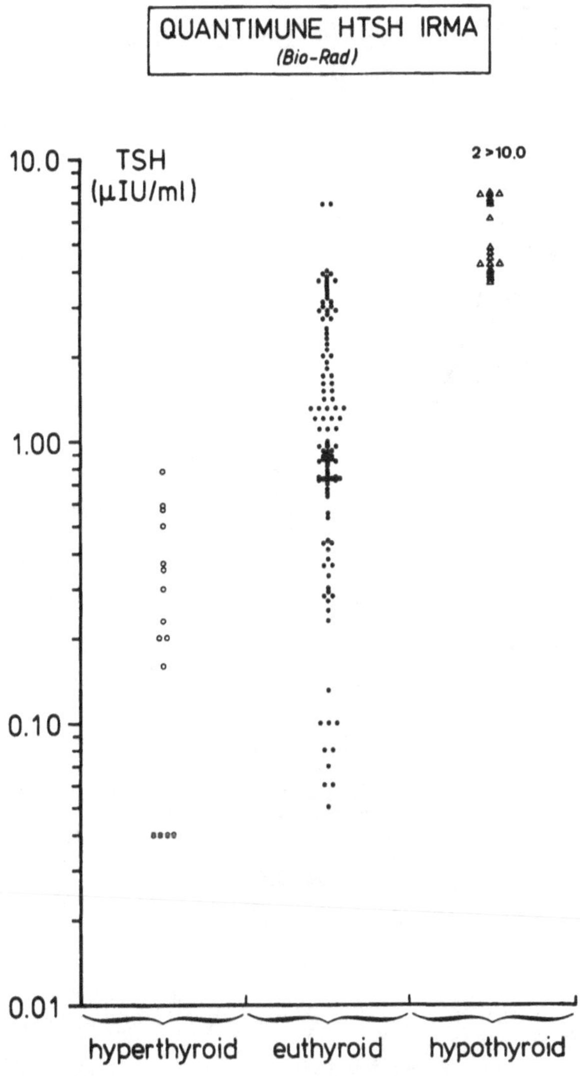

Fig. 7 TSH values using the HTSH IRMA from Bio Rad.

This may be caused by the different structure of the monoclonal antibodies and the fact that several antibodies are used. In addition, the second antibody (against the TSH-antibody-complex) is different in each test.

Another reason for these differences is a small deviation in the calibration of the standard sera in comparison to the international TSH standard preparation as well as variations in serum matrix and dilution buffer.

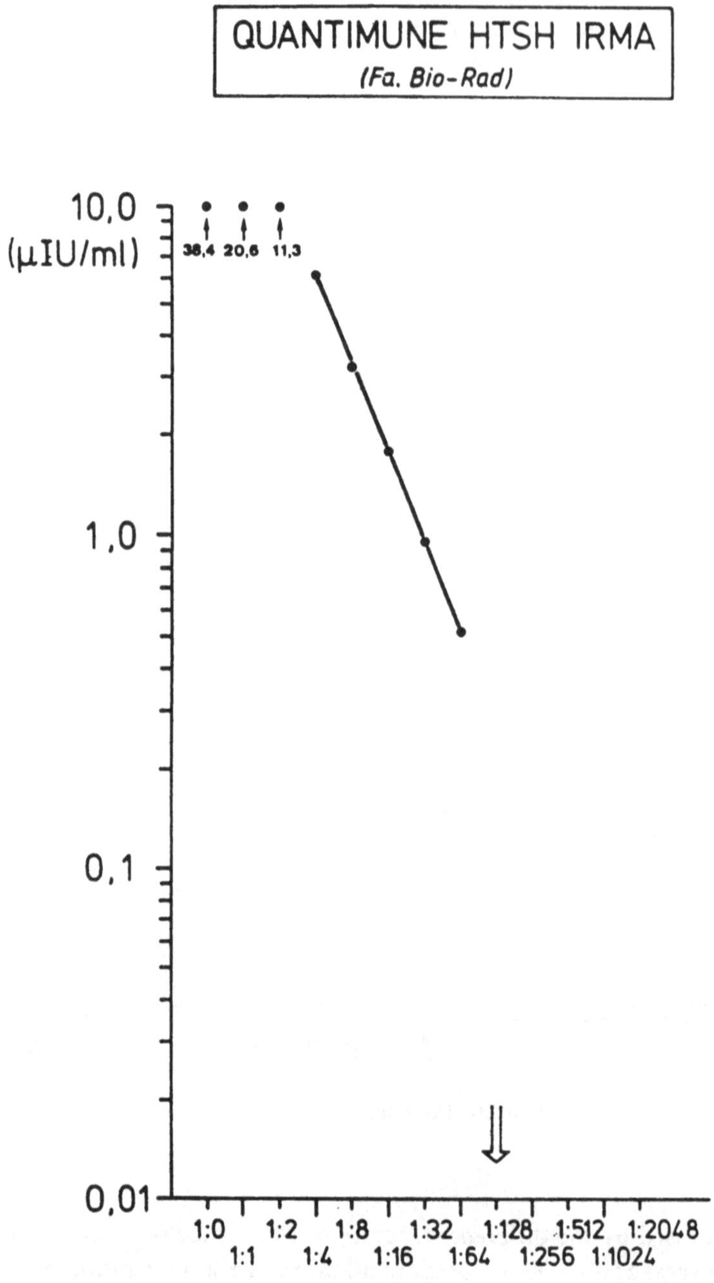

Fig. 8 Dilution study using the TSH IRMA from Bio Rad.

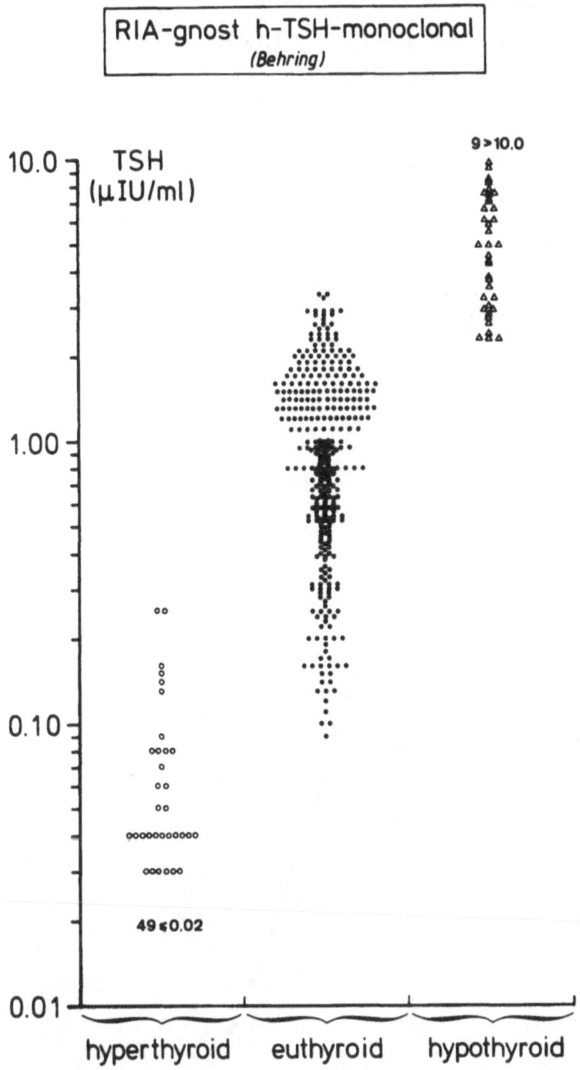

Fig. 9 TSH values using the hypersensitive IRMA test with monoclonal antibodies from Behring.

Furthermore the IRMA procedure itself is an important factor. The closer the TSH concentration comes to zero, the lower the radioactivity. Hyperthyroidism is usually accompanied by unmeasurable TSH or just small quantities of it. In these cases the result should be zero. However, small quantities of radioactive material and of enzymes, which are present in every individual, lead to an activity level marginally in excess of zero. Repeated measurements of sera containing no TSH show a coefficient of variation up to 185%. Therefore, the sensitivity limit

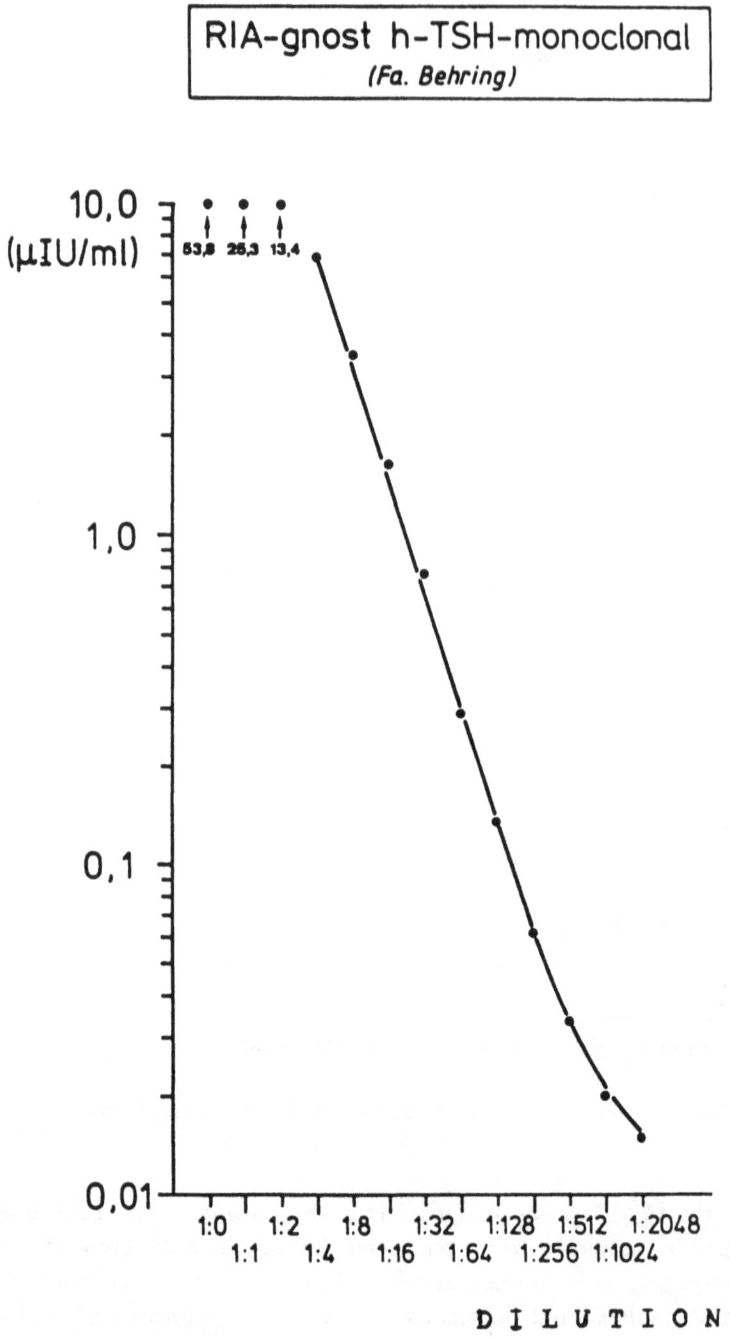

Fig. 10 Dilution study using the TSH IRMA with monoclonal antibodies from Behring.

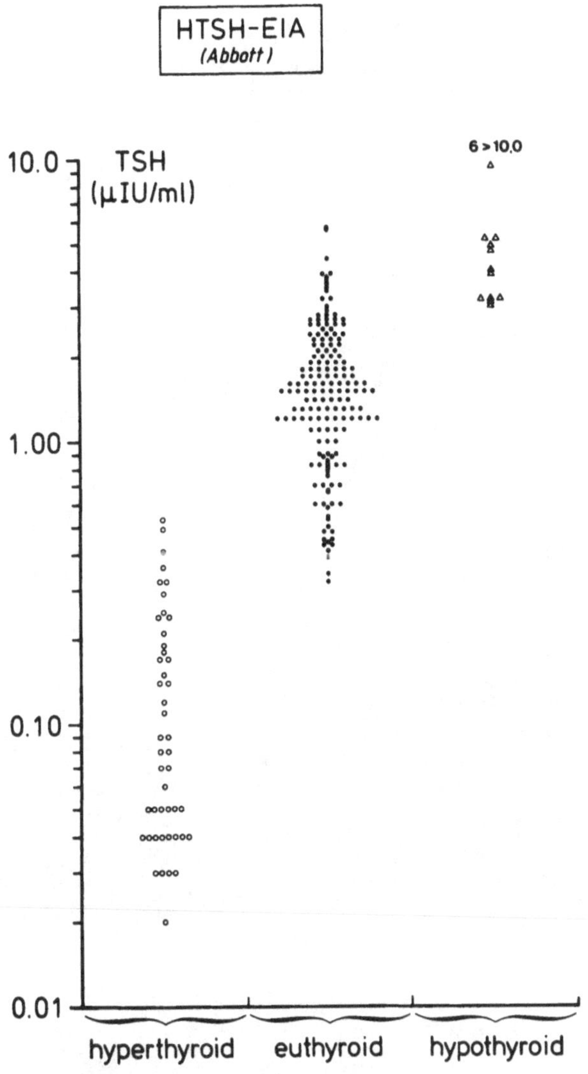

Fig. 11 TSH values using the immunoenzymometric assay with monoclonal antibodies from Abbott.

should be established as the mean value of a zero serum, measured in replicates plus two times and standard deviation.

The dilution studies carried out with the IRMA tests with monoclonal antibodies show differences in low-end sensitivity and precision between the various tests.

The investigations concerning the TRH tests show that the TRH test is no longer necessary, where TSH values are depressed or elevated. The TSH increase

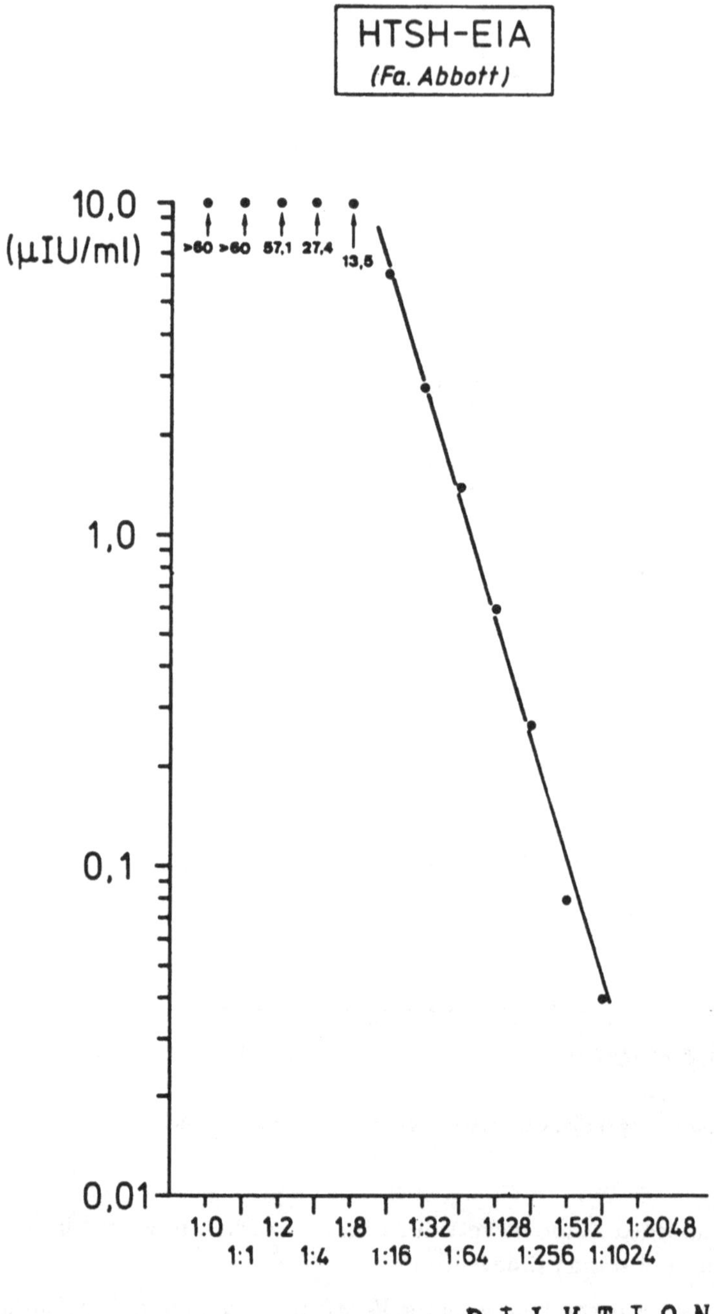

Fig. 12 Dilution study using the EIA with monoclonal antibodies from Abbott.

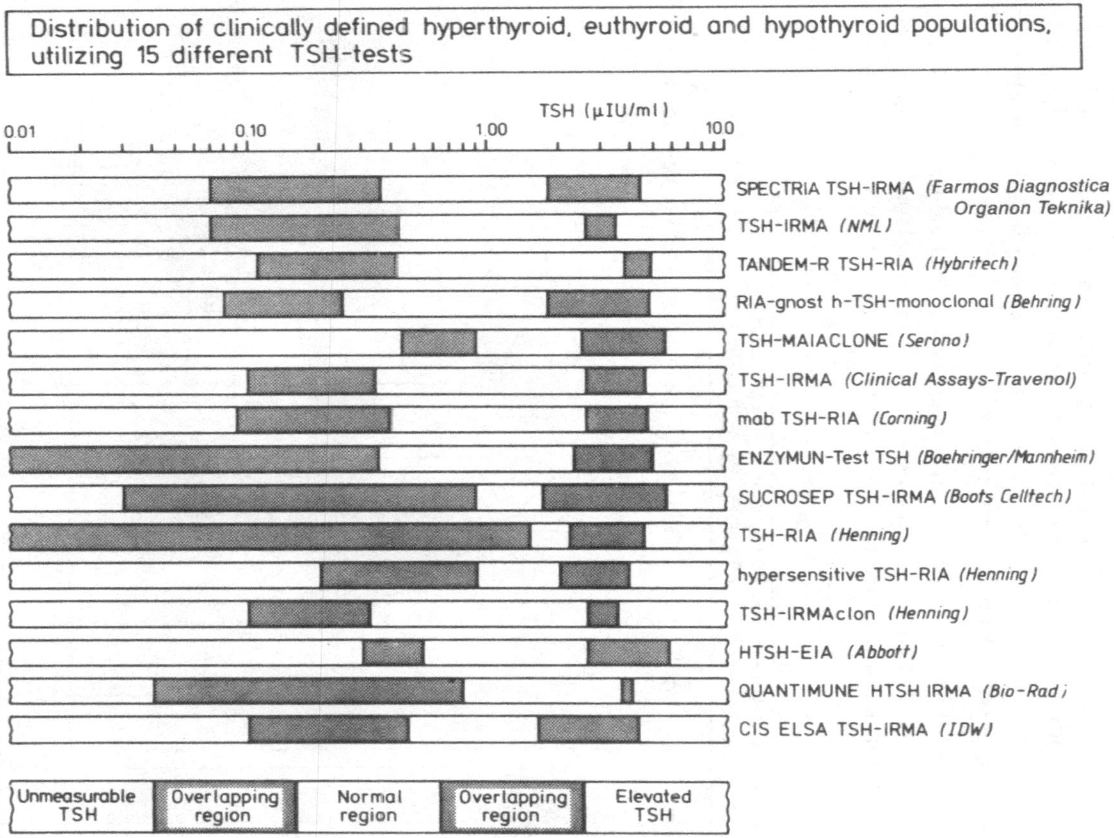

Fig. 13 Borderline values of the different regions seen in 15 TSH tests.

after TRH application varies in the different ranges. The CV for the different concentration ranges should be taken into consideration. Starting from a base of unmeasurable TSH the minimal amount of TSH increase observed range between 0.1 and 0.5 μIU/ml. In the "overlapping" region these values were found to be from 0.2 to 0.8 μIU/ml, in the normal range these values were found to be from 0.3 to 0.8 μIU/ml, in the next overlapping region (between normal and hypothyroid) they were found to be between 0.3 and 0.8 μIU/ml. For elevated TSH values they were greater than 0.5 μIU/ml.

Thyroxine substitution causes an adequate decrease of TSH values (figs. 14, 15). An optimal dose leads to values in the normal or lower overlapping region. The suppression dosage should move the TSH level to zero. For 25% of the patients

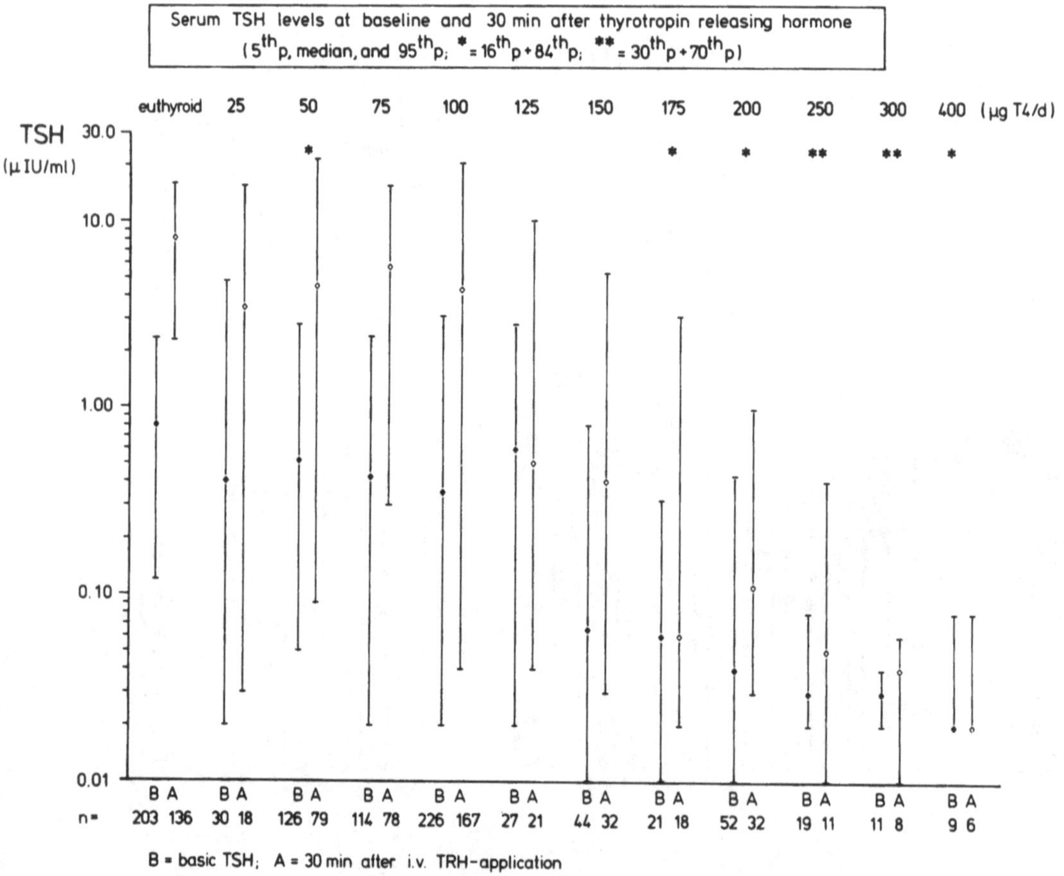

Fig. 14 TSH values before and after TRH application in euthyroid cases and seen in patients which take daily thyroxine in different doses.

	EU-THYROID	25	50	75	100	125	150	175	200	250	300	400 µg T4
	Basic TSH (µIU/ml)											
n	203	30	126	114	226	27	44	21	52	19	11	9
p 5% (or 16* or 30**%)	0.12	0.02	0.05*	0.02	0.02	0.02	0.01	0.01*	0.01*	0.02**	0.02**	
m	0.8	0.4	0.51	0.42	0.35	0.59	0.06	0.06	0.04	0.03	0.03	0.02
p 95% (or 70* or 84**%)	2.34	4.87	2.87	2.4	3.07	2.8	0.8	0.32**	0.43**	0.08*	0.04*	0.08**
$\bar{x}$	0.94	1.19	0.87	0.69	0.70	0.89	0.23	0.33	0.27	0.06	0.03	0.03
s	0.68	1.77	0.94	0.80	0.91	0.94	0.33	0.76	0.51	0.07	0.02	0.03
	TSH (µIU/ml) 30 min. after i. v. TRH-application											
n	136	18	79	78	167	21	32	18	32	11	8	6
p 5% (or 16*%)	2.3	0.03	0.09	0.3	0.04	0.04	0.03	0.02*	0.03*	0.01*	0.01*	
m	8.1	3.45	4.51	5.65	4.3	0.5	0.4	0.06	0.11	0.05	0.04	0.02
p 95% (or 84**%)	15.9	15.5	21.4	15.5	20.5	10.2	5.32	3.1**	0.98**	0.4**	0.06**	0.08**
$\bar{x}$	8.30	5.61	7.07	6.19	6.53	5.01	1.56	2.86	0.83	0.43	0.03	0.02
s	4.29	4.06	6.44	5.06	6.64	3.30	2.04	7.56	1.65	0.99	0.02	0.02

Fig. 15 Mathematic statistical values of the investigations from cases which are demonstrated in figure 14.

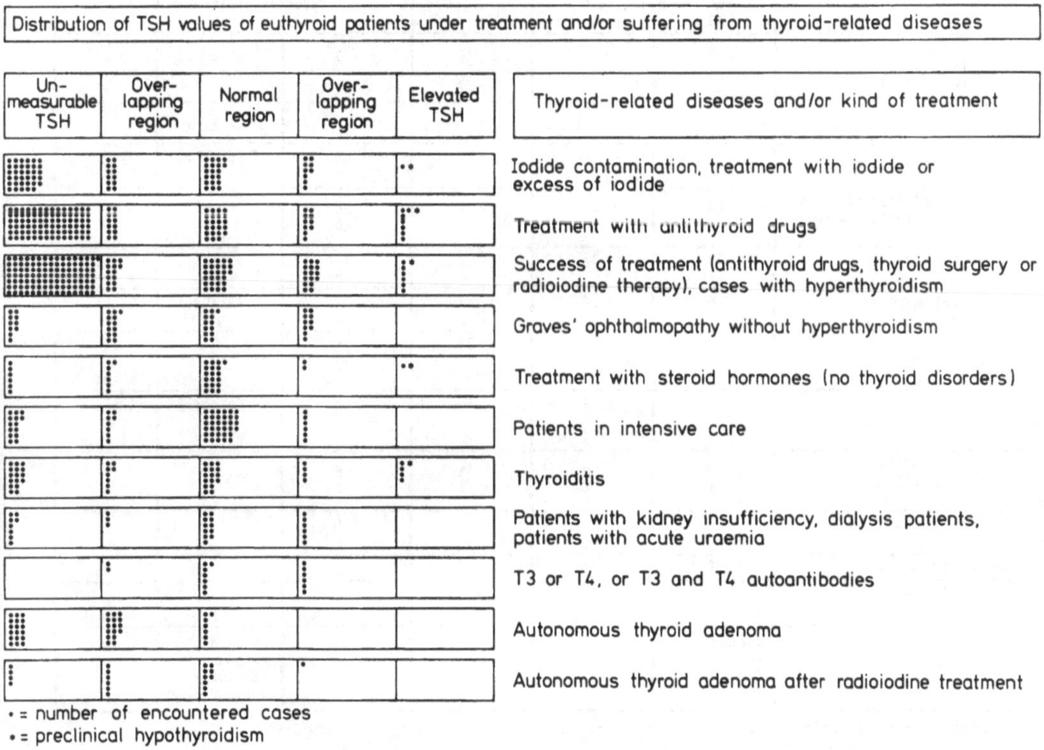

Fig. 16 The numerous possibilities to influence the TSH value.

a suppression was obtained by less than 150 µg T4/d, for 30% 150 µg T4/d were needed, for 9% 175 µg T4/d and for some cases even more (app. 1% 200 µg, 13% 250 µg and app. 22% 300 µg T4/d). Doses of 300 or 400 µg T4/D led to unmeasurable TSH values, but also led to a hyperthyroidism factitia [7].

The numerous possible influences on TSH values (figs. 16, 17) demonstrate the inadequacy of the TSH test for basic screening of the thyroid function. Unmeasurable TSH was also found in patients with iodine contamination, under treatment with thyroid hormones or antithyroid drugs, after successful treatment of hyperthyroidism, in patients with graves' ophthalmopathy, under treatment with steroid hormones without disorders of the thyroid, in patients in intensive

DISTRIBUTION OF TSH VALUES OF PATIENTS (CLINICALLY DEFINED THYROID STATUS) UNDER TREATMENT AND/OR SUFFERING FROM THYROID-RELATED DISEASES

THYROID-RELATED DISEASES AND/OR KIND OF TREATMENT	UNMEASURABLE TSH	OVERLAPPING REGION	NORMAL REGION	OVERLAPPING REGION	ELEVATED TSH	DIAGNOSIS
		EUTHYROID STATES				
	HYPERTHYROIDISM sec. hypothyroidism 13	 10		HYPOTHYROIDISM sec. hyperthyroidism		
Iodide contamination, treatment with iodide or excess of iodide	35 14	12 6	20	9	1 (precl.) 5	E - +
Treatment with thyroid hormones (see fig. 14)						
Treatment with antithyroid drugs	84 9	12 3	23 3	10 6	7 (precl.) 8	E -
Success of treatment (antithyroid drugs, thyroid surgery of radioiodine therapy), cases with hyperthyroidism	106 2	14	27	16 6	6 (precl.) 6	E -
Graves' ophthalmopathy without hyperthyroidism	10	13	19	10 2	 2	E -
Treatment with steroid hormones (no thyroid disorders)	6	7	21	2 2	1 (precl.) 2	E -
Patients in intensive care	14 79 2	8 54 2	34 73	6 14	 12	E - +
Thyroiditis	16 11	8 2 7	16	4 6	4 (precl.) 12	E - +
Patients with kidney insufficiency, dialysis patients, patients with acute uraemia	8 1	3 4	11 7	6 6	 6	E -
T3 or T4, or T3 and T4 auto-antibodies		2	7	6 7	 12	E -
Autonomous thyroid adenoma	24	16	7			E
Autonomous thyroid adenoma after radioiodine treatment	4	6	9	1		E
	unknown reasons TSH-auto-antibodies ??				unknown reasons TSH-auto-antibodies ??	E

E = euthyroid states; - = hypothyroidism; + = hyperthyroidism; (precl.) = preclinical hypothyroidism

Fig. 17 The numerous possibilities to influence the TSH value.

care, with thyroiditis, with kidney insufficiency, in dialysis patients, in patients with acute uremia, with autonomous adenoma, especially after treatment with radioiodine and in other patients not included in the above.

Acknowledgements

Mr. Schatz joined us in our investigations of the secondary hypothyroid cases. The measurements of the hypersensitive TSH RIA (Henning) were carried out by Mrs. Schirmer, those of the Boehringer-test by Mrs. Baumgärtner and those of the Bio Rad-test by Mr. Hartenstein.

References

[1] Biersack, H. J., et al.: Ermittlung der optimalen L-Thyroxin Dosis zur Behandlung der blanden Struma. Dtsch. Med. Wochenschr. **108** (1983) 1269.

[2] Caldwell, G., et al.: A new strategy for thyroid function testing. Lancet I (1985) 1117.

[3] Doepp, M., et al.: Eine Methode zur besseren Dosierung von L-Thyroxin in der Suppressionstherapie der Schilddrüse. Therapiewoche **28** (1978) 100.

[4] Doepp, M., et al.: Untersuchungen des TSH-Spiegels mit einem IRMA Ärzt. Lab. **24** (1978) 85.

[5] Doos, R. C., et al.: A highly sensitive non-isotopic assay for human TSH with extended clinical utility. Abstract presented at the international symposium on thyroid function tests, Maga 10, 1985. Ile de Bendor, France.

[6] Grebe, S. F.: Schilddrüsenhormon-Autoantikörper im Blut. Deutscher Ärzte-Verlag, Köln 1985.

[7] Grebe, S. K., et al.: Influence of different thyroxine doses on the TSH blood level measured by a hypersensitive TSH test. Nuc. Med. Commun. **6** (1985) 583.

[8] Hüfner, M., M. Grussendorf: Möglichkeiten und Grenzen des TRH-Tests. S.-M. **4** (1981) 45.

[9] Hunter, W. M.: Monoclonal antibodies in clinical chemistry. Proc. R. Soc. Edingurgh **81 B** (1982) 293.

[10] Hunter, W. M., et al.: Immunoassays for clinical chemistry. Sec. Ed. Churchill Livingstone, Edinburgh 1983.

[11] Joseph, K.: Erstdiagnostik und Verlaufskontrolle bei Schilddrüsenfunktionsstörungen mit der IRMA-TSH Bestimmung. Nuc. Compact **16** (1985) 240.

[12] Malter, J. S., et al.: Identification of hyperthyroid patients by means of a sensitive assay for thyrot. Clin. Chem. **31** (1985) G42.

[13] Pfannenstiel, P., et al.: Erfahrungen mit der Bestimmung von fT3 and fT4 sowie einem supersensitiven TSH-Assay bei lat. Schilddrüsenerkrankungen. Deutscher Ärzte-Verlag, Köln 1985.

[14] Rattle, S. J., et al.: New separation method for monoclonal immunoradiometric assay and its application to assays for thyrotropin and human choriogonadotropin. Clin. Chem. **30** (1984) 1457.

[15] Seth, J., et al.: A sensitive immunoradiometric assay for serum thyroid stimulations hormone: A replacement for the thyrotropin releasing hormone test. Br. Med. J. **289** (1984) 1334.

[16] Wevers, P., et al.: MAIAclone, Eine neue Generation immunoradiometrischer Assays. Labor Praxis in der Medizin **7** (1985) 1.

[17] Wood, W. G., et al.: An evaluation of six solid-phase thyrotropin (TSH) kits. J. Clin. Chem. Biochem. **23** (1985) 461.

Clinical comparison of 5 kits for sensitive TSH determination in hyperthyroidism and in non thyroidal illness

J. N. Talbot, M. L. Piketti, M. Michalski, G. Coutris,
S. Askienazy, G. Milhaud

Introduction

Several commercial kits are available for sensitive TSH determination whose aim is discrimination of hyperthyroid patients [1 – 3], as well as hypothyroidism. In order to determine the clinical significance of a low TSH level, we studied hyperthyroid patients (untreated or treated), central hypothyroid patients and patients suffering from non thyroidal illness (NTI) where TSH response to TRH has been demonstrated to be often diminished, such as elderly patients in poor condition [4, 5] or depressive patients [6].

Materials and methods

In order to compare the validity of 5 kits, each sample was assayed (in duplicate) using 2 to 5 of the following kits:

"A" = Ventrex distributed in France by Travenol, IRMA assay using monoclonal and polyclonal antibodies.
"B" = Behring, IRMA assay using to different monoclonal antibodies.
"C" = Corning, IRMA assay using monoclonal and polyclonal antibodies.
"D" = Pharmacia, IRMA assay using 2 polyclonal antibodies.
"E" = Abbot, IEMA assay using 3 different monoclonal antibodies.

Their technical characteristics are summarized in table 1.

The patients were distributed into 4 main groups:

- 91 untreated hyperthyroid patients,
- 60 treated hyperthyroid patients,
- 64 NTI, elderly patients, depression,
- and 3 patients suffering from untreated panhypopituitarism (Sheean's syndrome).

Thyrotropin

Table 1 Technical characteristics of the different assays

	Kit A	Kit B	Kit C	Kit D	Kit E
Calibrator	OMS 80/558	OMS 80/558	OMS 80/558	OMS 80/558	OMS 80/558
Matrix of the standards	Procine serum	Human serum	Human serum	Human serum	Porcine serum
Range covered (μU/ml)	0 – 100	0 – 50	0 – 100	0.1 – 50	0 – 60
Sample volume (μL)	200	200	200	100	100
Incubation time	1.30 h	2 h	2.30 h	3 h	2.30 h
Incubation steps	1	1	2	2	3
Washing steps	2	1	1	0	3 × 2
Radioactivity (kbq)	< 740	< 300	< 518	< 230	–

The diagnosis was assessed on clinical findings, T_3/TBG and T_4/TBG values and, in doubtfull cases (or central hypothyroidism), TRH challenge and captation ratio of ^{123}I by the thyroid gland.

T_3 and T_4 were determined using the Clinical Assays kits, TBG using the Behring kit. TRH was purchased from the Roussel-Uclaf Laboratory (Stimu TSH*) and ^{123}I from CIS.

Results

We obtained the following detection limits (defined as the lowest concentration of TSH which can be significantly differenciated from the zero standard).

Kit A = 0.06 mU/l
Kit B = 0.02
Kit C = 0.06
Kit D < 0.1
Kit E = 0.05

The "normal ranges", derived from more than 50 normal healty adults, are given in table 2.

Table 2 Normal range for TSH

Kit	A	B	C	D	E
n of controls	50	66	60	77	50
range (mU/l)	0.4 – 4.8	0.2 – 4.7	0.4 – 4.2	0.3 – 4.5	0.2 – 6.6

Table 3 TSH in untreated hyperthyroid patients

	Kit	A	B	C	D	E
Graves disease	n	44	40	63	33	26
	n of low TSH	44	40	63	30	26
Plummer's adenoma	n	3	2	4	5	2
	n of low TSH	3	2	4	5	2
Amiodarone induced	n	3	5	5	5	2
	n of low TSH	3	5	5	5	2
Iatrogenic (over treated hypo)	n	6	12	11	6	8
	n of low TSH	6	12	11	6	7
4 cases of discrepancy between the kits: TSH (mU/l)		0.11 0.07 0.13 –	– 0.05 – 0.16	< 0.06 0.11 0.06 –	0.41 0.32 0.31 –	– < 0.05 0 0.24

Table 3 illustrates the excellent sensitivity of sensitive TSH in untreated hyperthyroid patients regardless of the mechanism of hyperthyroidism (Graves' disease, Plummer's adenoma, Amiodarone induced or iatrogenic). However, TSH was 3 times within the normal range with the "D" kit and one time with the "E" kit but always very close to the boundary value.

Table 4: Central hypothyroidism is much rarer. In the 3 cases we studies, TSH values not only were detectable but they were borderline and even in the low normal values with some kits.

Table 4 TSH in 3 cases of untreated central hypothyroidism

Kit	A	B	C	D	E
TSH (mU/l)	0.36	0.3	0.46	0.45	–
	0.36	–	0.28	0.55	–
	0.23	0.22	0.29	< 0.1	–

Table 5: Treated hyperthyroids. When patient remains hyperthyroid under treatment, TSH remains low. But when patient returns clinically to euthyroidism with normalized T_3, TSH may also remain low. We have even observed 2 patients euthyroids for 2 years after stopping the treatment whose TSH is still low.

Table 5 TSH in carbimazole treated hyperthyroid patients

	Kit	A	B	C	D	E
Patients remanning hyperthyroid	n	13	10	22	21	10
	n of low TSH	13	10	22	20	10
Patients returned to euthyroids	n	14	28	33	24	14
	n of low TSH	5	11	14	10	8
2 cases of discrepancy between the kits: TSH (mU/ml)	1 hyper	–	–	< 0.06	0.39	< 0.05
	1 eu-	–	0.61	0.22	0.27	0.87

In elderly patients and in patients suffering from NTI, TSH is also very often diminsihed (tab. 6). This "low TSH syndrome" cannot be identified with the low T_3 syndrome. Low TSH was observed frequently in elderly patients whose T_3 was normal, in contrast TSH was sometimes normal in young NTI patients whose T_3 was low. Discrepancies between the kits are frequent in this group with a wide range of values observed for the same serum (for example from non detectable to .78, from .16 to 1).

Table 6 TSH in NTI and/or elderly patients

	Kit	A	B	C	D	E
NTI and/or Elderly patients	n	26	21	30	29	13
	n of low TSH	16	11	15	9	1
7 cases of discrepancy between the kits: TSH (mU/l)		–	–	0.16	1	0.86
		0.14	0.18	0.78	< 0.1	–
		–	0.60	0.20	0.85	–
		0.36	–	0.28	0.55	0.60
		0.34	0.56	0.64	0.36	–
		0.18	0.45	0.47	0.16	–
		0.28	–	0.31	0.31	–

Mean frequency of low values = 40%

In untreated depressive patients (tab. 7), TSH is low in almost half of the cases, regardless to the age of the patient. Discrepancies are also observed in this group.

Table 7 TSH in untreated depression

	Kit	A	B	C	D	E
Depression	n	24	27	25	20	27
	n of low TSH	12	12	9	7	12
3 cases of discrepancy between the kits: TSH (mU/l)		0.14 0.34 0.41	0.10 0.51 –	0.29 0.61 0.30	– 0.62 –	1.21 0.55 0.19

Mean frequency of low values = 40%

Discussion

Our study confirms the excellent sensitivity of sensitive TSH determination in the diagnosis of hyperthyroidism. These new techniques are definetly a progress compared to classical TSH determination. In hyperthyroid patients, TSH is low; there are only few discrepancies which can be related to lack of sensitivity of the "D" kit.

In hyperthyroid patients becoming euthyroid under treatment, low TSH levels are frequently encountered even long time after normalization of T_3 and T_4. The prognostic value of such persistence of low TSH levels remains to be determined. Low levels are also observed in elderly or NTI or depressive patients, as it was expected from low responsiveness to TRH described previously. Discrepancies are frequent in those groups. They partly can be due to unequal analytical performances of the kits (sensitivity, reproductibility in low values). For example, the "B" kit has the best slope in the low values and the best signal to noise ratio.

This hypothesis cannot explain the very large gaps we observed between the values in some cases. They might be elucidated if further information about the epitopes which are recognized by the monoclonal antibodies could be obtained.

Conclusions

Sensitive TSH determination can be used as the primary screenning test when searching for thyroid disfunction: In our experience, a normal TSH level excludes such a disfunction except in rare cases of central hypothyroidism where TSH can be in the low normal values.

But, at least in our hospital practice, TSH cannot be used alone to assess hyperthyroidism: There are too many circumstances where TSH is low and the patient euthyroid. It is therefore needed to determine free T_3 or T_3/TBG and, if borderline, to perform a two points TRH challenge (0 – 30 mn) when hyperthyroidism is suspected.

In the follow up of treated hyperthyroidism, TSH cannot be used as an index of antithyroid drugs efficacy, free T_3 or T_3/TBG determination is necessary.

Further studies are needed to determine the clinical significance and the possible prognostic value of low TSH in NTI, depression or in apparently cured hyperthyroidism.

References

[1] Seth, J., H. A. Kellet, G. Caldwell, et al.: A sensitive immunoradiometric assay for serum thyroid stimulating hormone: A replacement for the thyrotropin releasing hormone test? Br. Med. J. **289** (1984) 1334 – 1336.

[2] Semple, C. G., S, D. Slater, A. M. Reid, et al.: A sensitive immunoradiometric assay for serum thyroid stimulating hormone. Br. Med. J. **290** (1985) 69 – 70.

[3] Malter, J. S., S. E. Manotti, G. R. Knee, et al.: Identification of hyperthyroid patients by means of a sensitive assay for thyrotropin. Clin. Chem. **31** (1985) 642 – 644.

[4] Snyder, P. J., R. M. Utiger: Thyrotropin response to thyrotropin releasing hormone in normal females over forty. J. Clin. Endocrinol. Metab. **34** (1972) 1096 – 1098.

[5] Kissel, C., C. Jacques, M. Saint-Martin, et al.: Limites de l'intérêt du test à la thyrolibérine chez la personne âgée. Influence du sexe. La Presse Médicale **13** (1984) 681.

[6] Kirstein, L., M. S. Gold, A. L. C. Pottash, et al.: Thyrotropin releasing hormone test and male unipolar depression. Biol. Psy. **16** (1981) 819 – 824.

Comparison by receiver operating characteristics (ROC) analysis of three thyrotropin assays in the diagnosis of hyperthyroidism

P. Blockx, A. Vrancken, R. Speybrouck, R. Abs

Introduction

During the last two years, there has been a growing interest for high sensitivity TSH assays, mainly because they offer new possibilities in the diagnosis of hyperthyroidism [1 – 3]. This report describes the investigation of the relative diagnostic efficiency of three TSH assays in this clinical context.

In the first part of the study, we compared a "high sensitivity" TSH-assay with a classical TSH-assay. The second part consisted of the comparison of two high sensitivity TSH-kits.

First part of the study

The high sensitivity assay we investigated first was the RIA-gnost TSH coated tube kit, from Hoechst-Behring, FRG. The classical assay was the Amerlex TSH assay, from Amersham International plc, UK, which at that time was used as a routine procedure in our laboratory.

We assayed TSH-concentrations on the sera of 240 patients, of whom 83 were hyperthyroid and 157 were euthyroid. The classification in eu- or hyperthyroid was done according to the sum of information yielded by the direct assays of FT4 and FT3 (Amerlex, Amersham Int plc, UK) together with the clinical diagnosis and, eventually, the response to TRH stimulation.

In this population we determined, for both TSH-assays, the true negative and true positive ratios associated to all observed TSH concentrations. This allowed the plotting of a specificity (TNR) versus sensitivity (TPR) diagram, the Receiver Operating Characteristics (ROC) curve diagram [4] (fig. 1).

It can readily be observed that for any specificity level, the clinical sensitivity, i. e. the percentage of detected hyperthyroid patients, is far superior with the new, "highly sensitive" method. Indeed, at a specificity level of 97.5%, corresponding to

Thyrotropin

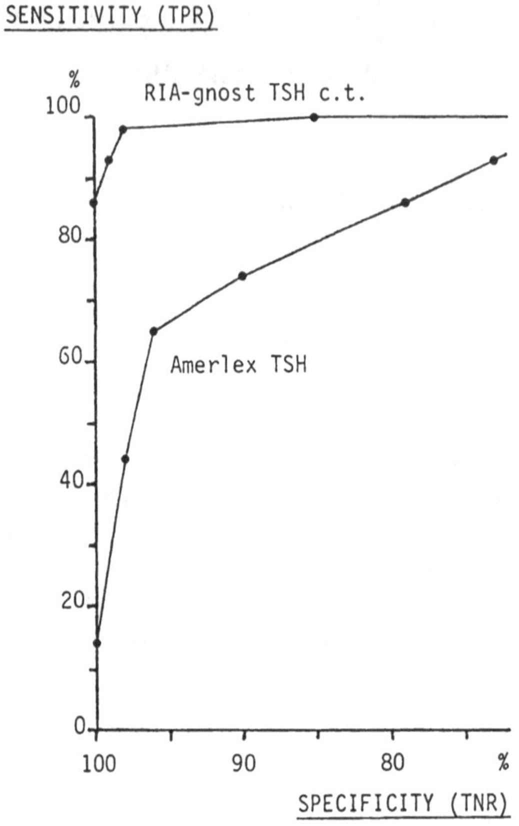

Fig. 1 ROC curves for Amerlex TSH and RIA-gnost TSH c. t.
Positive = hyperthyroid.

the lower limit of the normal range, a sensitivity of about 98% is found with the new method, compared to only 50% with the classical assay. Moreover, it should be mentioned that with the high sensitivity kit, about 80% of the hyperthyroid patients had even undetectable TSH serum levels.

We conclude that the diagnosis of primary hyperthyroidism can indeed be made by means of this high sensitivity TSH-assay. An essential condition to reach the desired clinical sensitivity, however, is that the outstanding analytical sensitivity of the method should not be degradated by careless manipulation or counting.

Second part of the study

Since the completion of this first evaluation, however, more new TSH assays, claimed to be have a high sensitivity, became available on the European market.

To investigate whether this claim was justified or not, we compared two "highly sensitive" TSH-assays.

The first kit was the same as analysed in the former part of the study, namely the RIA-gnost TSH coated tube assay, from Hoechst-Behring (FRG), which in the meantime we had chosen as the new routine TSH assay for our laboratory. The other high sensitivity assay was the more recent Pharmacia RIA TSH assay, from Pharmacia Diagnostics AB, Sweden.

Serum samples were obtained from 213 patients, of whom 116 were hyperthyroid and 97 euthyroid. Moreover, as we suspected the differences in clinical sensitivity would be very small, we tried to enhance them. Therefore, 75 out of the 213 patients were chosen because they had RIA-gnost TSH-levels between 0.03 and 0.5 μU/ml, to be representative of the borderline zone between the eu- and hyperthyroid range. A consequence of this selection, however, is that the investigated euthyroid group could not be considered as distributed in the same way as a true normal population.

Moreover, no patients with severe non-thyroidal illness were included in this study, because in these cases, a low TSH concentration is obviously not indicative of hyperthyroidism [5].

Using the reported population, ROC curves were obtained for both kits (fig. 2). It can clearly been seen that for an equal specificity (TNR) a higher sensitivity (TPR) is always attained with the Hoechst-kit.

The best separation between eu- and hyperthyroid patients was observed at 0.15 μU/ml for the Hoechst-kit, with a sensitivity of 99% (99.1%) for a specificity of 99%. With the Pharmacia-kit, the best separation was observed at 0.30 μU/ml, with a sensitivity of about 96% (95.7%) for a specificity of 92% (91.8%). Using these limits, the total number of misclassified patients amounted to about 1% for the Hoechst assay (2/213 = 0,9%), compared to 6% for the Pharmacia kit (13/213 = 6.1%).

These observations can be correlated with the overlap zone between eu- and hyperthyroid populations. Indeed, this zone ranges only from 0.14 to 0.15 μU/ml for the Hoechst kit (and contains only 1% of the tested population (2/213 = 0.9%)), but for the Pharmacia kit it extends from 0.1 to 0.59 μU/ml (containing 81/213 = 38% of the tested population).

This marked difference in overlap zone is obviously one of the reasons of the much higher clinical sensitivity of the Hoechst assay.

Another reason is to be found in the higher analytical sensitivity of the Hoechst method. Indeed, the typical detection limit we have found under routine conditions was 0.01 to 0.03 μU/ml. In the Pharmacia assay, however, the detection limit is much higher, due to the absence of a zero standard, and amounts to the concentration of the lowest standard, namely 0.1 μU/ml.

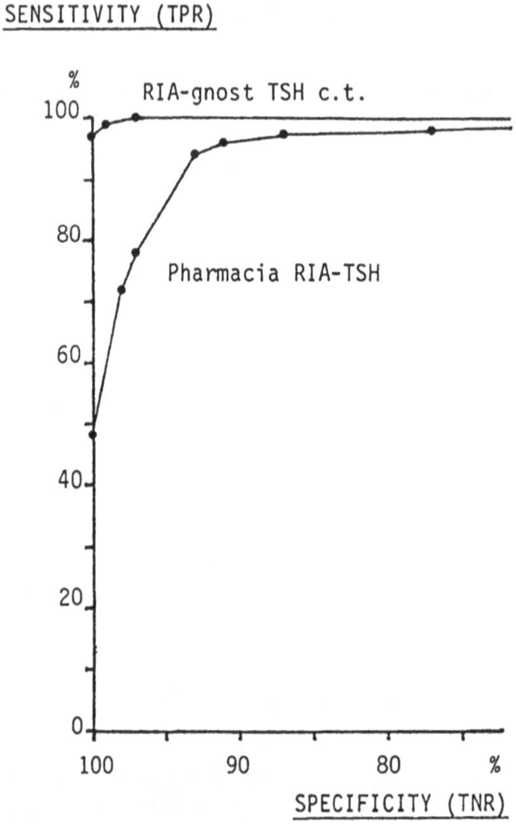

Fig. 2 ROC curves for RIA-gnost TSH c.t. and Pharmacia RIA-TSH.
Negative = euthyroid.

It should also be noted that, even with this very low detection limit, the percentage hyperthyroid patients with undetectable TSH levels was far higher with the Hoechst kit than with the Pharmacia kit: resp. 83% (96/116) and 66% (76/116).

Conclusion

These observations suggest that, although the high sensitivity TSH assays have a definite advantage over the classical TSH assays with respect to the diagnosis of hyperthyroidism, their clinical efficiency may differ quite a lot.

It is therefore essential, in order to achieve the best possible separation between eu- and hyperthyroid TSH levels, that the TSH assay would be chosen according to a critical evaluation, as suggested in this report.

Special care should be taken to obtain a very low detection limit, as well as the smallest possible overlap zone between eu- and hyperthyroidism.

References

[1] Wiersinga, W. M., E. Endert, M. D. Trip, et al.: Immunoradiometric assay for Thyrotropin in plasma: Its value in predicting response to Thyroliberin stimulation and assessing thyroid function in Amiodarone-treated patients. Clin. Chem. **32** (1986) 433–436.

[2] Bassett, F., C. J. Eastman, G. Ma, et al.: Diagnostic value of Thyrotropin concentrations in serum as measured by a sensitive immunoradiometric assay. Clin. Chem. **32** (1986) 461–464.

[3] Helenius, T., S. Tikanoja: A sensitive and practical immunoradiometric assay for Thyrotropin. Clin. Chem. **32** (1986) 514–518.

[4] O'Brien, P. C., M. A. Shampo, J. S. Robertson: Statistics for nuclear medicine; Part 6: Normal values, Evaluating a new procedure. J. Nucl. Med. **24** (1983) 535–541.

[5] Böttger, I., H. W. Schneck: Free thyroid hormones in patients with severe non-thyroidal illness. Nuc. Compact **6** (1985) 348–352.

Comparative evaluation of high sensitivity TSH kits*

A. D. Swift, S. E. Bruce, J. G. Ratcliffe

Introduction

From 1983 a new generation of commercial TSH assays started to become available in the United Kingdom. These assays uniformly used the two site immunometric principle with either isotopic (immunoradiometric) or non-isotopic labels (immunofluorometric, immunoenzymometric, immunochemiluminometric). Although immunoradiometric assays had been available earlier using specific antibodies purified from polyclonal antisera (notably the Corning Immophase TSH kit) the practicality of this approach was transformed by the development and application of monoclonal antibodies. Thus by 1985, at least 10 immunometric kit methods were in use in the United Kingdom. Several of the new generation of immunometric assays claimed significantly improved sensitivity over conventional radioimmunoassays thus offering the potential to discriminate subnormal from normal TSH levels. In addition the assays were rapid (completion within one working day) and had a wide working range (10 to 100 fold wider than radioimmunoassay).

Due to the potential significance of this development for clinical laboratories, it was considered important to evaluate independently those commercial kits which claimed high sensitivity. To this end, in 1984, the DHSS contacted all manufacturers who marketed, or were about to market, kits in the U. K. for the measurement of serum TSH. The kit manufacturers were asked a) if they produced a high sensitivity kit (for this purpose a detection limit of less than 0.5 mU/L was defined as high sensitivty) and b) whether they wished it to be included in a comparative evaluation of such kits supported by the DHSS. In all, 12 manufacturers expressed interest in such an evaluation.

It was decided that the study should proceed in two stages because of the large number of kits for evaluation (13 in all):

a) A preliminary trial to assess the sensitivity potential of the kits was started in September 1984. Particular attention was directed at their performance with

* This paper is abstracted from the final report on the Comparative evaluation of High Sensitivity TSH kits prepared by the authors on behalf of the DHSS.

sera containing low TSH concentrations including the recovery of low concentrations of TSH. The results of this preliminary trial were made available to NHS laboratories in February 1985.

b) A detailed assessment of the kits selected on the basis of results in the preliminary trial. These kits were: Boots Celltech Sucrosep, Serono MAIAclone, IQ BIO (Ltd), LKB Wallac Delfia, Amersham Amerlex-M, Hybritech Tandem and Hoechst RIAgnost. The results of the detailed evaluation on these seven kits is presented here. It should be noted that neither part of the trial was designed to assess performance at elevated TSH levels so that no conclusions should be drawn in either part of the trial as to the performance of the kits in the diagnosis of primary hypothyroidism.

Aims of the study

The evaluation protocol was designed to assess the following aspects of performance:

a) General features

The general features of each kit were compared with respect to overall duration of assay including "hands-on" time, technical ease of use, special equipment requirements and costs (if available).

b) Analytical

- Reproducibility (within and between assay, between reagent lots)
- Sensitivity (ie detection limit) and working range
- Bias (recovery of added TSH and performance on External Quality Assessment specimens)
- Parallelism of endogenous TSH with standard TSH
- Cross-reaction with structurally related glycoprotein hormones
- Effect of sample quality

c) Clinical

A limited assessment of clinical performance using specimens from defined and selected groups of subjects and patients was made. Particular emphasis was given to specimens containing low concentrations of TSH to assess base-line security, and discrimination of subnormal from normal values.

Design of the study

All the experimental work was conducted by the same technologist who at the outset of the study was inexperienced in immunoassay techniques. All the manufacturers were offered time to train the technician either within their own laboratories or within the University Department of Chemical Pathology at Hope Hospital. All of the manufacturers accepted this invitation. No time limit was placed upon the training period. Only when each manufacturer was satisfied with the competence of the technician with their method did the trial proceed.

Format of assays

All assays had the same general format:

Standards	(in duplicate)
3 QC samples	(in duplicate)
36 experimental samples	(in duplicate)
3 QC samples	(in duplicate)

Some of the internal QC samples were replaced by samples from the U.K. External Quality Assessment Scheme for Thyroid-related hormones when necessary.

Each kit was used in strict rotation whenever possible. A note was made of the lot number of the kit and the individual batch numbers of the component reagents.

Isotopic methods were counted on an LKB Wallac multigamma checking each well for contamination before and after each assay. Non-isotopic end-points were measured on equipment supplied by relevant the manufacturer.

Data from the isotopic methods were analysed by the computerised program of Raab and McKenzie using the 'raw' counts obtained from the LKB Wallac multigamma. Data from the non-isotopic methods were analysed by the software provided by the manufacturers themselves.

General kit review

General features of each of the kits which proceded onto the main study were reviewed. The contents and package inserts were compared with recommendations of the IFCC and tabulated. A review of the principles of each methodology can be obtained from the respective manufacturers and will not be included here.

Reproducibility

Reproducibility was assessed by repeating the same assay on at least 12 occasions for each kit. Every week for 12 consecutive weeks, seven assay runs were performed (i. e. one assay run for each kit in strict sequence whenever possible). Additional assays with identical format were subsequently run using reagents with different lot numbers.

Six test pools were used to assess reproducibility which were assayed six times in duplicate in each assay. The test pools were human serum containing endogenous concentrations of TSH covering the range 0.5 – 50 mU/L.

Results of the internal quality control pools were used to determine whether an assay should be rejected according to the following criteria: a) If values on more than two different pools were outside their 95% confidence limits or b) If values on the same pool were outside their 95% confidence limits twice in the same assay c) If there was significant drift on all pools between the beginning and end of the assay.

Within-assay imprecision was assessed from the quadratic mean of the within-assay coefficients of variation of each of the six pools. Between-assay imprecision was assessed from the between-assay coefficients of variation of the internal quality control samples and the first duplicate of each of the test pools in each assay. Between-lot imprecision was assessed from the first duplicate of each of the test pools in assays using different lots of reagents.

Sensitivity and working range

For comparative purposes sensitivity was defined as the TSH concentration at $\pm$ 2.5 S. D. of the zero dose as appropriate for the assay type (RIA or immunometric). The mean sensitivity and its 95% confidence limits were calculated for each kit.

The mean 'working range' of each kit (defined as that concentration range over which the coefficient of variation is less than 10% on individual within-assay imprecision profiles) was calculated.

Bias

Bias was assessed in two ways:

a) Recovery of added TSH.

Six individual donations of T_3-suppressed sera were divided into aliquots and spiked with known amounts of TSH (2nd IRP 80/558) to give final concentrations of 0.25, 0.50, 0.75, 1.0 and 2.0 mU/L. A further three individual donations of T_3-suppressed sera were divided into aliquots and spiked with known amounts of TSH (2nd IRP 80/558) to give final concentrations of 5.0, 10.0 and 20.0 mU/L. This study was aimed at identifying consistent under- or over-recovery or dose-dependent variation in recovery which might produce bias in patient results.

b) External quality assessment specimens.

From January 1985 samples were obtained from the U.K. EQAS for Thyroid related hormones on a monthly basis and these were assayed 'blind' and the results returned in the normal manner. EQAS was then able to calculate the cumulative running bias and variability of the bias of each method on a monthly basis. Only samples with greater than 5 mU/L were used in these calculations. The cumulative running bias and variability of the bias has been tabulated for comparative purposes.

Parallelism

Parallelism of test samples with standard TSH is a necessary though not sufficient test of identity of measured analyte with standard TSH and hence assay validity. Six euthyroid and two hypothyroid sera were diluted by factors of 2,4 and 8 in the diluent recommended by the manufacturer. If no diluent was recommended (LKB Wallac Delfia and I. Q. (BIO) Ltd) the dilutions were made in T_3-suppressed serum (previously shown to give an an undetectable value when assayed by that kit).

Cross reactivity

Cross-reactivity was assessed by preparation of calibration curves of TSH (2nd IRP 80/558) and structurally related glycoproteins in T_3-suppressed serum. The prepared TSH standard curve and the cross-reactant were assayed together. Highly purified preparations of the glycoproteins were used but it is not known whether all the preparation were devoid of immunoreactive TSH. The percentage cross-reaction was calculated from the ratio of mass of TSH and the mass of cross-reactant which gave the same percentage binding in the assay.

Patient samples

Sera were obtained from the following defined groups:

a) Euthyroid donors. Ninety nine sera were obtained from either laboratory personnel (32 donations) or from volunteers (of unknown age or sex) attending the Blood Transfusion Service to donate blood (67 donations). All laboratory personnel were clinically euthyroid and all donations from the Blood Transfusion Service were from healthy individuals who were eligible to donate blood. All sera had levels of total and free thyroxine, and triiodothyronine within the appropriate reference ranges for this laboratory.

b) Euthyroid pregnant volunteers. Sera were collected from women attending routine antenatal clinic during the first and second trimesters of their pregnancy (8 and 18 volunteers respectively). Sera from 18 women in the third trimester of their pregnancy were obtained from specimens taken for the measurement of serum oestriol for obstetrical reasons.

c) Euthyroid post menopausal samples. Sera were collected from seven women who were clinically post menopausal. All the routine thyroid function tests were found to be within the euthyroid reference ranges and their serum FSH concentrations were greater than 40 U/L.

d) T_3-suppressed serum. Sera were collected from 63 healthy euthyroid volunteers (who had been medically examined and had given informed consent) who had taken 80 µg T_3 daily in divided doses (20 µg q. i. d.) for five days prior to donation. Six of these volunteers also donated blood daily during T_3 administration in order to monitor serial changes in TSH. All volunteers had thyroid function tests within the euthyroid reference ranges prior to treatment.

e) Clinically and biochemically thyrotoxic. Specimens were obtained from patients attending a thyroid assessment clinic who were judged by at least two physicians to be clinically hyperthyroid. These specimens were assayed for total thyroxine, total triiodothyronine, free-thyroxine and free-triiodothyronine. All thyroid hormones were grossly elevated in 47 specimens and were included in this group.

f) Non-thyroidal illness. Six samples were obtained from hospital inpatients without any overt signs or symptoms of thyroidal disease but with subnormal total thyroxine and/or total triiodothyronine concentrations.

For comparative purposes the absolute euthyroid range and the 95th centile range were calculated for each kit. Samples which gave 'unexpected' TSH concentrations by more than two methods were assayed for TBG abnormalities or the presence of thyroidal antibodies (thyroglobulin and microsomal). Three samples from euthyroid subjects had thyroid antibodies and these have been excluded from the calculated euthyroid ranges but are identified on the respective figures.

Results

Results presented within this section will generally be shown in a comparative manner. In each section below there follows a brief description of the aspect studied, the relevant tables or figures and a brief comment on the results highlighting any general or important points.

Reproducibility

During the trial no assay was rejected because of either drift or more than two quality control samples falling outside the 95% confidence limits. The quadratic mean of the within-assay coefficient of variation and the between-assay coefficient of variation at each of the six doses studied are shown in table 1.

Table 1

		Nominal concentration of TSH (mU/l)					
	n	0.5	1.0	1.5	5.0	15.0	50.0
Boots Celltech	13	4.2 (7.8)	3.6 (5.1)	3.1 (3.3)	1.5 (2.8)	1.2 (2.8)	1.9 (3.4)
Serono	12	4.3 (5.7)	4.2 (3.9)	2.9 (2.5)	2.6 (2.4)	2.9 (2.1)	3.5 (5.8)
I.Q. (Bio)	13	3.6 (7.5)	4.8 (7.5)	3.9 (7.9)	4.2 (8.4)	4.6 (12.5)	* *
LKB Wallac	13	5.0 (14.4)	4.9 (4.3)	5.4 (6.1)	5.9 (13.1)	3.7 (12.0)	4.9 (10.1)
Amersham	12	4.9 (8.0)	5.2 (6.0)	3.1 (5.0)	2.2 (2.8)	5.2 (7.4)	7.2 (15.7)
Hybritech	11	9.7 (11.4)	7.5 (8.2)	4.9 (7.9)	2.9 (4.2)	2.9 (5.8)	2.6 (5.5)
Hoechst	14	3.3 (8.3)	6.3 (8.7)	2.1 (5.7)	2.5 (5.6)	2.3 (4.6)	2.4 (4.9)

n = number of assays used in calculation; * = outside working range; values mentioned without brackets = within assay coefficient of variation; values mentioned in brackets = between assay coefficient of variation.

Comment

All the kits yielded good within-batch precision with the Hybritech Tandem method showing some worsening at the lower values. Most showed some worsening of precision between-batch (eg I. Q. BIO (Ltd) and LKB Wallac Delfia) though the Serono MAIAclone and Boots Celltech Sucrosep retained excellent precision between-batch.

Sensitivity and imprecision

The mean sensitivities of the methods for the total number of assays performed and the mean 'working ranges' of the methods (defined as the mean concentration range over which the coefficient of variation is less than 10% on the within assay imprecision profile) are shown in table 2.

Table 2 Mean sensitivities and working range (mU/L)

Kit	Mean sensitivity	Range below 10% CV
Boots Celltech	0.07	0.4 – >HS (250.0)
Serono	0.19	0.6 – >HS (50.0)
I.Q. (Bio)	0.01	0.1 – >HS (25.0)
LKB Wallac	0.01	<0.1 – >HS (324.0)
Amersham	0.84	1.2 – >HS (25.0)
Hybritech	0.31	1.3 – >HS (100.0)
Hoechst	0.04	0.3 – >HS (50.0)

HS = Highest standard.

Comment

There are clear differences in the sensitivities achieved by the kits. The most sensitive systems appear to be the non-isotopic methods though the figures should be interpreted with caution in view of the possible differences in the methods of calculation. The most sensitive immunoradiometric methods are the Hoechst RIAgnost and Boots Celltech Sucrosep kits with both showing relatively tight error envelopes between-assay. Considerably less sensitive are the Amersham Amerlex-M and the Hybritech Tandem methods. All the immunoradiometric assays have wide working ranges extending in most cases to above their highest standard (> 50 mU/L). The Amersham Amerlex-M method showed a typical 'U' shaped imprecision profile with a much narrower working range, though the error envelope over this range is impressively tight.

Bias

The mean percentage recovery of each pool for each kit is shown in table 3. Cumulative statistics calculated and published by the U. K. EQAS are presented for each kit in table 4.

Table 3 BIAS – % recovery of exogenous TSH

	Theoretical TSH concentration (mU/l)							
Kit	0.25	0.5	0.75	1.0	2.0	5.0	10.0	20.0
Boots	72.0	87.0	89.4	94.6	98.6	94.4	91.0	89.8
Serono	118.8	112.2	114.0	114.8	110.2	97.5	95.9	93.6
I.Q.	87.9	89.4	88.7	90.7	95.6	76.0	76.0	75.8
LKB	88.3	81.2	94.9	90.5	88.1	78.1	76.5	77.5
Amer	37.3*	38.1*	47.2*	62.1	60.6	77.2	81.6	100.8
Hybr	45.8*	37.7	52.2	61.2	72.6	68.5	65.2	64.8
Hoe	74.0	75.6	70.7	73.0	71.0	76.9	77.1	76.2

* = below the kits lowest standard.

Table 4 Cumulative statistics from EQAS pools distributed from Jan. 1985

Month		Boots	Serono	I.Q. Bio	LKB	Amer	Hybrit	Hoechst
Feb	BIAS	N/A	−1.6	−11.0	−15.9	−2.9	−29.4	N/A
	VAR	N/A	7.0	6.8	9.8	18.9	9.6	N/A
Mar	BIAS	−13.4	−0.3	−12.6	−14.6	−3.8	−30.0	−15.2
	VAR	6.5	6.1	7.9	9.6	15.7	9.3	7.2
Apr	BIAS	−14.8	−1.0	−13.9	−14.9	−1.3	−31.7	−15.8
	VAR	8.1	6.0	9.0	9.2	17.2	12.2	7.8
May	BIAS	−18.7	−5.4	−15.0	−19.5	−4.8	−32.8	−16.3
	VAR	13.4	9.4	7.8	13.0	15.5	16.7	8.1
Jun	BIAS	−19.0	−5.4	−16.2	−18.3	−5.7	−35.2	−19.8
	VAR	11.1	8.5	11.1	10.4	15.5	15.5	14.0
Jul	BIAS	−17.2	−0.9	−12.8	−18.5	−0.2	−29.8	−10.5
	VAR	4.3	5.1	11.3	9.4	15.1	14.8	6.9

Comment

Table 3 shows that most of the methods tend to under-recover exogenous TSH added to T_3-suppressed sera. The Hybritech Tandem and Hoechst RIAgnost methods showed marked and consistent under-recovery whereas the Amersham Amerlex-M method showed dose related changes in recovery. Serono MAIAclone was exceptional in over-recovering at low TSH concentrations.

These trends arc also seen in the cumulative statistics (tab. 4) which relate only to specimens with an ALTM > 5mU/L. The relatively high variability of the bias for some methods may be in part related to the dose-related effect identified in the recovery experiments.

Parallelism

The mean recovery expressed as a percentage of the undiluted sample from 6 euthyroid sera and 2 hypothyroid sera when diluted with the diluent recommended by the manufacturer are shown in table 5. If no diluent was recommended by the manufacturer T_3-suppressed serum was used.

Comment

Within the limitations of this experiment all kits performed well on this test with no grossly unexpected results. Only a 2 fold dilution with the Amerlex-M kit was possible as the results obtained on further dilution were below the reliable detection limit of the method.

Table 5 Parallelism

	Dilution factor		
	2	4	8
Boots Celltech	95.8	95.3	75.5
Serono	101.7	86.5	102.0
I.Q. (Bio)	98.1	96.6	94.1
LKB Wallac	114.7	106.8	104.4
Amersham	95.7	*	*
Hybritech	102.6	102.8	90.9
Hoechst	109.3	108.6	112.4

Mean recovery (%) of TSH from 6 euthyroid and 2 hypothyroid sera. The value obtained in the undiluted sera is taken as 100%.

Cross-reactivity

The percent cross-reactivity of the peptides studied calculated from ratio of the mass of TSH and the mass of the cross-reactant which gave the same percentage binding in the assay is shown in table 6.

Table 6

Kit	LH	TSH	LH	FSH	TSH	FSH	HCG
Boots Celltech	none	0.40	0.42	4.35	0.02	0.22	none
Serono	none	0.23	0.12	2.95	0.06	0.18	none
I.Q. (Bio)	none	0.23	0.09	2.67	0.02	0.12	none
LKB Wallac	0.01	0.79	0.18	2.63	0.15	0.23	none
Amersham	0.01	0.50	0.14	4.27	0.03	0.23	0.03
Hybritech	1.73	>100	0.12	3.08	0.40	4.14	none
Hoechst	none	0.25	0.09	2.06	0.03	0.11	none

Comment

Although highly purified forms of the subunits and glycoprotein hormones were used we cannot be certain that all the preparations were devoid of immunoreactive TSH. The high cross-reaction of the kits with the FSH preparation may be attributed to a known contamination of this preparation of approximately 5–10% with TSH.

Patient samples

The clinical assessment of the kits was restricted to examining their behaviour with sera from a limited range of patient groups. Most attention was devoted to results from euthyroid subjects and patients with unequivocal thyrotoxicosis.

Samples from euthyroid donors (either blood donors or laboratory personnel) who were also biochemically euthyroid, with respect to total thyroxine and triiodothyronine, free thyroxine and triiodothyronine, were included in this group. Samples which gave apparently anomalous TSH results by two of the methods were further investigated biochemically with respect to thyroid hormone binding globulin levels and thyroid autoantibodies (microsomal and thyroglobulin). Three samples from the euthyroid group were positive for thyroid autoantibodies and these have been excluded from the quoted absolute euthyroid ranges and the mid 95th centile range (2.5 centile to 97.5 centile) (tab. 7).

Table 7 Euthyroid ranges (mU/l)

Kit	n	Absolute range	mid 95% centile	Median
Boots Celltech	97	0.2 – 5.53	0.45 – 5.25	2.0
Serono	99	0.5 – 5.64	0.54 – 4.58	1.9
I.Q. (Bio)	99	0.3 – 3.8	0.32 – 3.33	1.9
LKB Wallac	99	0.3 – 3.6	0.37 – 3.12	1.7
Amersham	99	0.6 – 3.9	1.0 – 3.15	1.3
Hybritech	98	U.D. – 3.0	0.25 – 2.85	1.2
Hoechst	97	0.3 – 3.8	0.30 – 3.70	1.3

U.D. = Undetectable.

Comment

There were some differences in the euthyroid ranges found with the kits. The ranges of the Boots Celltech Sucrosep and Serono MAIAclone methods were similar, and rather higher, than those found with I. Q. BIO, LKB Wallac Delfia and Hoechst RIAgnost. Hybritech Tandem had the lowest reference range with one value being below the limit of detection. The distribution of values with Amersham Amerlex-M was clearly different at the lower range due to the relative insensitivity of the method.

In sera from pregnant subjects the majority of values were within the respective euthyroid ranges for all methods. The third trimester values tended to be low normal with the Boots Celltech Sucrosep and Hoechst RIAgnost methods and values below the 2.5 centile were obtained on three and two samples respectively. None of the kits appeared to be grossly affected by haemolysis or lipaemia. The small number of sera from patients with non-thyroidal illness tended to give high normal results. Post menopausal values were within the euthyroid ranges.

With the exception of the Amerlex-M kit, the kits readily distinguished thyrotoxic and T_3-suppressed from euthyroid sera (tab. 8). Occasional detectable results were found with I. Q. BIO, LKB Wallac Delfia and Hoechst RIAgnost kits though

Table 8 Misclassification of toxic and T3-suppressed results into euthyroid ranges

	Manufacturers Suggested Range		Observed Range		Mid 95% centile range	
	TOXIC	T3-S	TOXIC	T3-SUP	TOXIC	T3-S*
Boots Celltech	1/43	1/63	0/43	0/63	0/43	0/63
Serono	0/46	0/63	0/46	0/63	0/46	0/63
I.Q. (Bio)	–	–	1/46	1/63	1/46	1/63
LKB	1/47	2/63	1/47	2/63	1/47	2/63
Amersham	5/45	11/63	19/45	11/63	5/45	11/63
Hybritech	0/46	0/63	0/46	0/63	0/46	0/63
Hoechst	1/47	2/63	0/47	1/63	0/47	1/63

* = T_3-suppressed sera.

rarely above 0.1 mU/L. The relative insensitivity of the Amersham Amerlex-M method was well demonstrated by the lack of suppression of TSH levels during T_3 administration. All the other kits showed convincing serial suppression of TSH levels. A point of potential concern for base-line security was the demonstration that many kits gave values below the 99% confidence limit of the zero calibrator (i. e. apparently "negative" results). This was especially pronounced with thyrotoxic sera. This highlights the difficulty of obtaining suitable matrices for the zero calibrant.

Conclusions

Five of the seven kits can be classified as high sensitivity according to the original study criteria (detection limit < 0.5 mU/L). They are Boots Celltech Sucrosep, Serono MAIAclone, I. Q. BIO (Ltd), LKB Wallac Delfia and Hoechst RIAgnost. All these methods use the two site immunometric principle and the kits with the highest sensitivities employed non-isotopic labels (I. Q. BIO, LKB Wallac Delfia). The most sensitive assays using radiolabels were Hoechst RIAgnost and the Boots Celltech Sucrosep both providing sensitivities an order of magnitude greater than achieved with current radioimmunoassays. The Serono MAIAclone assay was less sensitive than the above mentioned IRMAs. We consider these five kits have the potential to meet the sensitivity requirements for clinical diagnostic application.

The other two methods (Hybritech Tandem, Amersham Amerlex-M) were much less sensitive and do not meet the analytical requirements for high sensitivity assays. The Amersham Amerlex-M kit revealed the limitations of current RIA methods in having a narrow working range, long incubation time and inability to discriminate subnormal from normal TSH concentrations reliably. Nevertheless, it was rugged within its working range and had excellent reproducibility at the upper end of the euthyroid range. It showed pronounced dose-related under-recovery though was unbiased on EQAS specimens containing > 5 mU/L. The Hybritech Tandem method also gave good reproducibility at the the upper end of the euthyroid range and at higher levels than the Amersham Amerlex-M method. However it was severely negatively biased on EQAS specimens and under-recovered consistently throughout the dose range. The reference euthyroid range with the Hybritech Tandem kit was lower than those observed with other kits and there were occasional undetectable values. Despite these analytical limitations, the kit performed well in distinguishing sera from thyrotoxic and T_3-suppressed subjects from normal.

Trends in performance of clinical TSH assays as assessed by the United Kingdom EQAS for thyroid related hormones

A. D. Swift, J. G. Ratcliffe

The United Kingdom external quality assessment scheme (EQAS) for thyroid stimulating hormone (TSH) has been administered in its present form from Hope Hospital, University of Manchester, since 1982. The number of laboratories performing the TSH assay has increased over the years and is now the most widely performed endocrine measurement in the U.K. (tab. 1).

Liquid serum samples, generally five are distributed at four weekly intervals. The same samples are analysed for thyroxine, free-thyroxine, triiodothyronine and free triiodothyronine as well as TSH. The operating principles of the scheme dictate that results are returned to the EQAS office within 21 days of despatch. Results are analysed after logartihmic transformation and trimming and returned to the participants with the next sample distribution. Six monthly cumulative bias and variability of the bias tables are calculated and distributed.

Mainly euthyroid donor pools spiked with TSH (2nd IRP 80/558) are distributed. Some agarose-charcoaled material has also been prepared and circulated to check base-line security as has T_3-suppressed serum. Pathological material (hyper- and hypo-thyroid, TBG abnormalities, familial dysalbuminaemia, pregnancy, postmenopausal and thyroid antibodies) are used when sufficient is available. Each pool is distributed a minimum of two times.

As far as we are aware virtually all the laboratories with the U.K. that are performing TSH assays for patient care are returning results to EQAS. The increasing number of laboratories returning results EQAS represents a real increase in the number of laboratories performing thyroid function testing.

There has been quite a dramatic alteration in the methodologies used with the introduction of monoclonal antibody based immunometric kits onto the market. Upto mid 1985 the percentage of laboratories using in-house methodologies was constant at approximately 25%, however since then the percentage has decreased by half. Simultaneously the percentage of laboratories using kit radioimmunoassay methods has fallen but the number of laboratories using kit immunometric assays has increased (tab. 2).

Thyrotropin

Table 1 Participants

	1986*	1985	1984	1983	1982	1981
Total number of labs on file		288	269	249	232	216
a) UK Biochemistry labs		220	210	204	193	180
b) Endocrine laboratories		22	20	17	18	10
c) Uk Nuclear Medicine		12	12	12	13	16
d) Military Hospitals		7	6	2	2	2
e) Commercial firms		14	11	11	4	7
f) Non NHS Laboratories		13	10	3	2	1
Methods used						
RIA Kit Methods						
Amersham Amerlex	56	72	81	76	53	17
Becton Dickinson	3	3	3	5	5	3
NETRIA Reagents	1	5	7	13	–	–
Diagnostic Prods	2	4	5	3	–	–
Wellcome Daccel	3	8	11	15	13	10
IMA Kit Methods						
NETRIA Reagents	14	8	5	–	–	–
Corning Immophase	26	46	59	66	51	36
Corning MAGIC	3	3	3	–	–	–
Tandem Hybritech	12	12	6	3	–	–
Boots Celltech	32	19	9	1	–	–
Serono MAIAclone	61	37	21	–	–	–
Hoechst RIAgnost	5	2	–	–	–	–
I.Q. Bio LTD	1	1	–	–	–	–
LKB Delfia	8	2	–	–	–	–
In House Methods						
Double antibody	13	16	19	22	25	21
Peg assisted D/A	16	17	20	24	30	30
Solid phase D/A	7	8	7	2	3	–
IRMA	8	4	3	2	–	–

*April 1986.

Table 2

	Year				
	1986	1985	1984	1983	1982
% In-house RIA methods	11	15	18	19	25
% In-house IRMA	6	2	1	1	0
% Kit RIA methods	25	32	42	51	53
% Kit IRMA methods	58	51	39	29	22

Surveys of EQAS participants over the previous years have indicated both an increase in the total number of laboratories performing TSH analyses and an increase in the number of patient samples analysed (0.73 million in 1982 to 1.5 million in 1985).

The initial strategy of the U. K. EQAS for TSH was to substantiate and validate a target value against which individual performance of laboratories (and methods), in terms of bias and variability of the bias, could be assessed. It was hoped to validate a target value by spiking normal euthyroid serum and serum from volunteers who had taken T_3 for five days prior to serum donation with known amounts of TSH. Quantitative mean recovery of the exogenous TSH would at least suggest that the All Laboratory Trimmed Mean (ALTM) was a reliable target value. Initially between-laboratory coefficients of variation were generally greater than 30% and sometimes greater than 60% and although most assays were poor in terms of base-line security, recovery and precision within the euthyroid range, the mean recovery was quantitative in samples which contained more than 5 mU/L TSH. In addition we were able to demonstrate that this ALTM was stable for upto 9 months when pools were recirculated. It was therefore indicated that the ALTM was a satisfactory target value (for samples containing more than 5 mU/L) and six monthly cumulative statistics tables were produced.

The first annual report of the U. K. EQAS (in 1982) showed that there were severe method-related problems with both bias and variability of the bias. For the first time, in the U. K., laboratories were able to assess objectively whether the method that they used gave satisfactory results, judged against target values that were at least validated with respect to recovery of exogenous TSH. After

Table 3 Six-monthly cumulative performance (figures indicate % labs in each category)

	Year					
	1982	1983	1984	1985	1985*	1986*
BIAS						
< ± 10%	58.1	78.4	69.5	75.4	49.0	43.1
> ± 10.1 – 25%	37.3	18.1	26.4	21.1	37.2	49.0
> ± 25.1%	4.6	3.5	3.5	4.1	13.8	7.8
Variability of the BIAS						
< 10%	18.9	38.5	26.7	40.2	5.1	31.2
> 10.1 – < 25%	59.0	52.9	63.9	53.6	58.9	60.9
> 25.1%	22.1	8.6	9.4	6.2	36.0	7.8

* Using all samples with an ALTM above 1 mU/L.

the first report many laboratories changed their method to a more reliable one (tab. 1). By the time of the second annual report (in 1983) there had been a significant improvement in performance with respect to bias and variability of the bias (tab. 3).

The recent introduction of high sensitivity methods for TSH provides the opportunity to improve the most recalcitrant problems of bias at low levels (< 5 mU/L). Many of the new methods claim sensitivities of 0.1 mU/l and extend the working range upto 100 mU/L and more. These advances in technology prompted EQAS to examine recoveries of low TSH levels (0.5 – 5.0 mU/L) from T_3-suppressed sera. Such experiments have shown that the new generation of immunometric assays are less prone to base-line insecurity and that commonly used monoclonal IRMAs give approximately quantitative mean recovery of low levels of TSH. This was an important development and our Steering Committee advised that target values can be extended downwards to include samples with an ALTM between 1 mU/l and 5 mU/L for calculation of the cumulative statistics. The appropriate target value in this range is the subset of laboratories which use the high sensitivity immunometric assays shown to give quantitative recovery rather than the ALTM (tab. 4).

Table 4 Recovery of exogenous TSH from agarose-charcoaled serum, T_3-suppressed sera or euthyroid sera by selected high sensitivity TSH IRMAs

	pool	TSH concentration	% recovery of group (IRMA)	No of labs
Agarose charcoaled serum	basal	0.45	–	
	+ 0.5 mU/l	0.94	98.0%	54
	+ 1.0 mU/l	1.48	103.0%	62
T_3-suppressed serum	basal	0.0	–	
	+ 0.5 mU/l	0.5	100.0	61
	+ 1.0 mU/l	1.0	100.0	62
	+ 1.5 mU/l	1.5	100.0	65
Euthyroid serum	basal	1.5	–	
	+ 1.0 mU/l	2.5	100.0	64
	+ 2.0 mU/l	3.5	100.0	62
	+ 5.0 mU/l	6.4	98.0	65
	+ 10.0 mU/l	11.4	99.0	65

At levels above 5 mU/L the ALTM will be continue to be used. This change meant that laboratories with an unrealistic detection limit moved rapidly into the unacceptable performance category (bias > ± 25% or var. bias > 25%) (tab. 3) and the apparent worsening of performance in the second half of 1985 was due to the inclusion of results from pools with TSH values > 1 mU/L rather than > 5 mU/L. It was hoped that this would improve as laboratories changed to high sensitivity TSH methods or revised their reliable limit of detection upwards. This has been borne out by the number of laboratories changing to the newer methods recently (tab. 1, 2) and by fewer laboratories now falling into the unacceptable performance category (tab. 3).

The second major problem highlighted repeatedly by EQAS in the past has been poor base-line security. Between 28% and 40% of laboratories have positive bias clearly demonstrated on T_3-suppressed sera or agarose-charcoaled sera and a few have gross positive bias reporting values higher than 3 mU/L on such sera (tab. 5). The use of the new IRMA assays has virtually removed the base-line insecurity within these methods.

Table 5 Method-related base-Line security

Range of results reported from a T_3-suppressed sample	Methods 1	2	3	4	5	6	7	8
'0' or undetectable	17	18	0	6	13	17	7	11
0 – 0.5 mU/l	3	5	0	0	1	7	0	0
0.51 – 1.0 mU/l	24	6	0	0	0	0	0	0
1.0 – 2.0 mU/l	12	10	3	0	0	0	3	2
2.1 – 3.0 mU/l	2	2	0	0	0	0	1	1
> 3.0 mU/l	0	0	1	0	0	0	1	0

Methods 1 – 3 are commercial RIA kits; 4 – 6 are commercial IRMA kits; 7 and 8 are in-house RIA methods.

The introduction of these new immunometric assays has halved the between assay between laboratory coefficients of variation on samples containing below 5 mU/L. Between laboratory within method (i. e. all laboratories using the same method) coefficients of variation have been greatly improved by the IRMA methods with CV's in the order of 5 – 10% compared with 20 – 30% for RIA. These data suggest that these assays are a good deal more rugged than the previously available RIA methods. However the between method agreement has not been significantly improved by the new assays. This is highlighted by the two most commonly selected commercial IRMA kits which differ by over 20% in the results that they obtain on the same samples. This highlights the difficulty in standardisation and/or obtaining the correct composition of the matrix in which the standards are prepared to reflect the correct concentrations in patient samples.

In conclusion the U. K. EQAS for TSH, by establishing valid target values, has been able to demonstrate to participants that some methods give better performance with respect to bias, variability of the bias and base-line security. It is encouraging that overall analytical performance has improved significantly in recent years. By illustrating the strengths and limitations of certain methods it is hoped that the U.K. EQAS for TSH will continue to contribute to improved analytical performance and, hence, patient care.

III TSH in non-thyroidal illness

Thyroidal and extrathyroidal influences on TSH before and after TRH stimulation

C. R. Pickardt, C. Bernutz, K. Horn

Introduction

TSH determination by conventional radioimmunoassays before and after TRH stimulation is a highly sensitive tool to gain an overall information on thyroid function. Due to the negative feedback regulation, variations of the concentrations of free thyroid hormones result in a modulation of the TSH levels. Since the TSH determination is widely used for primary diagnostics in thyroid diseases, extrathyroidal influences on TSH response to TRH have been intensively investigated during the early seventeens.

The diurnal variations of TSH had been described, using conventional double antibody TSH radioimmunoassay [38, 43]. The use of highly sensitive immunoassays led to the detection of a pulsatility of the TSH secretion in normal human beeings also [4]. The thyrotropic activity of the pituitary is under an inhibitory control of somatostatine [44] and dopamine [6, 8, 10, 14, 15, 23, 26, 34, 37, 46, 48]. Dopamine modulates the diurnal variation of TSH secretion [38, 43]. In states with increased hypothalamic dopamine turnover the tonic inhibition of TSH is thought to be enhanced [39]. It is well known that the TSH response to TRH is modulated by estrogens in females and in males [11]. This modulation is due to increasing binding sites of pituitary cells for TRH under estrogen influence, which can be partly antagonized by thyroid hormones [25]. In Cushings syndrome is respective the pathogenesis and during glucocorticosteroid pharmacotherapy basal TSH and TSH response to TRH may be blunted or suppressed [10, 24 – 26, 27, 42, 46, 47, 48], normalizing after successful treatment of hypercortisolism. In contrast, in Addisons disease moderately elevated basal TSH levels have been observed. In patients with hypersecretion of growth hormone TSH response to TRH may be blunted [7], whereas a hyperresponsiveness of TSH has been observed in GH deficiency. Moreover hypercalcemia may induce a diminished TSH response [19].

From these facts it can easily be understood, that TSH may be blunted in patients with extrathyroidal endocrine diseases and those under dopamine or glucocorticosteroid therapy, whereas it may be exaggerated during metoclopramide treatment. Other influences, such as advanced age, total fasting and

Thyrotropin

realimentation [2, 41] and severe acute or chronic non thyroidal illness [45], which can induce a blunted TSH response to TRH are less well understood.

TRH test in diagnosis of hypothalamo-pituitary diseases

Patients with hypothyroidism of hypothalamic origin have a TSH response to TRH, which is often delayed or exaggerated [3, 9, 11 – 13, 17, 28, 29, 32, 40]. In patients with pituitary tumors, suprasellar extension and visual field impairment TSH response to TRH has been found to be normal or elevated despite low thyroxine levels unexspectedly. Impaired bioactivity of this TSH radioactivity has been discussed mainly by the group of Faglia [11, 12, 13, 28]. In none of our own patients with pituitary tumors the TSH response to TRH was completely absent before pituitary surgery and in only in some of them postoperatively [17, 29, 30, 31]. From these data, we suggested, that the increase of TSH levels after TRH indicates a suprasellar cause of secondary hypothyroidism, probably in partial portal vessel occlusion which prevents the endogenous TRH from reaching the remaining pituitary thyrotrophs. Thus, the failure of the TRH test to differentiate between hypothalamic and pituitary insufficiency has been documented.

TRH test in diagnosis of thyroid diseases

In euthyroid men basal TSH levels as measured by conventional radioimmunoassay are undetectable in about 30%. Thus by means of basal TSH we cannot distinguish between normal and suppressed TSH secretion. Therefore, TRH unresponsiveness of TSH offers more information on the thyroid function in cases of borderline hypothyroidism, in "euthyroid" Graves disease, in cases with autonomously functioning solitary or multiple nodules and in nodular goiters. For instance, using the TRH test for routine purposes in patients with goiter we observed in our hospital in 273 out of a total of 668 patients with TRH unresponsiveness of TSH with otherwise undetected preclinical hyperthyroidism [16, 33]. Out of these approximately 40% had elevated total iodine levels when compared to thyroxine iodine, indicating exogenous iodine contamination. Thus, patients at risk of hyperthyroidism were more easily detected by the TRH test in areas with nutritional iodine deficiency and endemic goiter with the characteristic increased prevalence of autonomously functioning thyroid tissue. By the combination of TRH stimulation test and scintiscans, thyroid autonomy can be classified more exactly [32, 35].

In primary thyroid failure, exaggerated TSH response may indicate thyroid insufficiency long before thyroid hormone levels are decreased and before clinical signs of thyroid hormone deficiency become obvious. This situation concerns nearly 20% of our patients with endemic goiter. For economical reasons, German thyroidologists recommend the use of TRH test because of its amplifying potency as the first step diagnostic tool.

The availability of methods to measure TSH with a sensitivity of 0.01 – 0.1 mU/l induced the reevalutation of the diagnostic use of TSH mainly under the question whether TRH-test can be omitted or not. An overview over the different test systems will be given by Doctor Wood [49]. From our experience [2, 3] we conclude that the test systems have to be handled with a high degree of accuracy, an internal quality control is necessary; the interpretation of the test results has to be made very careful and should be done by the doctor who knows the clinical situation of the patient under investigation. Inappropriate TSH secretion can be easier disclosed, since heterophilic antibodies crossreacting with rabbit serum are not interfering in these tests [1, 18].

Our present experience depends on different test systems [2, 3]. All systems used differentiate clearly the basal TSH levels of patients with overt or only shortly treated hyperthyroidism, who are unresponsive to TRH stimulation, from the basal TSH levels of clearly euthyroid patients with goiter and a normal TSH response to TRH. No overlap of basal values was found, when only these clearly defined patient groups were compared. This finding has been repeatedly published for different tests [5, 36] and led to the recommendation, to omitt the expensive TRH stimulation test. We agree to this recommendation only when the question is either to exclude hyperthyroidism or to confirm normal thyroid function. But as depicted in figure 1 there is a group of patients with basal levels in between those of normals and those of hyperthyroid patients. Most of them had thyroid autonomy.

Diagnostic reliability of basal TSH levels in thyroid autonomy

Earlier, we have observed that patients with functional autonomy of the thyroid may have a blunted, but measurable TSH increase after TRH stimulation [35]. In nearly all these cases, the basal TSH level was below the lower limit of detection. When the TSH response to TRH was suppressed by triiodothyronine, the residual paranodular 131 J uptake decreased, indicating normally suppressible parts of thyroid tissue. The degree of suppressibility was correlated to the initial TSH response to TRH [35].

Using the sensitive TSH method, we investigated 121 patients with scintigraphically proven uni- and multinodular thyroid autonomy. 41 patients had classical 20 had T3-hyperthyroidism whereas 63 patients had normal thyroid hormone levels and basal TSH levels below the normal range (fig. 1, 2). Only 9.8% of the

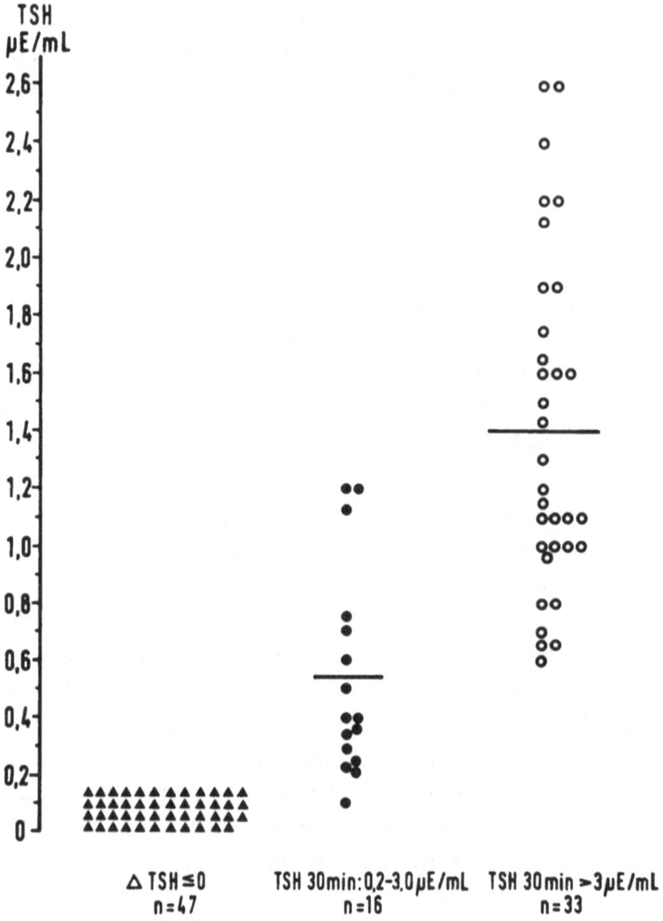

Fig. 1 Basal TSH levels, measured by a sensitive method in patients with hyperthyroidism (n = 47; ▲), diminished TSH response (n = 16; ●) and those with normal TSH response to TRH (n = 33; ○).

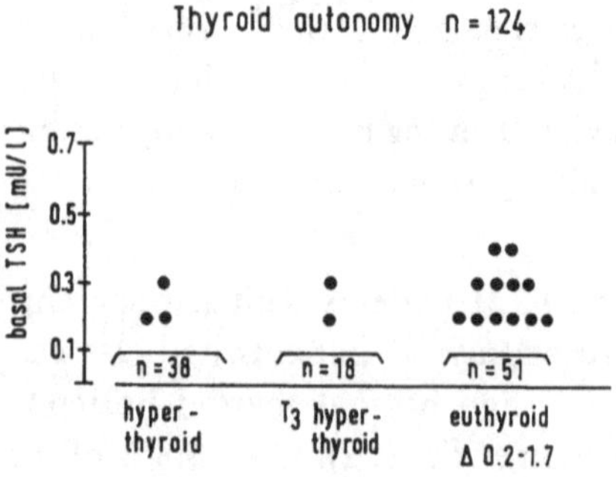

Fig. 2 Basal TSH levels in patients with thyroid autonomy: Hyperthyroidism with elevated T4/TBG ratio (n = 41); T3-hyperthyroidism (n = 20); normal peripheral thyroid hormone levels incompletely suppressed TSH response to TRH (n = 63).

hyperthyroid patients had measurable basal TSH levels in the range of 0.2 – 0.3 mU/l but none of them had a significant TSH increase after TRH stimulation. In contrast 19% of the 63 "euthyroid" patients had subnormal TSH levels in the range of 0.2 – 0.5 mU/l, all of them had a blunted TSH response to TRH in the range of 0.2 – 1.7 mU/l. Another 24 patients with proven euthyroid autonomy, selected by basal TSH levels of 0.2 – 0.7 mU/l were found to have a normal TSH increase in 46%, whereas 54% had a subnormal or absent TSH increase after TRH (fig. 3).

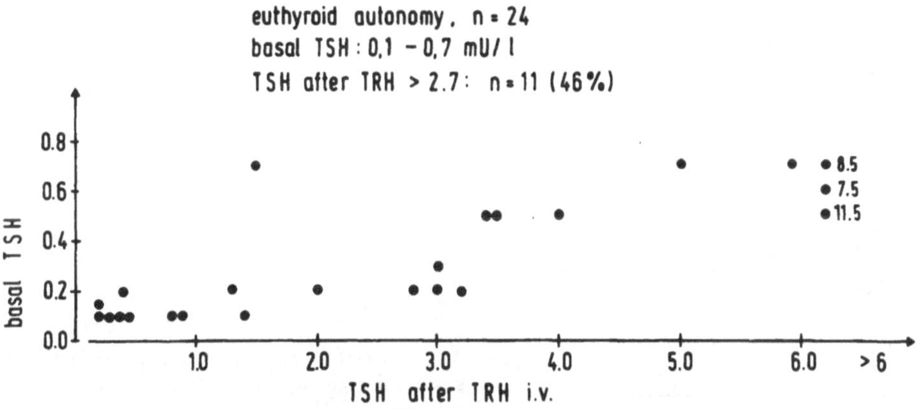

Fig. 3 Basal TSH and TSH response to TRH in 24 patients with proven regional thyroid autonomy.

In 29 patients, in which regional autonomy was suspected by scintiscan with lowered technetium uptake in the surrounding thyroid tissue who had normal thyroid levels, the basal TSH levels were clearly above 0.4 mU/l. In this patient group the increase of TSH after TRH was normal also (fig. 4). This indicates that patients with a socalled compensated autonomy (unsuppressible regions within the thyroid and normal peripheral thyroid function) are indistinguishable from euthyroid patients with multinodular goiter without autonomy. These data document that basal TSH levels in the range of 0.2 – 0.5 mU/l have to be interpreted as an index of a disturbed thyroid function [20], whereas normal basal TSH levels do not exclude autonomy. Taken all these data together, the basal TSH levels as measured by a sensitive method gives the same diagnostic information as does the TRH test using conventional radioimmunoassays. But without the stimulation test the second information of an incomplete suppression of the TSH secretion is lacking, which makes the interpretation more difficult. Therefore, the users have to accept measurable but subnormal TSH levels as a pathological finding even when the thyroid hormone concentration in serum is normal.

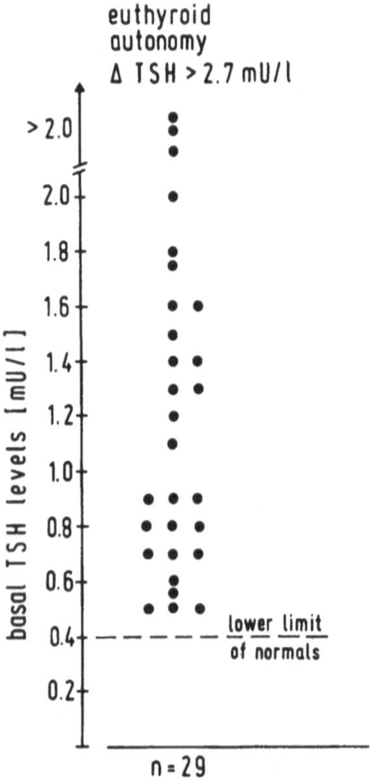

Fig. 4 Basal TSH of 29 patients with euthyroidism and suspected regional autonomy, but normal TSH response to TRH.

Sensitive basal TSH levels in patients with Cushings syndrome and in severely ill patients

As mentioned above, TSH response to TRH may be blunted in patients with Cushings syndrome and in those under glucocorticosteroid treatment and in severely ill patients without thyroid diseases. The sensitive TSH assay applied to 6 patients with active Cushings syndrome due to ACTH producing adenoma or ectopic ACTH secretion revealed TSH levels in the range of below 0.1 – 3.6 mU/l. There was no obvious correlation between the severity of the disease or ACTH and cortisol levels and the basal TSH levels. Thus, hypercortisolism is not "a priori" accompanied by low TSH levels. In critically ill patients without thyroid diseases, we and others [22] found basal TSH levels in the range of 0.1 – 2.4 mU/l independent on presence or absence of a low T3 syndrome. Most of them had an inadequate low TSH increase after TRH stimulation. Thus, also under the condition of a severe extrathyroidal illness basal TSH can be normal, below normal or completely suppressed without giving any further information concerning the thyroid function.

Sensitive basal TSH and borderline hypothyroidism

Using the sensitive TSH methods, the recognition of borderline hypothyroidism by means of basal levels seems to be an unresolved problem. Since we saw in a pilot investigation that TSH levels in the range of 5 mU/l and more were estimated

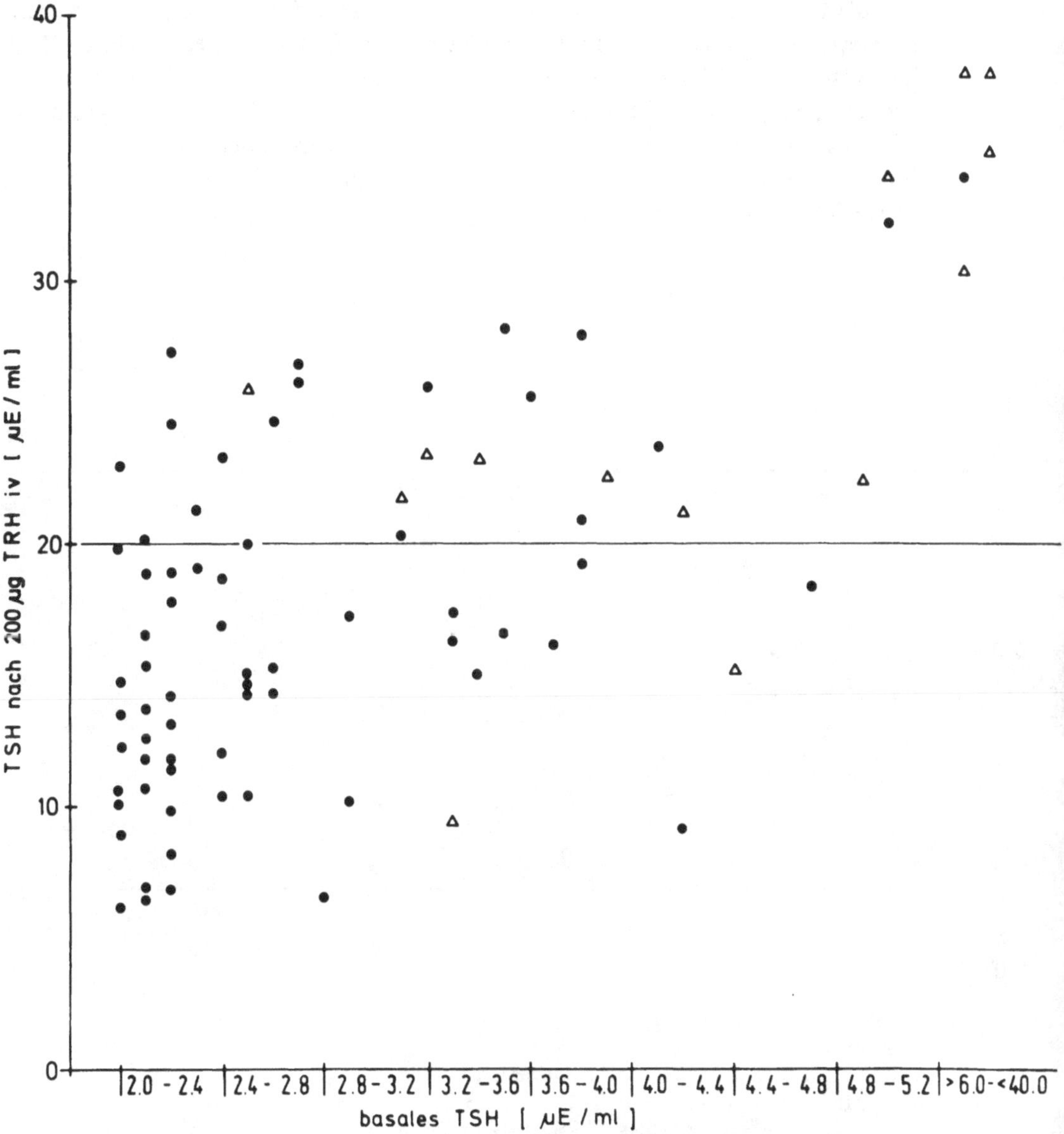

Fig. 5 TSH response to TRH (ordinate) in 86 patients with borderline or elevated basal TSH levels (abszissa). ●: patients with goiter; △: patients with a known thyroid disease (n = 14).

identically by conventional and sensitive TSH assays we used the upper limit of the TSH increase after TRH as measured by the conventional assay to determine upper limit of normal to 20 mU/l. Using this criterium of normality, we investigated the TSH increase after TRH in 79 patients with borderline basal TSH levels in the range of 2.0 – 5.0 mU/l. 63% of these patients had a normal TSH response to TRH, whereas 37% exhibited an elevated TSH response after TRH stimulation. In contrast, all patients with basal TSH of 5 mU/l and more exhibited an elevated response after TRH stimulation (fig. 5). Only when the basal TSH levels were 5 mU/l and more, a decrease of T4/TBG ratio could be observed (fig. 6). Thus, basal TSH levels of 5.0 mU/l and more indicate hypothyroidism, whereas preclinical hypothyroidism may be present in patients with basal TSH levels of more than 2 and less than 5 mU/l. In questionable cases, performance of the TSH stimulation test is necessary.

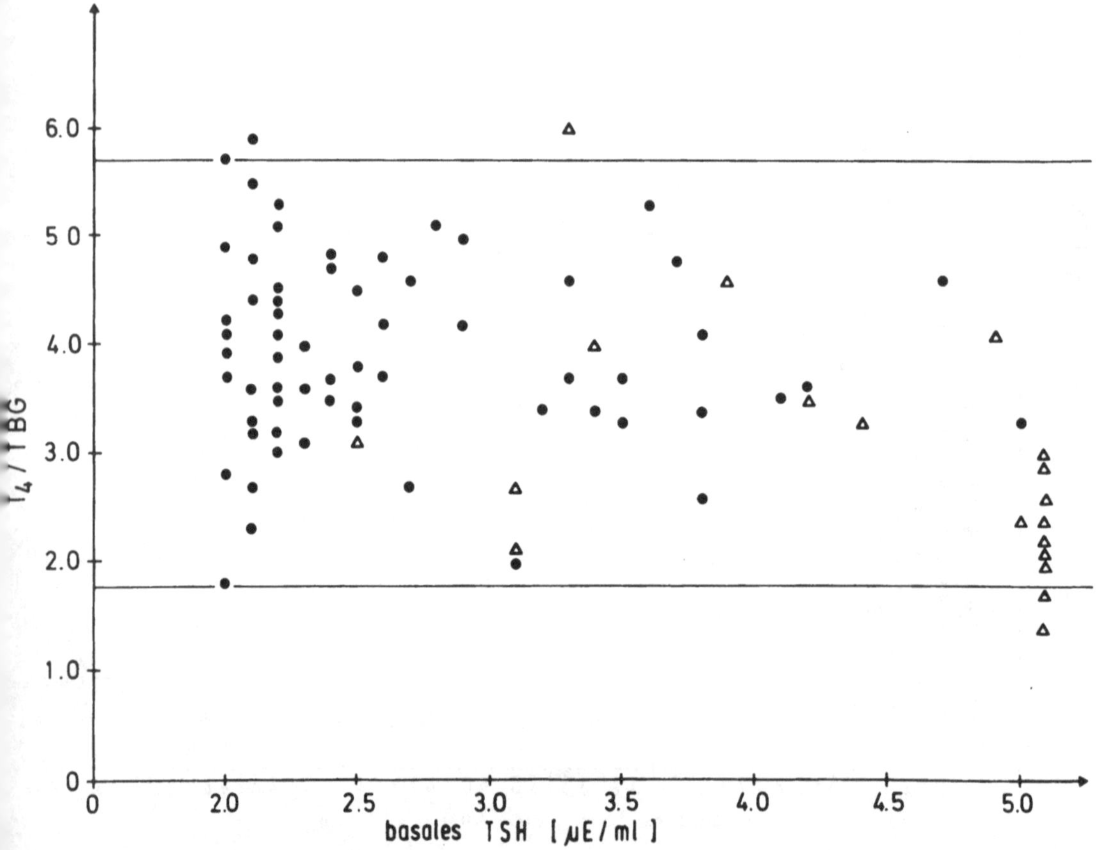

Fig. 6 T4/TBG ratio (ordinate) and basal TSH levels in patients of figure 5.

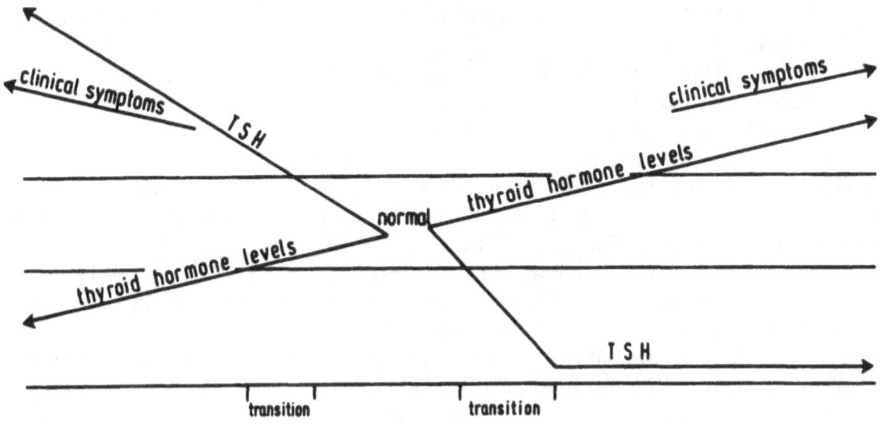

Fig. 7 Scheme of the transition of thyroid function from normal to hyperthyroidism (right) and to hypothyroidism (left). This concept was drawn together with R. D. Hesch, Hannover.

The use of the more sensitive TSH assays stimulated us to a schematic presentation of the functional transition from normal to hyperthyroidism and from normal to hypothyroidism on the other hand. In both situations thyroid function increases or decreases slowly (fig. 7). In response to these variations of the thyroid function, TSH decreases or increases early before the thyroid hormone levels cross the limits of the normal range. Thereafter, the manifestation of the clinical symptoms comes up with a further delay. Therefore, if the patient is under investigation because of thyroid enlargement only, the functional test results may be found in between the normal and the pathological ranges. When we use a sensitive TSH test system and the determination of the basal TSH level only the second which is usually the confirming information, such as a blunted or an exaggerated TSH response, is lacking. Therefore, we have to interprete our basal levels very careful with respect to the possibility, that the patient is on the way to develop a thyroid disease with hyper- or hypothyroidism just in the moment of the diagnostic procedure. In doubtful cases, the TRH stimulation test should be performed before therapeutic consequences can be drawn.

References

[1] Beck-Peccoz, P., G. Piscitelli, G. Medri, et al.: Thyroid test Strategy. Lancet I (1985) 1456.

[2] Bernutz, C., K. Horn, A. König, et al.: Advantages of sensitive assays for thyrotrophin in the diagnosis of thyroid disorders. J. Clin. Chem. Clin. Biochem. Vol. *23* (1985) 851–856.

[3] Bernutz, C., K. Horn, A. König, et al.: Detection of thyroid disorders by use of basal thyrotropin values Determined with an optimized "sandwich" Enzyme immunoassay. Clin. Chem. 31/2 (1985) 289–292.

[4] Brabant, G., K. Ocran, U. Ranft, et al.: The effect of glucocorticoid on the circadian and episodic secretion of thyrotropin in man. Acta Endocrinol. Suppl. 274 (1986) 37.

[5] Caldwell, G., S. M. Gow, V. M. Sweeting, et al.: A new strategy for thyroid function testing, Lancet I (1985) 1117–1119.

[6] Chen, H. J., J. Meites: Effects of biogenic amines and TRH on release of prolactin and TSH in the rat. Endocrinology **96** (1975) 10–22.

[7] Cobb, W. E., S. Reichlin, I. M. D. Jackson: Growth hormone secretory status is a determinant of the thyrotropin response to thyrotropin releasing hormone in euthyroid patients with hypothalamic pituitary diseases. J. Clin. Endocrinol. Metab. 52 (1981) 324–329.

[8] Cooper, D. S., A. Klibanski, E. C. Ridgway: Dopaminergic modulation on TSH and its subunits: In vitro studies. Clin. Endocrin. **18** (1983) 265–275.

[9] Faglia, G., P. Beck-Peccoz, B. Ambrose, et al.: Prolonged and exaggerated elevations in plasma thyrotropin (HTSH) after thyrotropin releasing factor (TRF) in patients with pituitary tumors. J. Clin. Endocrinol. Metab. **33** (1971) 999–1002.

[10] Faglia, G., C. Ferrari, P. Beck-Peccoz, et al.: Reduced plasma thyrotropin response to thyrotropin releasing hormone after dexamethasone administration in normal subjects. Horm. Metab. Res. **5** (1973) 289–292.

[11] Faglia, G., C. Ferrari, A. Paracchi, et al.: Triiodothyronine response to thyrotrophin releasing hormone in patients with hypothalamic-pituitary disorders. Clin. Endocrinol. **4** (1975) 585–590.

[12] Faglia, C., L. Bitensky, A. Pinchera, et al.: Thyrotropin secretion in patients with central hypothyroidism: Evidence for reduced biological activity of immunoreactive thyrotropin. J. Clin. Endocrinol. Metab. **48** (1979) 989–998.

[13] Faglia, G., P. Beck-Peccoz, M. Ballabio, et al.: Excess of β-subunit of thyrotropin (TSH) in patients with idiopathic central hypothyroidism due to the secretion of TSH with reduced biological activity. J. Clin. Endocrinol. Metab. **56** (1983) 908–914.

[14] Feek, C. M., J. S. A. Sawers, N. S. Brown, et al.: Influence of the thyroid status on dopaminergic inhibition of thyrotropin and prolactin secretion: Evidence of an additional feedback mechanism in the control of thyroid hormone secretion. J. Clin. Endocrinol. Metab. **51** (1980) 585–589.

[15] Foord, St. M., J. R. Peters, C. Dieguez, et al.: Dopamine receptors on intact anterior pituitary cells in culture: Functional association with inhibition on prolactin and thyrotropin. Endocrinology **112** (1983) 1567–1577.

[16] Habermann, J., B. Leisner, A. Witte, et al.: Iodine contamination as a cause of hyperthyroidism or lack of TSH response to TRH stimulation (results based on a screening investigation). J. Endocrinol. Invest. 5 (1982) 153–156.

[17] Hall, R., B. J. Ormston, G. M. Besser, et al.: The thyrotrophin-releasing hormone test in diseases of the pituitary and hypothalamus. Lancet I (1972) 754–763.

[18] Hamburger, J. I., A. Meier, W. E. Szpuna: Factitious elevation of thyrotropin in euthyroid patients. N. Engl. J. Med. **313** (1985) 267–268.

[19] Hiramatsu, K., K. Hashizume, T. Aizawa, et al.: Thyrotropin secretion in patients with hyperparathyroidism or hypoparathyroidism: Effect of serum calcium on thyrotropin release. J. Clin. Endocrinol. Metab. **56** (1983) 623–626.

[20] Hörmann, R., B. Saller, E. Moser, et al.: Thyroid test strategy. Lancet I (1985) 1455–1456.

[21] Hugues, J.-N., A. G. Burger, D. Grouselle, et al.: Evidence of a thyrotropin-releasing hormone dependent increase in plasma thyrotropin during refeeding of starved rats. Endocrinology **112** (1983) 715–719.

[22] Kirkegaard, C., C. Bregengard, K. Feldt-Rasmussen, et al.: Thyroid test strategy. Lancet I (1985) 1455.

[23] Köbberling, J., A. Darragh, E. del Pozo: Chronic dopamine receptor stimulation using bromocriptine: Failure to modify thyroid function. Clin. Endocrinol. **11** (1979) 367–370.

[24] Kuku, S. F., D. F. Child, S. Nader, et al.: Thyrotrophin and prolactin responsiveness to thyrotrophin releasing hormone in Cushings disease. Clin. Endocrinol. **4** (1975) 437–442.

[25] Labrie, F., J. Drouin, L. Ferlang, et al.: Mechanism of action of hypothalamic hormones in the anterior pituitary gland and specific modulation of their activity by sex steroids and thyroid hormones. Recent Prog. Horm. Res. **34** (1978) 25 – 93.

[26] Massara, F., F. Camanni, A. Amoroso, et al.: Increased thyrotrophin and prolactin secretion induced by domperidone in hypothyroid subjects. Acta Endocrinol. (Copenh.) **97** (1981) 48 – 53.

[27] Otsuki, M., M. Dakoda, S. Baba: Influence of glucocorticoids on TRH-induced TSH-response in man. J. Clin. Endocrinol. Metab. **36** (1973) 95 – 102.

[28] Petersen, V. B., A. M. McGregor, P. E. Belchetz, et al.: The secretion on thyrotrophin with impaired biological activity in patients with hypothalamic-pituitary disease. Clin. Enocrinol. **8** (1978) 397 – 402.

[29] Pickardt, C. R., W. Geiger, R. Fahlbusch, et al.: Stimulation der TSH-Sekretion durch TRF-Belastung bei hypothalamischen und hypophysären Krankheitsbildern. Klin. Wochenschr. **50** (1972) 42 – 52.

[30] Pickardt, C. R., F. Erhardt, R. Fahlbusch, et al.: Portal vessel occlusion: A cause for pituitary insufficiency in patients with pituitary tumors? Eur. J. Clin. Invest. **3** (1973) 262.

[31] Pickardt, C. R., F. Erhardt, R. Fahlbusch, et al.: The diagnostic significance of the stimulation of TSH secretion by thyrotropin releasing hormone (TRH) administration in desease of the hypothalamus and pituitary. Excerpta Med. (Amsterdam) ICS **306** (1973) 105 – 107.

[32] Pickard, C. R., P. C. Scriba: TRH: Pathophysiologic and clinical implications. Acta Neurochir. (Wien) 75 (1985) 43 – 48.

[33] Pickardt, C. R., A. Witte, G. Busch, et al.: Die Bedeutung exogener Jodkontamination für die Manifestation von Hyperthyreosen. In: Schilddrüse, pp. 303 – 310. G. Thieme, Stuttgart, New York 1985.

[34] Refetoff, S., V. S. Fang, B. Rapoport, et al.: Interrelationships in the regulation of TSH and prolactin secretion in man: Effects of L-Dopa, TRH and thyroid hormone in various combinations. J. Clin. Endocrinol. Metab. **38** (1974) 450 – 457.

[35] Ribka, A., B. Mayr, U. Büll, et al.: Wertigkeit nulearmedizinischer und endokrinologischer Methoden zur Klassifizierung autonomer Schilddrüsenadenome. Med. Klin. **74** (1979) 511 – 515.

[36] Roddis, K. J., K. J. Burrin, A. Johannssen, et al.: Serum thyrotropin: A first line discriminatory test of thyroid function. Lancet I (1985) 277 – 278.

[37] Scanlon, M. F., D. R. Weightman, D. J. Shale, et al.: Dopamine is a physiological regulator of thyrotropin (TSH) secretion in normal man. Clin. Endocrinol. **10** (1979) 7 – 15.

[38] Scanlon, M. F., A. D. Wechman, M. Lewis, et al.: Dopaminergic modulation of circadian thyrotrophin rhythms and thyroid hormone levels in euthyroid subjects. J. Clin. Endocrinol. Metab. **51** (1980) 1251 – 1256.

[39] Scanlon, M. F., M. D. Rodriguez-Arnao, A. M. McGregor, et al.: Altered dopaminergic regulation of thyrotrophin release in patients with prolactinomas: Comparison with other tests of hypothalamic-pituitary function. Clin. Endocrinol. **14** (1981) 133 – 143.

[40] Scriba, P. C., T. Erhardt, H. G. Heinze, et al.: Anterior pituitary and TSH. In: Regulation of thyroid function (Klein, E., D. Reinwein, eds.), pp. 35 – 46. Schattauer, Stuttgart – New York 1976.

[41] Scriba, P. C., M. Bauer, D. Emmert, et al.: Effects of obesity, total fasting and re-alimentation on L-thyroxine (T4) 3,5,3-L-triiodothyronine (T3) 3,3,5,-L-triiodothyronine (rT3), thyroxine binding globulin (TBG), cortisol thyrotrophin, cortisol binding globulin (CGB), transferrin, a2-haptoglobin and complement C3 in serum. Acta Endocrinol. (Copenh.) **91** (1979) 629 – 643.

[42] Sowers, J. R., H. E. Carlson, N. Brautbar, et al.: Effect of dexamethasone on prolactin and TSH responses to TRH and metoclopramide in man. J. Clin. Endocrinol. Metab. **4** (1977) 237 – 241.

[43] Sowers, J. R., R. A. Catania, J. M. Hershman: Evidence for dopaminergic control of circadian veriations in thyrotropin secretion. J. Clin. Endocrinol. Metab. **54** (1982) 673 – 675.

[44] Urmann, S., C. Critchlow: Long term elevations in plasma thyrotropin but not growth hormone concentrations associated with lesion-induces depletion of median eminence somatostatin. Endocrinology **112** (1983) 659 – 644.

[45] Wartofsky, L., K. D. Burmann: Alterations in thyroid function in patients with systemic illness: The "euthyroid sick syndrome". Endocr. Rev. **3** (1982) 164 – 217.

[46] Wenzel, K. W.: Pharmacological interference with in vitrotests of thyroid. Metabolism **30** (1981) 717 – 732.

[47] Wenzel, K. W., J. Döring: Lack of influence of the antidopaminergic drug domperidone on basal and TRH-stimulated TSH-serum levels after oral administration. Acta Endocrinol. (Copenh.) **101** (1982) 550 – 554.

[48] Wilber, J. F., R. D. Utiger: The effect of glucocorticoids on thyrotropin secretion. J. Clin. Invest. **48** (1969) 2096 – 2103.

[49] Wood, W. G., D. Waller, U. Hantke: An evaluation of six solidphase thyrotropin (TSH) kits. J. Clin. Chem. Clin. Biochem. **23** (1985) 461 – 471.

Parameters of thyroid function in patients on hemodialysis

E. Leicht, H. Albersmeyer, G. Biro, R. Lipecky, R. Bambauer, Chr. Marx

In patients with chronic renal failure, low values of total thyroxine (TT4) and total triiodothyronine (TT3) in serum have been repeatedly reported. In these patients, symptoms as dry skin with increased desquamation or hyperlipoproteinemia are frequently encountered, which are also typical for hypothyroidism, although other symptoms may not suggest subnormal thyroid function.

In an attempt to get more information on the cause of the low values of total thyroid hormones in patients with chronic renal failure, we studied 50 male subjects aged 30 – 50 years, who had been treated by hemodialysis for 3 months to 17 years. The patients were selected in 3 centres of hemodialysis. Good general state of health except for renal function was a prerequisite for entering the study. The patients were being dialyzed 3 times a week. Blood samples were taken 48 hours after the last hemodialysis. The control group consisted of 20 age-matched members of the medical staff of our clinic.

Total T4, total T3 and prolactin in plasma were assayed by radioimmunoassay kits of Corning, free T4, free T3 and thyroxine binding protein (TBG) by radioimmunoassay-kits of Henning/Berlin, TSH with a highly sensitive immunoradiometric kit of Henning/Berlin, T3-uptake by a kit of the ZER company, growth hormone, parathyroid hormone, calcitonin, calcium, inorganic phosphorus, albumin and cholesterol by routine methods of our laboratory.

Plasma concentrations of TT4 and TT3 were considerably lower in the patients' group; TT4 was definitely subnormal in 20 patients, TT3 in 9 patients. No difference between the two groups was found with regard to thyroxine binding globulin. T3-uptake was slightly lower in patients on hemodialysis and FT4-index (TT4 X T3-uptake) was considerably lower (tab. 1). Basal TSH, although in the normal range, was slightly but significantly higher in the patients' group, the TSH surge 30 min. after intravenous TRH however, was lower. Free T4 and free T3, when measured with the Henning kits, were definitely lower in the patients' group (tab. 1). No surge of total T3 or free T3 30 min. after TRH could be detected in normals or in patients. Prolactin, calcitonin and GH were elevated in the patients' group, but there was no significant correlation of these or other routinely measured values with parameters of thyroid function.

Thyrotropin

Table 1 Parameters of thyroid function in normal persons and in patients on hemodialysis. Free T_4 values lower in the patient's group than in normal persons when measured with the analogue tracer method, higher than in normal persons with the Spac-ET-kit

	normal persons ($\bar{x} \pm s\bar{x}$)	patients ($\bar{x} \pm s\bar{x}$)		normal values
TT4 (μg/dl)	7,87 ± 0.32	5,37 ± 0,23	$p < 0{,}001$	5 – 12,5
TT3 (ng/ml)	1,37 ± 0.03	0,98 ± 0,04	$p < 0{,}001$	1,0 – 2,2
TBG (mg/l)	17,3 ± 0,81	17,5 ± 0,56	n.s.	20,1 – 6,0
T3-uptake (%)	50,8 ± 0,94	46,8 ± 0,9	$p < 0{,}01$	45 – 55
fT4-index	3,9 ± 0,13	2,4 ± 0,10	$p < 0{,}001$	
TSH 0 min. (μU/ml)	0,8 ± 0,07	1,2 ± 0,09	$p < 0{,}05$	0 – 4,5
TSH 30 min. (μU/ml)	6,8 ± 0,61	4,0 ± 0,33	$p < 0{,}001$	<25
f-T4 (pg/ml)	15,8 ± 0,52	10,2 ± 0,33	$p < 0{,}001$	10 – 19 (Henning)
f-T3 (pmol/l)	4,6 ± 0,11	2,6 ± 0,13	$p < 0{,}001$	3,0 – 9,5 (Henning)
f-T4 (pg/ml)	10,6 ± 0,02	12,2 ± 0,03	$p < 0{,}01$	Spac-ET Mallinckrodt

If we suppose these results to be true, we should have to assume that a considerable number of our patients suffer from hypothyroidism. However, the elevation of basal TSH is minimal and the TSH surge after administration of TRH is blunted instead of elevated. It could be discussed, that the slight elevation of basal TSH is inadequate for the low values of total and free thyroid hormones, as a consequence of hypophyseal-hypothalamic failure [3]. Moreover it cannot be excluded, that the elevation of basal TSH represents an accumulation of immunoreactive TSH fragments in renal failure without adequate biological activity, as it is in part true for parathyroid hormone.

According to Stockigt et al. and Ooi et al. [5, 2] analogue tracer methods for free T4 depend on albumin concentration. These methods are known to yield low free T4 concentrations in severe nonthyroidal illness [4]. In our patients, who were in good general health, except for renal function, plasma albumin was only slightly lower than in normales. There was a slight correlation between free T4 values and plasma albumin in the control group, not, however, in patients. We therefore measured free T4 with another method, the Spac-ET-kit of Mallinckrodt. This method provides TT4-values, which were in fairly good correlation with those measured with the Henning kit ($r = 0.82$). There was, however, a profound difference in fT4-concentrations, which were slightly but significantly ($p < 0.01$) lower in the control group (10.6 ± 0.02 pg/ml) than in patients (12.2 ± 0.03 pg/ml), when the correction factor recommended by the manufacturer was a applied. This was opposite to what we have found with the analogue tracer method (tab. 1).

On the basis of our results we cannot decide, which of the two sets of free T4 values should be preferred. None of the methods yielded a significant negative correlation between total T4 or free T4 and basal or stimulated TSH. None of the methods was free of the influence of TBG. There was a positive correlation between free T4 and total T4 with the analogue tracer method, which seems to be more reasonable (fig. 1) than the negative correlation between these two

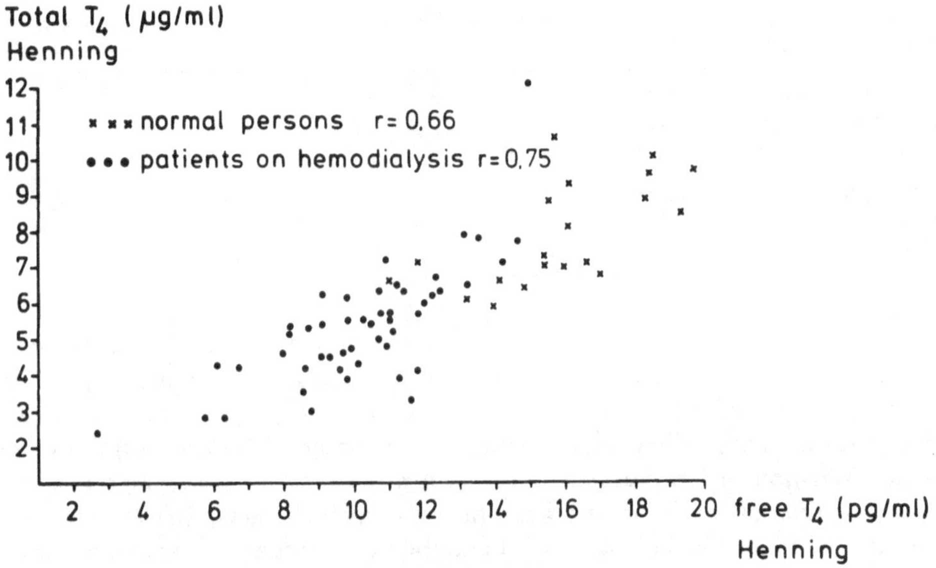

Fig. 1 Positive correlation between total T4 and free T4 (analogue tracer method).

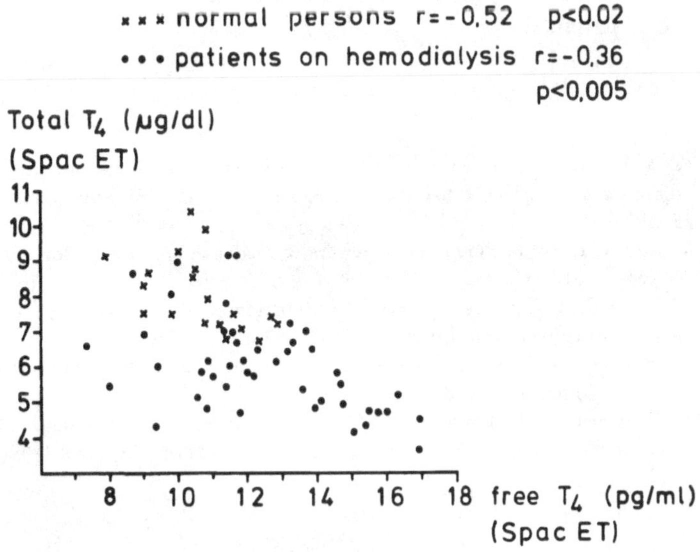

Fig. 2 Negative correlation between total T4 and free T4 (Spac-ET method of Mallinckrodt).

parameters with the Spac-ET-kit (fig. 2, tab. 2). Free T4 results of the Spac-ET method would seem to fit more the clinical status of our patients, none of whom had overt thyroid problems. However, we cannot settle the issue of some of our patients suffer from hypothyroidism.

Table 2 Correlations of the free T_4 values measured by two methods with relevant parameters of thyroid function

f-T4 "Henning kit"	– TSH basal	r = 0,04	n.s.
f-T4 "Henning kit"	– TBG	r = 0,50	p < 0,02
f-T4 "Henning kit"	– TT4 "Henning-kit"	r = 0,66	p < 0,002
f-T4 "Spac-ET-kit"	– TSH basal	r = 0,16	n.s.
f-T4 "Spac-ET-kit"	– TBG	r = −0,77	p < 0,001
f-T4 "Spac-ET-kit"	– TT_4 "Spac-ET-kit"	r = −0,52	p < 0,02

As mentioned, T3 resin uptake was lower in the patients' group than in normal persons (tab. 1). One would expect the opposite in case of an impaired protein binding of thyroid hormones. However, we have not a great confidence to this parameter. According to Felicetta and coworkers T3-uptake leads to an underestimation of free hormone levels, when the resin uptake is high and an overestimation of free hormones when the resin uptake is low [1]. The Spac-ET-kit also yields an uptake value, a T4-antibody coated-tube uptake, which was higher in patients than in controls. Further parameters seem to be necessary for assessing the thyroid status of patients with chronic renal failure. At present we are doing a bioassay in order to clarify the meaning of the slightly elevated basal levels of TSH in our patients.

References

[1] Felicetta, J. V., W. L. Green, L. B. Haas, et al.: Thyroid function and lipids in patients with chronic renal disease treated by hemodialysis: With comments on the "Free thyroxine index". Metabolism **28** (1979) 756–763.

[2] Ooi, D. S., A. Sorisky: Effect of albumine on results of analogue type assays for thyroxine. Clin. Chem. **30** (1984) 1109–1110.

[3] Ramirez, G., W. O'Neill, W. Jubiz, et al.: Thyroid dysfunction in uremia: Evidence for thyroid and hypophyseal abnormalities. Ann. Intern. Med. **84** (1976) 672–676.

[4] Spencer, C. A.: The comparative clinical value of free T4-estimation using different methodological approaches. Nuc. Compact **16** (1985) 321–327.

[5] Stockigt, J. R., V. Stevens, E. L. White, et al.: "Unbound analogue" radioimmunoassays for free thyroxin measure the albumin-bound hormone fraction. Clin. Chem. **29** (1983) 1408–1410.

TSH-Immunoradiometric assay (IRMA) in geriatric patients*

I. Szabolcs, Chr. Ploenes, J. Herrmann, W. Bernard, M. Beyer, H. L. Krüskemper

Introduction

The most recently developed immunoradiometric assay (IRMA) using monoclonal antibodies are sensitive enough to discriminate small TSH quantities from normal values, a thing which was not possible by the conventional RIA-s. Discrepancies between TSH-IRMA and RIA values are most probable in patients with suppressed or diminished TSH secretion. Several authors investigated the value of TSH-IRMA in subclinical and overt hyperthyroidism [1–4].

The aim of this study was to compare TSH IRMA and RIA methods in a geriatric group where low TSH levels could be related to thyroid autonomy as well as to old age.

Patients and methods

134 geriatric patients (> 60 years old, 81 females and 53 males) without any severe illness were screened for thyroid disorders by estimating serum total T_4, T_3 (Corning-RIA), free T_4 (Travenol-RIA), TBG (Behring-RIA) and TRH test (200 μg TRH i. v.). TSH was measured by both a traditional double antibody RIA (Corning, normal ranges: 0–6 μU/ml, intraassay variation: 5.3%, interassay variation: 9.3%), and a more sensitive IRMA using monoclonal antibodies (Behring, normal ranges 0.5–3.5 μU/ml, intraassay variation: 5.8%, interassay variation: 5.0%). The patients were classified according to the TRH tests as euthyroid (positive test, TSH increase more than 2.0 μU/ml), "hyperthyroid" (negative TRH tests, TSH increase less than 2.0 μU/ml) and hypothyroid (elevated basal TSH level) as indicated in table 1.

* This work was supported by the A. v. Humboldt Stiftung.

Thyrotropin

Table 1 Classification of geriatric patients (134 TRH tests) using TSH IRMA and TSH RIA

	euthyroid (ΔTSH > 2.0 µU/ml)	"hyperthyroid" (ΔTSH < 2.0 µU/ml)	hypothyroidism (TSH IRMA > 3.5 µU/ml) (TSH RIA > 6.0 µU/ml)
TSH IRMA Behring	97	32	5
TSH RIA Corning	80	47	7

Results

In the same geriatric group fewer negative TRH tests could be found using IRMA than RIA (tab. 1). Both mean basal and evoked (30') TSH-IRMA values in positive as well as in negative TRH tests were less than the corresponding RIA values (fig. 1), the increases (Δ TSH) being very similar (positive tests: Mean ± SE Δ TSH-IRMA: 5.44 ± 0.28 µU/ml, Δ TSH-RIA: 5.18 ± 0.35 µU/ml; negative tests: Δ TSH-IRMA: 0.67 ± 0.11 µU/ml, Δ TSH-RIA: 0.69 ± 0.09 µU/ml). Morover, if positivity of a TRH test was defined by TSH-IRMA alone, mean Δ TSH-IRMA (5.44 ± 0.28 µU/ml) was even greater than Δ TSH-RIA (4.47 ± 0.35 µU/ml, n = 97, $p < 0.05$). Using the TSH-IRMA a much better correlation between basal and delta TSH values could be shown both for patients with positive TRH tests and for those with negative tests (tab. 2).

The euthyroid geriatric patients with positive TRH test (IRMA, n = 97) had a significantly lower mean basal TSH value than a control group of 57, 20 to 40

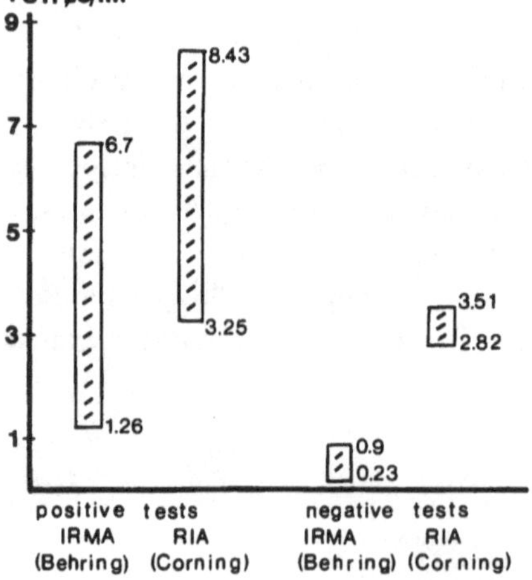

Fig.1 TRH tests (n = 134) in geriatric patients.

Table 2 Correlation of basal and delta TSH in geriatric patients (n = 134)

	positive TRH test	negative TRH test
TSH IRMA Behring	r = 0.66	r = 0.73
TSH RIA Corning	r = 0.30	r = 0.36

Table 3 Basal TSH in euthyroid geriatric patients and healthy controls

	geriatric patients (n = 97)		healthy young controls (n = 57)
TSH IRMA Behring (μU/ml)	1.27 ± 0.06	$p < 0.05$	1.57 ± 0.11
TSH RIA Corning (μU/ml)	3.49 ± 0.14		3.22 ± 0.11

year old healthy volunteers. Using the RIA method the corresponding values showed no significant difference (tab. 3).

Discussion

Most of the data show the advantage of TSH-IRMA: The fact that less negative TRH test were seen in the same geriatric population using IRMA is a sign of greater sensitivity, but this depends on the quality of both the IRMA (Behring) and RIA (Corning) used, and can not be taken for a rule for all TSH IRMA-s and RIA-s. (As a matter of fact, comparing recently TSH-IRMA Behring to another RIA we could not observe this difference of the occurence of negative TRH tests.)

Using TSH IRMA a decreased mean basal TSH value could be found in euthyroid geriatric patients. Diminished pituitary TSH reserve capacity in geriatric population is well established by estimating TSH release in the TRH test [5–7], but the IRMA method was necessary to show also a diminished basal value, most probably being a sign of decreased TSH secretion.

The great number of negative TRH tests in our geriatric group seems to be not only the result of age. We think, that negativity of the TRH test in geriatric patients is more frequently related to thyroid autonomy, medication, or nonthyroidal illness, than to the old age per se.

The good correlation of basal and delta TSH values is a valuable advantage of TSH-IRMA as compared to RIA. Since TSH-IRMA with monoclonal antibodies has been developed, the main question is how far the TRH test can be replaced by the basal TSH IRMA [1 – 4]. Correlation of basal and delta TSH-IRMA in geriatric patients is significant but in our opinion not close enough to make the TRH test redundant. A more detailed study of this topic determining specificity, sensitivity and predictive value of basal TSH-IRMA in geriatric patients in relation to the TRH test outcome is necessary.

Abstract

134 geriatric patients were screened for thyroid disorders by the TRH test, TSH being measured by both a traditional RIA (Corning) and a more sensitive IRMA using monoclonal antibodies (Behring). In the same geriatric group fewer negative TRH tests could be found using IRMA than RIA. Both mean basal and evoked TSH-IRMA values were less than the corresponding RIA values, the increases (Δ TSH) being very similar. Using the TSH IRMA a much better correlation between basal and delta TSH values could be shown both for patients with positive TRH tests and for those with negative tests. The euthyroid geriatric patients with positive TRH test (IRMA) had a significantly lower mean basal TSH value than a control group of young healthy volunteers. The data show the advantage of use of TSH-IRMA in geriatric patients.

References

[1] Abbott, S., I. Wright, S. Daniel, et al.: A simple, sensitive TSH immunoradiometric assay for the discrimination of thyroid function. Wissenschaftlicher Informationsdienst, Röhm Pharma, Edinburgh 1984.

[2] Alexander, W. D., D. J. Kerr, M. M. Ferguson: First line test of thyroid function. Lancet Sept. 15 (1984) 674.

[3] Caldwell, G., H. A. Kellett, S. M. Gow, et al.: A new strategy fot thyroid function testing. Lancet, May 18 (1985) 1117 – 1119.

[4] Joseph, K.: Schilddrüsen-Estdiagnostik: TSH immunradiometrisch. Diagnose und Labor 35 (1985) 133 – 149.

[5] Wenzel, K. W., H. Meinhold, M. Herpich, et al.: TRH-Stimulationstest mit alters- und geschlechtsabhängigen TSH-Anstieg bei Normalpersonen. Klin. Wochenschr. 52 (1974) 722 – 727.

[6] Szabolcs, I., G. Szilágyi, M. Góth, et al.: Plasma triiodothyronine response to thyrotropin releasing hormone, thyrotropin and propranolol in old age. Exp. Geront. 16 (1981) 309 – 316.

[7] Harman, S. M., R. E. Wehmann, M. R. Blackman: Pituitary-thyroid hormone economy in healthy aging men: Basal indices of thyroid function and thyrotropin responses to constans infusions of thyrotropin releasing hormone. J. Clin. Endocrinol. Metab. 58 (1984) 320 – 325.

Low T_3 syndrome and pituitary thyrotrophin function in diabetes mellitus in relation to type of diabetes and metabolic control – a review

Ch. Schnack, G. Schernthaner

Alterations of serum thyroid hormone concentrations in clinically euthyroid patients with severe, chronic – non-thyroidal diseases have been described in a number of studies [1]. In most of these subjects a low T3 syndrome with markedly reduced serum T3 concentrations, elevated rT3 values with mildly decreased T4 levels was observed. This phenomenon could be explained by an inhibition of peripheral conversion of thyroxine to triiodothyronine [1].

In patients with diabetes mellitus similar alterations of thyroid hormone concentrations have been described in a number of studies [2–9]. However, in some reports abnormalities of the pituitary thyrotroph function – possible influencing the peripheral thyroid hormone concentrations were observed [2, 3].

A low T3 syndrome in diabetic ketoacidosis associated with a blunted TRH induced TSH secretion has been observed by Naeije et al. [2] (tab. 1). Changes of peripheral thyroid hormone concentrations were at least partly reversible with shortterm correction of hyperglycemia and ketosis, whereas the blunted TSH response to TRH persisted over 5 days, suggesting a pituitary defect induced by the decompensated diabetic state. Furthermore, a dysfunction of pituitary thyrotroph axis has been described in streptozotocin diabetic rats [10, 11]. Lower levels of TSH associated with a decreased rate of iodide uptake by the thyroid (in vitro) were observed in diabetic rats compared to controls, as well insulin as TSH administration could normalize these alterations [10]. Wilber et al. [11] reported reduced TSH and TRH concentrations associated with low T3 and T4 levels in the peripheral blood of diabetic rats. As TRH binding capacities of the pituitary plasma membranes were normal, it was concluded that diabetes mellitus induces a downward resetting of the hypothalamic pituitary thyroid axis. Both studies [10, 11] were performed in streptozotocin induced acute diabetes with a duration of only a few days.

Data concerning TRH induced TSH secretion in diabetic patients are conflicting as most of the studies were performed in patients with a different degree of metabolic control and duration of disease. A blunted TSH response to TRH was observed in diabetic ketoacidosis [2] and – recently in newly discovered obese

Thyrotropin

type-II diabetics [3]. It could be shown that TSH response returned to normal after 8 – 12 weeks of normalized metabolic control in type-II diabetics [3].

A normal TRH induced TSH secretion was reported in type-I diabetics without ketoacidosis [12, 14] and in uncomplicated diabetes mellitus (type-I and type-II) with a different duration of disease [13]. Our own recent results [16] could not detect any significant changes in TSH response to TRH in long-standing type-II diabetics with normal body weight before and after insulin treatment (tab. 1).

Thus, it may be concluded that the alterations of pituitary thyrotroph function in diabetes are associated either with acute onset of diabetes or with severe metabolic derangement such as diabetic ketoacidosis. In long-standing diabetes (type-I and type-II) even with moderate metabolic control TRH induces TSH secretion seems to be unchanged compared to controls.

The reduction of basal TSH levels described in some reports [6, 8, 14] in diabetic patients seems to be independent from the TSH response of the thyrotroph cells to TRH stimulus [14] and cannot explain the divergent changes of T4, T3 and rT3 in diabetics [6]. A disturbance of the negative feedback relationship between thyroid hormones and the pituitary with rT3 occupying the pituitary binding sites of T3 might explain this phenomenon as it was discussed by Carter et al. [1].

Most of the studies performed in type-I and type-II diabetic patients described reduced T3 and elevated rT3 levels with only slight changes of T4 concentrations.

A close relation of T3 concentration to peripheral blood glucose utilization rate in IDDM was observed, whereas an inverse correlation was described for T3 levels and plasma ketone bodies concentrations [6].

In thyroid hormone turnover studies Pittmann et al. [4] documented a reduced peripheral T4 deiodination to T3 in close relation to metabolic control in diabetics and in an other report a significant correlation between T4 deiodination and peripheral blood glucose utilization was observed [5].

Consequently a close relation of rT3 to the fasting blood glucose which was negative correlated to T3 levels [7] and a correlation of HbA1c to rT3 concentrations was reported [9].

Short-term improvement of metabolic control not always completely corrects alterations of thyroid hormone concentrations [2, 8, 15]. Alexander et al. [15] have shown that the duration of the preexisting katabolic state (ketoacidosis) in type-I diabetics might influence the reversibility of thyroid hormone alterations.

In obese newly discovered type-II diabetics a low T3 syndrome, not influenced by improved metabolic control by dietary treatment for 6 weeks was observed [8], however, the postprandial blood glucose and HbA1 concentration remained

Table 1 Studies on TRH-induced TSH secretion in diabetes

Study [Lit.]	type of diabetes	duration of diabetes resp. age	number of patients	results	follow-up	remarks
Naeije et al. 1978 [2]	type-I type-II	age: 47 ± 20 SD years	19	depressed TSH secretion rate	5 days: no alteration of depressed TSH secretion after improved metabolic control	diabetic ketoacidosis
Morley et al. 1977 [12]	type-I	age: 12 – 63 years dur.: 3 months to 8 years	14	no significant alteration of TSH secretion compared to controls		poor metabolic control without ketoacidosis
MacFarlane et al. 1982 [14]	type-I	age: 17 – 35 years	7	no alteration of TSH secretion compared to controls	1. 4 – 6 days 2. 6 – 8 weeks } no alteration of TSH secretion	poor metabolic control (HbA1: 15,4 ± 3,4) at begin of the study
Leroith et al. 1980 [13]	type-I type-II	age: 24 – 52 years	15	no alteration of TSH secretion in type-I or type-II		uncomplicated diabetes
Kabadi et al. 1984 [3]	type-II	newly discovered type-II diabetics age: 45 – 64 years	29	depressed TSH secretion	8 – 12 weeks: normalization of TSH secretion with improved metabolic control	obese patients
Schnack and Schernthaner 1986 [16]	type-II	dur.: 11 ± 7,9 years age: 70,8 ± 8,8 SD years	12	no alteration of TSH secretion compared to controls	1. 10 days 2. 3 months } no alteration of TSH secretion	patients with normal body weight before and after insulin treatment

in the hyperglycemic range. Adequate correction of hyperglycemia for 8 – 12 weeks completely corrects changes of peripheral thyroid hormone concentrations in newly discovered type-II diabetics [3]. In long-standing type-II diabetics [16] the alterations of thyroid hormones are at least partly reversible by improved metabolic control.

Summarizing it appears that the low T3 syndrome in diabetes mellitus is caused by an altered peripheral deiodination of T4 to T3 with increased production of rT3, which is influenced by the degree of hyperglycemia and ketoacidosis.

The alterations of thyroid hormone concentrations are at least partly reversible with correction of metabolic control.

The disturbance of the pituitary thyrotroph function seems to be a transient phenomenon observed at the onset of diabetes and in severe ketoacidosis.

References

[1] Carter, J. N., C. J. Eastman, J. M. Corcoran, et al.: Inhibition of conversion of thyroxine to triiodothyronine in patients with severe chronic illness. Clin. Endocrinol. **5** (1976) 587.

[2] Naeije, R., J. Goldstein, N. Clumeck, et al.: A low T4 syndrome in diabetic ketoacidosis. Clin. Endocrinol. **8** (1978) 467.

[3] Kabadi, U. M.: Impaired pituitary tyhrotroph function in uncontrolled type-II diabetes mellitus: Normalization on recovery. J. Clin. Endocrinol. Metab. **59** (1984) 521.

[4] Pittman, C. S., A. K. Suda, J. B. Chambers, et al.: Abnormalities of thyroid hormone turnover in patients with diabetes mellitus before and after insulin therapy. J. Clin. Endocrinol. Metab. **48** (1979) 854.

[5] Pittman, C. S., A. K. Suda, J. B. Chambers, et al.: Impaired 3,5,3'-triiodothyronine (T3) production in diabetic patients. Metabolism **28** (1979) 333.

[6] Saunders, J., S. E. H. Hall, P. H. Sönksen: Thyroid hormones in insulin requiring diabetes before and after treatment. Diabetologia **15** (1978) 29.

[7] Kabadi, U. M., B. N. Premachandra, M. Maayan: Low serum 3,5,3'-triiodothyronine (T3) and raised 3,3',5'-triiodothyronine (reverse T3, or rT3) in diabetes mellitus: Normalization on improvement in hyperglycemia. Acta Diabetol. Lat **19** (1982) 233.

[8] Sheppard, M. C., D. B. Ramsden: Thyroid hormones in non-insulin-dependent diabetes before and after dietary treatment. Clin. Endocrinol. **18** (1983) 593.

[9] Notarbartolo, A., G. Rini, G. Licata, et al.: Correlation between different degree and duration of metabolic control and thyroid hormone levels in type 1 and type 2 diabetics. Acta Diabetol. Lat **20** (1983) 341.

[10] Jolin, T., C. Conzalez: Thyroid iodine metabolism in streptozotocin-diabetic rats. Acta Endocrinol. **88** (1978) 506.

[11] Wilber, J. F., A. Banerji, C. Prasad, et al.: Alterations in hypothalamic-pituitary-thyroid regulation produced by diabetes mellitus. Life Sci **28** (1981) 1757.

[12] Morley, J. E., C. Klein, W. J. Kalk, et al.: Pituitary responsiveness to thyrotropin releasing hormone in insulin-dependent diabetes mellitus. Horm. Metab. Res. **10** (1978) 231.

[13] Leroith, D., M. Shapiro, R. Luboshitsky, et al.: The hypothalamic-pituitary axis in diabetes mellitus. Horm. Metab. Res. **12** (1980) 608.

[14] MacFarlane, L. A., M. C. Sheppard, S. Gilbey, et al.: Thyroid stimulating hormone secretion in type I (insulin-dependent) diabetic patients: Influence of metabolic control. Diabetologia 23 (1982) 471.
[15] Alexander, C. M., E. M. Kapstein, S. M. C. Lum: Pattern of recovery of thyroid hormone indices associated with treatment of diabetes mellitus. J. Clin. Endocrinol. Metab. 54 (1982) 362.
[16] Schnack, C., G. Schernthaner: Pituitary thyrotroph function and thyroid hormones in long-standing type-II diabetes mellitus before and after insulin treatment (submitted for publication).

TRH test and diagnostic of undefined secondary amenorrhea

B. Schurz, R. Fitz, B. Grubek, J. Huber, J. Spona

There are only few references an literature to the frequency of diseases of the thyroid as a cause of secondary amenorrhea and the incidence of the condition is stated to be less than 1%. The pathophysiological mechanism which triggers of anovulation, oligomenorrhoe or amenorrhea in hyper- or hypothyroidism lies in the change of the steroid metabolism through thyroxine [2]. A hyperthyroid metabolism increases SHBG and thus leads to a reduction in the metabolic clearance of androgens and estrogens. In case of hypothyroidism, SHBG is reduced. Here also, androstenedion is increasingly converted to testosterone, estradiol and estriol. The peripheral steroids-increased in this manner-disturb the ovarial-thyroid feedback mechanism and thus also gonadotropin fluctuation. At the same time, the thyroid sensitivity to TRH is reactively increased in any hypothyroid condition. As TRH also increases the prolactin level, hypothyroidism can at the same time also lead to mild hyperprolactemia [1, 4]. Determination of T4 in the blood is a suitable method for the detection of hyperthyroidism, but hypothyroidism, on the other hand, is ascertained by the TRH test, even in its latent form. After the administration of 200 microg. of TRH, the TSH is measured after 20 and 40 minutes. If the value of 18 is exceeded after 20 minutes, hypothyroidism is indicated.

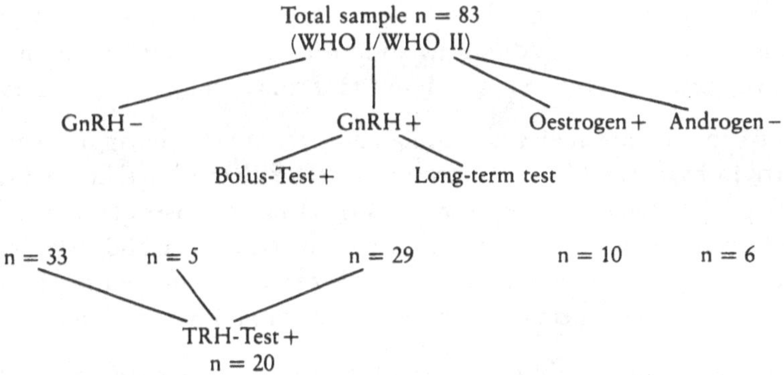

We carried out the TRH test with 83 patients suffering from secondary amenorrhea in the framework of a thorough endocrinological examination. The forms

Thyrotropin

of amenorrhea corresponding to WHO groups I and II. Six woman had endocrinologically established hyperandrogenemic ovarial insufficiency and in 10 women it was possible to normalize gonadotropin fluctuation by exogenously administered estrogen. In 34 cases, gonodotropin stimulation with substitution of GnRH was successful, gonadotropin release being induced in 5 cases on administration of GnRH bolus but in 29 cases not until after prolonged GnRH-infusion. In 33 cases, a GnRH refractory pituitary was diagnosed. Excessive TSH release and thus also hypothyroid metabolism was found in 20 women from among the last two groups mentioned. The prolactin level was raised in two cases in the hypothyroid group and in only one case in the euthyroid group.

It was demonstrated experimentally that after thyroidectomy in female rats with primarily intact ovaries the LH and FSH synthesis in the pituitary was suppressed and steroid formation in the ovaries was disturbed [2]. Leyendecker has also described the connection between cyclic disturbance of undefined origin and dysfunction of the thyroid in humans [3]. In women with normal thyroid activity, the thyroid hormones inhibit TSH and prolactin. The question whether the hypothyroid metabolism diagnosed is causally related to amenorrhea or ist perhaps only a consecutive secondary effect is in the final analysis answered by the result of therapy. If the menstrual cycle begins to stabilize on administration of substitution therapy with Thyroxin, a direct causal connection can be assumed. In the case of 7 of the 20 patients whom we began to treat with a thyroid hormone after diagnosis, we were in fact able to restore the normal cyclic pattern. It is possible to conclude from this fact, that the thyroid hormones and sex hormones influence each others' effects.

In a second group of patients with hirsute complaints, we were also able to gather our first experience with the TRH test. In 30 hirsute women whose androgen levels lay in the normal range or were only slightly raised, we investigated the thyroid reaction and found a pathologically increased TRH test in 7 cases. It is known that in addition to androgens and receptors; the androgen-binding carrier protein SHBG plays an important role in the etiology of hirsutism.

The patients' endocrine balance is modulated by the thyroid hormones thyroxine (T_4) and triidothyronine (T_3). A depressed level of thyroid activity reduces the SHBG. The proportion of the free testosterone is thus increased. Despite normale overall androgen values, there is an increase in the free active androgen fraction. It can penetrate the cell wall and occupy the cytosomal androgen receptor. This is possibly due to the connection between hirsutism and hypothyroidism.

Hypergonadotropic amenorrhea in a sexually mature woman represents a particular challenge to endocrinologists. It is especially worthy to mention that we succeeded in restoring the ovarial function in 3 of our patients despite the presence of hypergonadotropism (of the WHO III type). Thorough endocrinological examination revealed the additional existence of a hypothyroid metabolism in all three. After unsuccessful hormone treatment, the women hat to undergo a thyroid-substitution therapy with Thyroxin. After 4–8 weeks of treatment, normogonadotropy was achieved, with follicle maturation and ovulation. The connection between hypergonadotropism and a hypothyroid metabolism can be discussed. A scientific explanation has not been found yet.

Both in the case of secondary amenorrhea and hisutism, the unexplained forms that are hormonally apparently normal still play an important role. By the exact determination of the thyroidogenic reaction forms, the number of these so-calles "essential" forms of hirsutism and also of amenorrhea can be reduced.

Abstract

In 50 secondary amenorrheic patients the TRH-test was performed during an untreated peroid. Normal results were found in 26 times; in 24 patients a hypothyroid reaction type was confirmed. These results seem to prove the interaction between thyroid and sex hormones. After a short peroid of thyroxin treatment normal menses started in five cases. In three times a hypergonadotropic amenorrhea corresponding to WHO III was confirmed in correlation with a hypothyroid reaction type. After thyroxin treatment there was a normalisation of the gonadotropins and subsequently ovulation was observed after clomifen treatment. Further results: Five hypothyroid patients showed hirsutism with normal values for androgens. In two cases thyroxin treatment reduced complaints such as abnormal hair growth.

References

[1] Gooren, L. M., E. A. van der Veen, H. an Kessel, et al.: The effect of endogenous and exogenous gonadotropin-releasing hormone on the prolactin response to TRH. Clin. Endocrinol. 20 (1984) 281–288.

[2] Larochelle, F. F., M. E. Freeman: Superimposition of thyroid hormone regulation on gonadotropin secretion. Endocrinology 95 (1974) 379–386.

[3] Leyendecker, G., L. Wildt, E. J. Plotz: Die hypothalamische Ovarialinsuffizienz. Gynäkologe 14 (1981) 84–103.

[4] Rezai, P., F. Nora: Triplet gestation following thyroid replacement in a patient with infertillity hyperprolactinaemia, and enlarged sella secondary to hypothyroidism. Fertil. Steril. 42 (1984) 486–488.

Value of an immunoradiometric assay for thyrotropin in non-thyroidal illness

G. Caldwell, S. M. Gow, A. Elder, G. M. Bell, V. M. Sweeting, G. J. Beckett, J. Seth, A. D. Toft

Thyroid dysfunction is suspected in a wide range of clinical settings and consequently requests for thyroid function tests constitute an important part of the workload of any Clinical Chemistry Department. However, acute and chronic non-thyroidal illness can have profound effects on the results of thyroid function tests, seen usually as low thyroid hormone levels, an increase in reverse T_3 and some blunting of the TRH test [1, 2, 4].

We conducted a study to assess the value of radioimmunoassays (RIA) for total thyroxine (TT_4), total triiodothyronine (TT_3), free thyroxine (fT_4), free triiodothyronine (fT_3) and an immunoradiometric assay (IRMA) for thyrotropin as a screening test in the presence of non-thyroidal illness. In-house RIAs were used for TT_4 and TT_3, the Amersham kit for fT_4, the Beckton-Dickinson kit for fT_3 and the Boots-Celltech IRMA for TSH.

We have previously shown that the highly sensitive and specific IRMA for TSH can replace a TRH test in out-patients at diagnosis [3]. The first group of patients studied was 264 acute admisssions to a general medical unit. There were 137 males and 127 females, ages 16 – 96 years. Thyroid dysfunction was not identified in their discharge summaries, none had a goitre and none was being treated for thyroid dysfunction.

The principal discharge diagnoses were cardio- and cerebro-vascular 39%, respiratory 19%, gastrointestinal and liver 8%, diabetes and endocrine 6%, renal 4% and other 15%. A high proportion of abnormal low thyroid hormone results were recorded varying from 8% with TT_4 to 49% with fT_3 (tab. 1). A few elevated thyroid hormone levels were noted (< 1%). Only 1% of TSH (IRMA) levels were low but 4% of levels were elevated. Inappropriately high TSH levels have been recorded in non-thyroidal illness but only in the recovery phase of severe acute illness and we believe that these were truly elevated TSH levels consistent with subclinical hypothyroidism. TRH tests were conducted in 74 of these patients and analysed by RIA, 72 tests were normal and in all these patients detectable basal TSH (IRMA) levels were found. In two moribund patients, subnormal TRH tests (increment of < 1 mU/l at 20 minutes) were recorded with

Thyrotropin

Table 1 The number of patients with abnormal thyroid function tests

	Group I (264 patients)		Group II (35 patients)	
Result	Low	High	Low	High
T_4	21 (8%)	3 (0.1%)	15 (43%)	0 (–)
FT_4	40 (15%)	2 (< 0.1%)	24 (69%)	0 (–)
T_3	50 (19%)	0 –	10 (29%)	0 (–)
FT_3	128 (49%)	2 (< 0.1%)	25 (71%)	0 (–)
TSH IRMA	3 (1%)*	15 (6%)	0 (–)	1 (3%)

* undetectable

detectable basal TSH (IRMA) levels. Thyroid hormone levels were normal or low in these patients.

We also studied 35 patients, treated by haemodialysis for chronic renal failure. There were 15 males and 20 females, ages 14–70 years. Again, low thyroid hormone levels were common, ranging from 29% with TT_3 to 72% with free T_3, whereas an abnormally high TSH (IRMA) level was found in only one patient.

In conclusion, the rapid, highly sensitive and specific immunoradiometric assay for TSH gives a low false positive rate in clinically euthyroid patients with acute and chronic non-thyroidal illness and is the most suitable initial investigation for suspected thyroid dysfunction in the presence of nonthyroidal illness.

References

[1] Chopra, I. J., J. M. Hersham, W. M. Pardridge, et al.: Thyroid function in non thyroidal illness. Ann. Intern. Med. **98** (1983) 946–957.

[2] Wenzel, K. W., R. Ekins, T. Jackson: Thyroxine analogne assays in clinical medicine. Lancet II (1985) 181–182.

[3] Seth, J., H. A. Kellett, G. Caldwell, et al.: A sensitive immunoradiometric assay for serum thyroid stimulating hormone: A replacement for the thyrotropin releasing hormone test. Br. Med. J. II (1984) 1334–1336.

[4] Bacci, V., G. C. Schusser, T. B. Kaplan: The relationship between serum triiodothyronine and thyrotropin during systemic illness. J. Clin. Endocrinol. Metab. **54** (1982) 1229–1235.

IV TSH in clinical diagnostics

Thyrotropin – clinical relevance of sensitive TSH-assays

P. Pfannenstiel, N. Panitz, E. Rummeny

During the last 25 years there have been major advances in laboratory analysis and assays for both the total and free forms of thyroxine (T4) and triiodothyronine (T3). Also thyroid stimulating hormone (TSH) has become essential to the investigations of thyroid dysfunction [5, 18, 31, 35, 36, 44]. The aim of this clinical overview is to summarize the role of thyrotropin in diagnosis of thyroid disorders including our own recent data.

A few pathophysiological data will be recalled first: The maintenance of normal T3 and T4 secretion and an euthyroid metabolic state depends upon normal release from the hypothalamus of thyrotropin releasing hormone (TRH) and normal responsiveness of the anterior pituitary thyrotrophs to both the stimulatory action of TRH and the inhibitory effect of elevated thyroid hormone levels (fig. 1). TSH plays a central role in controlling the hypothalamic-pituitary-thyroid axis [25, 37, 38, 43, 48].

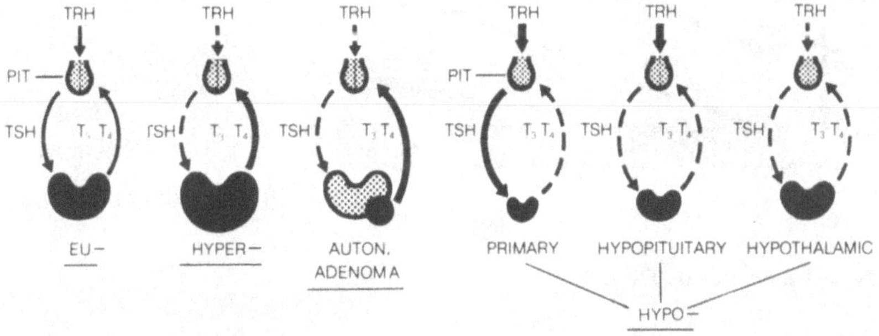

Fig. 1 The interrelationship of the hypothalamus, pituitary and thyroid glands in the most common defects of the thyroid function.

In euthyroid states T3 and T4 are within normal limits. In hyperthyroidism T3 and T4 are elevated and TSH is decreased in both Graves' disease and toxic adenoma. Thyroid hormone concentrations are decreased in hypothyroidism, but in primary hypothyroidism TSH is elevated and in secondary hypothyroidism (due to pituitary or hypothalamic disease) it is decreased.

Thyrotropin

A reduction of circulating thyroid hormones causes a rise in serum TSH-concentrations, while an increase of serum-T3 and serum-T4 is followed by suppression of TSH secretion except for the rare TSH-secreting tumors [21].

TSH measurements reflect the cellular and metabolic impact of free thyroid hormones which cannot always be interpreted from steady-state free thyroid hormone determinations. Thus, the serum TSH-determination provides a more precise evaluation of thyroid function.

For many years thyroidologists were looking for sensitive TSH-measurements enabling us to differentiate between true normal, suppressed and elevated TSH levels in serum [4, 39, 40, 45]. From a physiological viewpoint and from the experiences with TRH-tests (fig. 2), this was expected to be more sensitive for the differentiation of euthyroidism, hyperthyroidism and hypothyroidism than the determination of total or free T4 and/or total or free T3 serum levels. Most previous sensitive TSH-assays were cumbersome and time consuming and could not be employed on a routine basis.

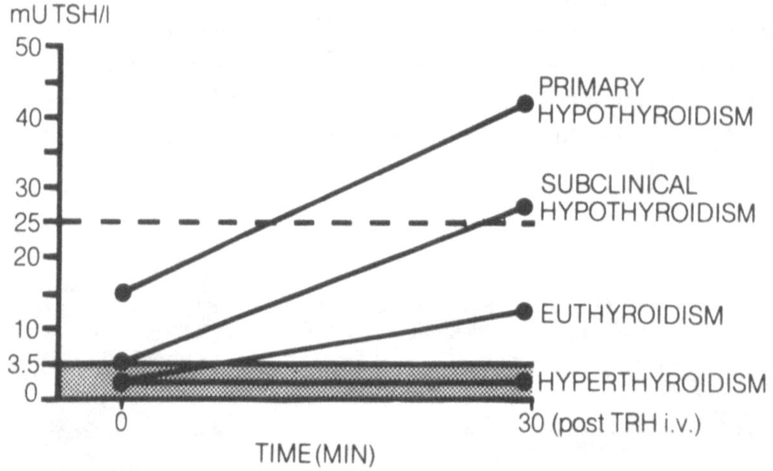

Fig. 2 Typical responses to TRH.

We, therefore, became interested in a sensitive TSH-IRMA* two years ago, attracted by the claim, that by using this assay one could separate hyperthyroid and euthyroid patients without a TRH stimulation test [18, 19, 21, 22]. We now have evidence, as do many other investigators, that the true basal values of TSH in untreated thyrotoxicosis are generally less than 0.1 mU/l serum [1, 2, 6, 8, 10, 13, 17, 19, 28–30, 34, 42, 50].

* SUCROSEP-TM-TSH-IRMA by Boots-Celltech, England is distributed in Germany by Röhm-Pharma GmbH, Weiterstadt, FRG.

The higher sensitivity and speed of the IRMA-technique is due to the use of excess reagents, while the higher specifity is related to the combination of two distinct anti-TSH monoclonal antibodies. Similar results have been recently reported using other methods such as immunochemiluminometric assay [47] or an enzyme-amplified assay [32].

The much higher sensitivity of these assays with respect to conventional RIA methods, suggested the possibility that the basal measurement of TSH alone often might allow to distinguish between suppressed, elevated and normal TSH values without the need of a TRH stimulation.

In this present report we will summarize our experience during the last two years using the TSH-IRMA.

Our over-all conclusions are that the TSH-IRMA is accurate and highly sensitive, with an excellent intra- and interassay precision, displaying a wide working range from 0.02 to over 200 mU TSH/l serum.

The TSH-IRMA method has a very high sensitivity. Detectable serum TSH-concentrations are found in almost all normal subjects by the IRMA-technique, but in only about 75% by the RIA-technique [22]. The discrimination of TSH-changes to TRH-stimulation is much more distinct using TSH-IRMA tests as compared to TSH-RIA-tests.

Since the TRH-test involves a certain amount of physician's time, a good deal of patients and nursing time, and no small expense for synthetic TRH and the two TSH determinations before and after stimulation, we decided to determine in which situations the TRH test may be redundant for excluding patients with thyrotoxicosis and for identifying those who need further work-up.

First, we correlated the basal TSH values in 170 patients (140 women and 30 men) with the final clinical diagnosis established by special history, physical examination and evaluating all available data such as laboratory tests, ultrasonography and/or radionuclide scanning of the thyroid gland.

The data (tab. 1) revealed, that in untreated patients the stimulated TSH values are strongly related to the result of the sensitive TSH measurements.

The following statements can be derived from more than 30000 measurements of TSH by the sensitive IRMA-technique during the last two years as well as from our recent evaluation (tab. 1) and our overall clinical experience:

- True basal TSH values above 0.3 mU/l serum are able to predict a positive TSH response to TRH stimulation (which we routinely performed with 400 µg TRH intravenously). There is a good correlation between basal TSH concentrations and the pituitary TSH reserve. A normal TSH response to TRH was observed in virtually all patients with detectable basal serum TSH.

Table 1 Basal TSH values (mU/l) in patients with euthyroidism, under levothyroxine medication, with manifest or latent hyperthyroidism, manifest or latent hypothyroidism and in patients after iodine contamination and clinical euthyroidism

diagnosis		hyperth. ≤ 0.1	grey zone > 0.1 ≤ 0.3	euthyr. > 0.3 ≤ 3.5	hypoth. > 3.5	n
euthyroid		5	10	18	1	34
	under L-T_4	32	18	10	–	60
hyperthyroid	manifest	14	5	1	–	20
	latent	26	7	4	–	37
hypothyroid	manifest	–	–	–	14	14
	latent	–	–	1	1	2
euthyroid	iodine-contamin.	1	2	–	–	3
n		78	42	34	16	170

- The normal range for the sensitive TSH assay is 0.3 to 3.5 mU TSH/l serum for euthyroid persons. TSH-values in this range suggest an euthyroid metabolic condition, also in patients where total T4-values are elevated, for instance, in states of altered thyroxine binding capacity of the serum.
- Only very few thyroid patients have suppressed TSH values of 0.1 to 0.3 mU TSH/l serum. These borderline low TSH values require a thyroid hormone determination and more important a TRH test to be performed to dinstinguish euthyroidism and hyperthyroidism.
- In about 50% of these cases no TSH response to TRH stimulation was found. Not all causes are known. In these patients not only a TRH stimulation test but, also thyroid scanning before and, if necessary, after suppression with thyroid hormones is still indicated to demask a possible cause of this situation, the compensatory autonomy of the thyroid gland, which is very common in endemic iodine deficient goiter areas.
- If these patients, however, do not have any clinical symptoms as well as normal (F)T3 and (F)T4 values, the borderline biochemical laboratory data of latent hyperthyroidism should not always be "treated", since TSH-concentrations were reported as "undetectable" not only for hyperthyroid patients, but also for a considerable portion of euthyroid subjects. Consequently confirming a hyperthyroid hormone situation in borderline cases, one has to look at the TSH response to TRH-stimulation [33].
- Basal TSH values below 0.1 mU/l serum are associated with negative TRH tests in untreated patients with hyperthyroidism, either due to thyroidal

autonomy or Graves' disease. The data obtained is as expected: very low basal TSH values, no response to TRH, elevated (F)T4 and especially elevated (F)T3 values. However, in 3% of suppressed basal TSH-values still a slight increase of TSH after TRH-stimulation with an increase of basal TSH of more than 1.5 mU/l was found (tab. 2).

Table 2 Basal TSH value (mU/l) in correlation to the result of the TSH response after TRH stimulation

n = 1098	hyperthyroid		grey zone		euthyroid		hypothyroid	
	⩽ 0.1		> 0.1	⩽ 0.3	> 0.3	⩽ 3.5	> 3.5	
TRH-test	+	–	+	–	+	–	+	–
patient numbers	6	198 97%	38	47 55%	717 99%	4	88	
valuation	f.p.	r.p.			r.p.	f.n.	r.p.	f.p.

+ = positive TSH result; – = negative TSH result; f.p. = falsely positive; r.p. = right positive; f.n. = falsely negative; r.n. = right negative.

- Patients on sufficient suppressive thyroid hormone replacement therapy generally also exhibit TSH concentrations below 0.1 mU/l serum and do not respond to TRH stimulation. The (F)T4 and (F)T3 values are normal or borderline high. Therefore, in patients with TSH-values below an arbitrary cut-off of 0.1 mU/l serum the determination of (F)T4 or (F)T3 levels should follow, so that either hyperthyroidism or suppressed thyrotropic activity caused by replacement therapy can be categorized.
- Also in cases of sek. (hypopituitary) and tert. (hypothalamic) hypothyroidis, low TSH-values (0.3 – 3.5) are expected. Therefore the determination of (F)T4 or (F)T3 levels and TRH-Stimulation is necessary for differentiation.
- In cases of primary hypothyroidism, the basal TSH values are elevated with further increase after TRH stimulation. With unequivocally raised TSH values over 10 mU/l serum a TRH test is not necessary, but the severity of the disease should be assessed by measuring thyroid hormones.
- In contrast, we all have little experience with latent hypothyroidism, which is difficult to define. With borderline high TSH values over 3.5 mU/l a TRH test may be necessary to diagnose such subclinical hypothyroidism with normal or even elevated thyroid hormone levels.

Since in patients undergoing treatment no clear-cut correlation could be made during follow-up studies, we retrospectively investigated the response of TSH to stimulation with TRH in 1098 out-patients. All had determinations of FT3, FT4 as well as a TRH test. Also in all patients ultrasonography and/or radionuclide scanning of the thyroid gland was performed.

The clinical diagnosis was made by asking the patient appropriate questions, by carefully examining the patient and by applying the previously mentioned diagnostic tests.

Between the clinical diagnosis and the result of the determination of the basal TSH values in the serum, no clear-cut correlation was possible. Therefore, we investigated whether a basal TSH result determined by the TSH-IRMA is a reliable predictor of the response to TRH (tab. 2).

- The data indicated that the expected responses of TSH after TRH stimulation can be predicted in almost all cases by the basal TSH concentration. Only in 0.6% of patients with normal TSH-values no response of TSH was found, i. e. 4 false negative cases.
- In none of the cases with normal basal TSH-values the TSH response to TRH was exaggerated as seen in patients with latent hypothyroidism.
- Only borderline low TSH values from 0.1 to 0.3 mU/l require – as previously mentioned – a TRH test to distinguish euthyroidism and hyperthyroidism. In this "grey zone" a positive TRH test may be expected in 50% of the cases. Even in 3% of TSH-values smaller than 0.1 mU/l a slight increase of TSH after TRH-stimulation was observed, i. e. 6 "false positive" cases.
- With borderline high TSH values over 3.5 mU/l serum a TRH test may also be necessary to define the so called subclinical hypothyroidism.
- The TSH-IRMA with these cut-off limits, has a sensitivity of 98.5% and a specifity of 99.1%, the requirements of a screening test. Therefore, a basal TSH result determined by sensitive IRMA techniques is in 96% of the cases a reliable predictor of the TSH response to TRH.

It follows, that when an excess or deficiency in thyroid hormone production occurs, the TSH-IRMA surpasses all previously used methods in thyroid hormone determination for screening, by distinguishing between patients at the lower end of normal and those with hyperthyroidism [12, 14–16].

We believe that the approach to thyroid function testing strategy now has to change. We propose a new strategy shown in figure 3 and as others, we are using this strategy with a TSH-IRMA as a first-line thyroid function test in our laboratory [9, 12, 24, 26–29, 41, 42, 46].

The possibility of replacing the TRH-stimulation test with a highly sensitive TSH assay has been raised by many investigators, given that the later is less expensive, less time consuming and certainly more convenient to the patient [1, 2, 5, 8–12, 14–16, 18, 20, 22–24, 26–30, 32, 33, 35, 38, 41, 42, 45–47].

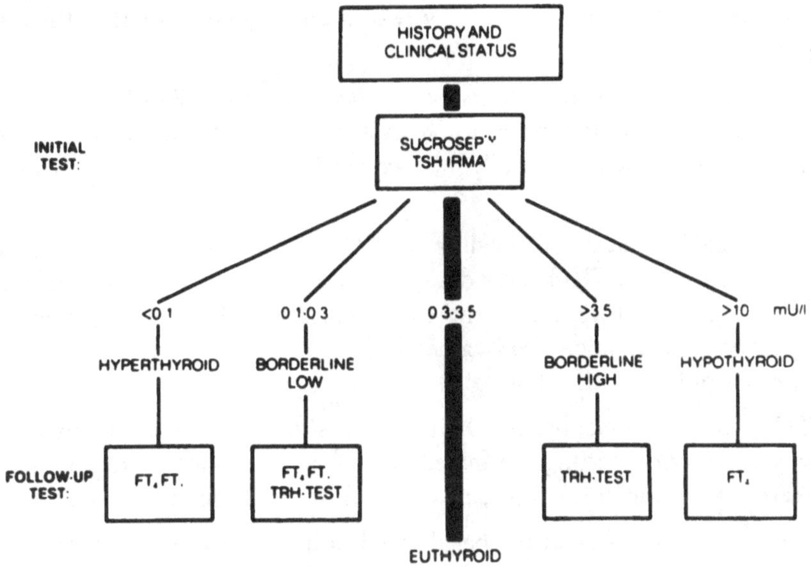

Fig. 3 Proposed strategy for diagnosis of thyroid disease based on TSH IRMA as a first-line test.

This approach provides an appropriate balance between clinical findings and a basic step-by-step work-up of laboratory tests. It should especially help general practioners to diagnose patients with suspected thyroid diseases or even more important, to exclude thyroid dysfunction. Only in elderly patients compensated thyroidal autonomy might be overseen by this approach.

Whether what we and others have shown so far remains valid in a wider context, e. g. for elderly or hospitalized patients or those with severe non-thyroidal illnesses or low T4- or low T3-syndroms, can only be determined by further studies. In the outpatient framework, however, we believe it is time to reexamine the way in which thyroid dysfunction is diagnosed, since basal TSH measurements by IRMA categorize nearly all functional situations in clinical diagnosis.

In our experience, the sensitive TSH assay also proved to be useful in monitoring thyroid replacement therapy, in fine tuning hormone dosage in goiter treatment, in post-operative prophylaxis, suppressive therapy of thyroid carcinoma and in monitoring antithyroid drug therapy in thyrotoxicosis [5, 20, 49].

However, we would like to stress that a complete clinical information is still needed in interpreting TSH results in patients undergoing treatment. Also, in apparent remission from antithyroid drugs, caution is necessary since both may have low TSH values. This caution is advised especially for follow-up studies of treated thyrotoxic patients with normal or low circulating thyroid hormones, since the suppression of the thyrotropic function may result in undetectable TSH levels by IRMA tests, even several weeks after remission of the disease took place.

In conclusion: we and many others believe, that the TSH-IRMA is an important addition to our current laboratory tests for a more economical approach to evaluate thyroid function. The TSH has the following potentials in diagnosis and treatment:

- A basal TSH result determined by the IRMA-technique is a reliable predictor of the response to TRH. Our data, and those of others, suggest that it is no longer necessary to perform the timeconsuming TRH test in patients with hyperthyroidism, since TSH-values below 0.1 mU/l serum are indicative of hyperthyroidism with a high probability.
- TSH determinations by the IRMA-Test should become the first step in thyroid function testing, followed by TRH-tests and/or thyroid hormone determinations in some diseases, i. e. in those with questionable results.
- The strategy of measuring basal TSH followed by total or free thyroid hormones is more economical than an approach using thyroid hormone determinations as a first line test of thyroid function.
- The TSH IRMA-Test proved also to be useful in monitoring medical treatment of thyroid diseases.

Therefore, we consider the sensitive TSH IRMA as an excellent first line test, both for excluding patients with thyrotoxicosis and for identifying those who need further work-up. Thus, cost-benefit and reliability considerations recommend this assay as a "screening test", to be followed by TRH-stimulation only in borderline cases.

Summary

Since we now have evidence that the true basal TSH values determined by sensitive TSH-IRMA tests in untreated thyreotoxicosis are generally less than 0.1 mU/l serum, we correlated the basal TSH values in 170 patients (140 women and 30 men) with the final clinical diagnosis. The data revealed that in untreated patients the stimulated TSH values are strongly related to the result of the sentitive TSH basal measurements. Since, however, in patients under treatment no clear-cut correlation could be made during follow-up studies, we investigated retrospectively the response of TSH to stimulation with TRH in 1098 patients. The most important result was that TSH values in the "new" normal range of 0.3 – 3.5 mU/l serum were sufficient to define euthyroidism. There was no need to perform further thyroid hormone measurements. TSH values below an arbitrary cut-off of 0.1 mU/l should be followed by (F)T4 or (F)T3 to categorize either hyperthyroidism or suppressed thyrotropic activity caused by replacement therapy. Borderline low TSH values of 0.1 – 0.3 mU/l require a thyroid hormone determination or a TRH test to be carried out to distinguish euthyroidism and hyperthyroidism. Clinical hypothyroidism patients with TSH-levels < 0,2 require determination of (F)T3, (F)T4 and a TRH-Test to rule out or differentiate the hypopituitary of hypothalamic hypothyroidism. With borderline high TSH values over 3.5 mU/l a TRH test may be necessary to define sublinical hypothyroidism. With unequivocally raised TSH values over 10 mU/l a TRH test is not necessary, but the severity of the disease should be assessed by measuring thyroid hormones.

These cut-off limits with a sensitivity of 98.5% and a specifity of 99.1% fulfill the requirements of a screening test. Therefore, a basal TSH result determined by sensitive IRMA-techniques is in 96% of the cases a reliable predictor of the TSH response to TRH. The strategy of measuring first TSH by sensitive assays, followed by total or free thyroid hormones is more economical than an approach using thyroid hormone determinations or the time-consuming TRH test as first-line tests. The sensitive TSH assay also proved to be useful in monitoring thyroid replacement therapy, in fine tuning hormone dosage in goiter treatment, in post-operative prophylaxis, in suppressive therapy of thyroid carcinoma and in monitoring anti-thyroid drug therapy in thyrotoxicosis. However, in all instances a good clinical information is still needed in interpreting TSH results on primary or on follow-up examinations of patients.

References

[1] Alexander, W. D., D. J. Kerr, M. M. Ferguson: First-line test of thyroid function. Lancet *II* (1984) 647.

[2] Allen, K. R., D. Watson: Thyrotropin as the initial screening test for thyroid disease. Clin. Chem. **30** (1984) 503.

[3] Bernutz, C., K. Horn, H. König, et al.: Advantages of sensitive assays for thyrotropin in the diagnosis of thyroid disorders. J. Clin. Chem. Clin. Biochem. **23** (1985) 851 – 865.

[4] Bitensky, L., J. Aleghband-Zadeh, J. Chayen: Studies on thyroid stimulating hormone and the long acting thyroid stimulating hormone. Clin. Endocrinol. **3** (1974) 363 – 374.

[5] Börner, W., J. Hermann, M. Hüfner, et al. (eds.): Wertigkeit von in-vitro-Testverfahren zur Schilddrüsendiagnostik. Akt. Endokr. Stoffw. **5** (Suppl. 1) (1984) 1 – 134.

[6] Böttger, I., W. Pabst, R. Senekowitsch, et al.: Performance of two new solid-phase ligand assays for TSH using monoclonal antibodies. Nuc. Med. Comm. **6** (1985) 195.

[7] Bretzel, R., K. F. Federlin: Neuer TSH-Radioimmunoassay als Optimierungshilfe einer Suppressionstherapie mit L-Thyroxin bei Patienten mit verschiedenen Schilddrüsenerkrankungen. Klin. Wochenschr. Suppl. IV (1985) 203.

[8] Mc Bride, J. H., R. V. Thibeault, D. O. Rodgerson: Thyrotropin as measured by a sensitive immunoradiometric assay. Clin. Chem. **31** (1985) 1865 – 1867.

[9] Caldwell, G., H. A. Keller, S. M. Gow, et al.: A new strategy for thyroid function testing. Lancet II (1985) 1117 – 1119.

[10] Cobb, W. E., R. P. Lamperton, I. M. D. Jackson: Use of a rapid sensitive immunoradiometric assay for thyrotropin to distinguish normal from hyperthyroid subjects. Clin. Chem. **30** (1984) 1558.

[11] Durham, A. P.: The upper limit of normal for thyreotropin is 3 or 4 milli – int units/l. Clin. Chem. **31** (1985) 296 – 298.

[12] Joseph, K.: Erstdiagnostik und Verlaufskontrolle bei Schilddrüsenfunktionsstörungen mit der immunoradiometrischen TSH-Bestimmung. Nuc. Compact **16** (1985) 240 – 254.

[13] Joseph, K.: TSH by immunoradiometric assay as a screening test for thyroid disease. Med. Lab. **14** (1985) 3 – 19.

[14] Kerr, D. J., W. D. Alexander: Is the TRH test usually necessary? Lancet II **17** (1984) 1161.

[15] Kirkegaard, C., S. D. Slater, A. M. Ried, et al.: A sensitive immunoradiometric assay for serum thyroid stimulating hormone. Br. Med. J. **290** (1985) 69.

[16] Kirkegaard, C., C. Bregengard: Is the TRH test necessary? Lancet **26** (1985) 222.

[17] Klinger, W., P. Ball: Die Bestimmung des Thyreotropin (TSH) im Serum mit einer sensitiven immunometrischen Methode. Ärztl. Lab. **31** (1985) 219 – 223.

[18] Mahlstedt, J.: Alleinige Aussagekraft der radioimmunologischen TSH-Bestimmung. Nucl. Med. **21** (1982) 164 – 168.

[19] Mahlstedt, J., A. Hotze: Erste Erfahrungen mit einem ultrasensitiven TSH-Assay. Nuc. Compact **16** (1985) 72 – 76.

[20] Mardell, R. J., T. R. Gamlen, M. R. J. Winton: High sensitivity assay of thyroid stimulating hormone in patients receiving thyroxine for primary hyperthyroidism and thyroid carcinoma. Br. Med. J. **190** (1985) 355.

[21] Morley, J. E.: Neuroendocrine control of thyrotropic secretion. Endocr. Rev. 2 (1981) 396 – 434.

[22] Mortino, E., G. Bambini, L. Bartalena, et al.: Human serum thyrotropin measurement by ultrasensitive immunometric assay as a first-line test in the evaluation of thyroid function. Clin. Endocrunol. **24** (1986) 141 – 148.

[23] Panitz, N.: A german evaluation of a TSH-IRMA. In: A simple sensitive TSH immunoradiometric assay for the discrimination of thyroid function." Proc. Int. Symp. Edinburgh, March 1984.

[24] Panitz, N., E. Rummeny, P. Pfannenstiel: Thyreotropes Hormon im Serum – klinische Beurteilung sogenannter "ultrasensitiver" TSH-Assays. Int. Welt (in press).

[25] Pfannenstiel, P.: Strategy of thyroid function tests with special reference to measurements of serum TSH. In: Radioimmunoassay of hormones, proteins and enzymes, pp. 114 – 123. Proc. Int. Symp., Gardone, Riviera, May 8 – 10, 1980 (A. Albertini, ed.). Excerpta Medica, Amsterdam – Oxford – Princeton 1980.

[26] Pfannenstiel, P., N. Panitz: Clinical evaluation of a sensitive TSH-IRMA in the assessment of thyroid dysfunction. Proc. Symp. in conjunction with the 4th Joint Meeting of the Brit. Endoc. Soc., Oxford, March 1985.

[27] Pfannenstiel, P.: Significance of supersensitive TSH-determinations and its relationship to free T4 and free T3. Nuc. Compact **16** (1985) 396 – 398.

[28] Pfannenstiel, P., N. Panitz: Erste Erfahrungen mit einem hochsensitiven immunometrischen TSH-Assay zur Diagnostik von Schilddrüsenfunktionsstörungen. Nuklearmediziner **2** (1985) 185 – 189.

[29] Pfannenstiel, P., N. Panitz: Erfahrung mit der Bestimmung von FT3 und FT4 sowie einem supersensitiven TSH-Assay bei latenten Schilddrüsenkrankheiten. In: Freie Schilddrüsenhormone in der klinischen Diagnostik (O. Eber, W. Langsteger, eds.), pp. 159 – 180. Deutscher Ärzteverlag, Köln 1985.

[30] Pinchera, A., E. Martino, L. Bartalena, et al.: Radioimmunoassay utilization in the assessment of thyroid status. In: Cost-Benefit and Predicting Values of Radioimmunoassays. A. Albertini, R. P. Ekins, K. S. Galen, eds.), pp. 151 – 160. Elsevier Science Publishers B. B., Amsterdam 1984.

[31] Reinwein, D., G. Benker: Stufendiagnostik "Schilddrüse" – epidemiologische und methodische Voraussetzungen, Internist **26** (1985) 155.

[32] Roddis, M. J., J. M. Burrin, A. Johanssen, et al.: Serum thyrotropin: A first-line discriminatory test of thyroid function. Lancet I (1985) 227 – 278.

[33] Schmidt, R., K. Michl, R. Lipecky, et al.: Validity of the TRH-Test in the diagnosis of thyroid disease using a hypersensitive TSH methodology. Acta Endocrinol. **111**, Suppl. 274 (1986)36 – 37.

[34] Schmidt, R., K. Michl: Comparison of new assays for the estimation of thyrotropin in serum using monoclonal antibodes. J. Clin. Chem. Biochem. **23** (1985) 627.

[35] Seidel, Ch., D. Ziegelitz, K. Sydow, et al.: TSH-Basiswerte in der Diagnostik von Schilddrüsenerkrankungen. Dt. Gesundheitswesen **34** (1979) 2029.

[36] Seidel, Ch., D. Ziegelitz, J. Rademacher, et al.: Basale TSH-Konzentrationen bei gesunden Personen. Nuc. Compact. **11** (1980) 125 – 129.

[37] Seidel, Ch., G. Heller, W. Rohde: Methodische Vergleiche zur radioimmunologischen Bestimmung basaler TSH-Spiegel im Serum. Endokrinologie **78** (1981) 205 – 218.

[38] Seidel, Ch., D. Ziegelitz, H.-J. Correns: Zur klinischen Eingruppierung supprimierter und niedrignormaler TSH-Basalspiegel bei Euthyreose. Nuc. Compact **12** (1981) 2 – 7.

[39] Seidel, Ch., D. Ziegelitz, A. Weber, et al.: Zum klinischen Stellenwert eines empfindlichen TSH-RIA. Endokrinologie **80** (1982) 181.

[40] Seidel, Ch., H. J. Correns: Optimization of incubation time for precise and sensitive measurement of serum TSH by radioimmunoassay. Nuc. Compact **14** (1983) 10 – 16.

[41] Semple, A., S. D. Slater, A. M. Ried, et al.: A sensitive immunoradioimetric assay for serum thyroid stimulating hormone. Br. Med. J. **290** (1985) 69.

[42] Seth, H., H. A. Kellet, G. Caldwell, et al.: A sensitive radioimmunometric assay for serum thyroid stimulating hormone: A replacement for the thyrotropin releasing hormone test? Br. Med. J. **289** (1984) 1334.

[43] Stahl, T. J.: Radioimmunoassay and the hormones of thyroid function. Semin. Nucl. Med. **5** (1975) 221 – 246.

[44] Staub, J. J.: Der TRH-Test: Seine Bedeutung für die Praxis. Schweiz. Rundschau Med. (Praxis) **662** (1977) 33 – 36.

[45] Wehrmann, R. E., H. A. Rubinstein, B. C. Nisula: A sensitive convenient radioimmunoassay procedure, which demonstrates that serum TSH is suppressed below the normal range in thyrotropic patients. Endocr. Res. Comm. **6** (1977) 249 – 255.

[46] Wehrmann, R. E., H. A. Rubinstein, M. Pugeat, et al.: Extended clinical utility of a sensitive and reliable radioimmunoassay of thyroid-stimulating hormone. Med. J. **76** (1983) 969.

[47] Weeks, I., M. Sturgess, K. Siddle, et al.: A high sensitivity immunochemilumimetric assay for human thyrotropin. Clin. Endocrinol. (Oxf.) **20** (1984) 489 – 495.

[48] Wenzel, K. W.: Überlegenheit des TRH-Testes als rationelle und rationale Schilddrüsendiagnostik. Nuklearmedizin 2 (1979) 37 – 39.

[49] Wilber, J.: Regulation of TSH release: Clinical implications of replacing FT4 and FT3 estimations by ultrasensitive TSH assays. Nuc. Compact **16** (1985) 393 – 395.

[50] Wood, W. G., D. Waller, U. Hantke: An evaluation of six solid-phase thyrotropin (TSH) kits. J. Clin. Chem. Clin. Biochem. **23** (1985) 461 – 471.

TSH response to TRH as a function of basal serum TSH – new aspects in pituitary-thyroid regulation

I. G. Böttger, H. W. Pabst, G. Bienhaus, Ch. Seidel

Introduction

Early studies of the relationship between basal and TRH-induced TSH serum concentrations revealed a positive yet not very close correlation on high dose oral administration of TRH [3, 6]. Following technical improvement of radioimmunological TSH determination by increasing assay sensitivity and precision such a positive correlation of basal and TRH-stimulated TSH could also be demonstrated by i. v. administration of 500 µg of the releasing hormone [11]. This finding could be confirmed by use of an even lower i. v. dose of 200 µg TRH.

A further improvement of the TSH assay enabled for the first time a discrimination between suppressed and normal TSH concentrations being separated by a "gray zone". Furthermore, it could be shown that, in general, suppressed basal TSH levels correlated with a suppressed TSH response following i. v. administration of 200 µg TRH (TSH < 0.2 mU/l) only in a few cases reaching detectable concentrations (< 1.0 mU/l). Normal basal TSH levels, however, were associated with stimulated concentrations between 2.5 and 25 mU/l. For the latter range a linear correlation and a respective regression equation was calculated which, however, did not continue into the range of subnormal, yet still detectable basal TSH levels being consistent with the above mentioned "gray zone" [14]. These findings were fully confirmed by other authors [8].

During the last three years a new generation of supersensitive TSH assays has been developed by combination of IRMA and monoclonal antibody technology [10] which have been shown to influence thyroid routine in vitro diagnostics [1, 2, 4] by superior precision and specificity besides clearly increased sensitivity [5, 7, 9]. The aim of this study was to reevaluate the relationship between basal and TRH-stimulated TSH concentrations by use of one of these new supersensitive TSH IRMAs.

Thyrotropin

Patients and methods

All TRH tests of a radioimmunological-radiochemical laboratory being performed within a period of six weeks were reviewed retrospectively. In general, patients (n = 761) originated from the Nuclear Medicine Clinic and Policlinic, occasionally also from other Clinics of the Technical University of Munich. There was no dominance of a certain age range in either sex group or basal TSH range. The TRH tests were performed by i. v. administration of 200 µg TRH the second blood sample being drawn 30 min p. i. TSH serum concentrations (n = 1522) were determined by use of a supersensitive TSH IRMA, TSH-IRMAclon®, Henning-Berlin GmbH, in duplicates in a total of 18 assays. Logarithmic transformation of TSH concentrations was achieved by means of a modified Curve Fitter Program (P. K. Warme, Interactive Microware) with an Apple II^R computer. The lower detection limit (B_0 + 3 s) was found to be 0.03 mU/l, yet the studies were based upon a stable lower detection limit derived from all individual assays (n = 18) of 0.07 mU/l.

Results

The relationship of basal and corresponding TRH-induced TSH levels in patients regardless of age, sex, diagnosis and treatment is depicted in figure 1. 78 of the 761 TRH tests (10.8%) revealed basal TSH levels beneath 0.07 mU/l, the TSH response being also suppressed in 51 cases (65.4%). In 25 instances TRH-induced TSH was in the range of 0.07 – 0.20 mU/l and in two other cases at 0.3 and 0.8 mU/l.

Before mathematical work-up of the whole group the above mentioned 78 pairs with basal TSH levels < 0.07 as well as another 14 TRH tests (1.8%) with basal TSH > 20 mU/l (range 20 – 70 mU/l), too small a group, were eliminated. Therefore, 669 TRH tests (87.9%) non selected in respect to the basal TSH range of 0.07 – 20 mU/l and to the range of TRH-stimulated TSH of 0.08 – 100 mU/l, remained for calculations. As also demonstrated by figure 1 the relationship between basal and TRH-induced TSH levels would be described only insufficiently by applying a linear correlation. Therefore, in order to obtain a mean curve a least-square fit of a polynomial type was performed.

The mean curve received is continuous and demonstrates three turning points (fig. 2). There is a very good correlation with r = 0.962. This curve is described by the following equation I:

$$z = (\ln x)$$

$$\ln y = 0.013099\, z^6 - 0.035196\, z^5 - 0.115136\, z^4 + 0.329864\, z^3 + 0.038486\, z^2 + 0.532402\, z + 1.988057 \qquad \text{(I)}$$

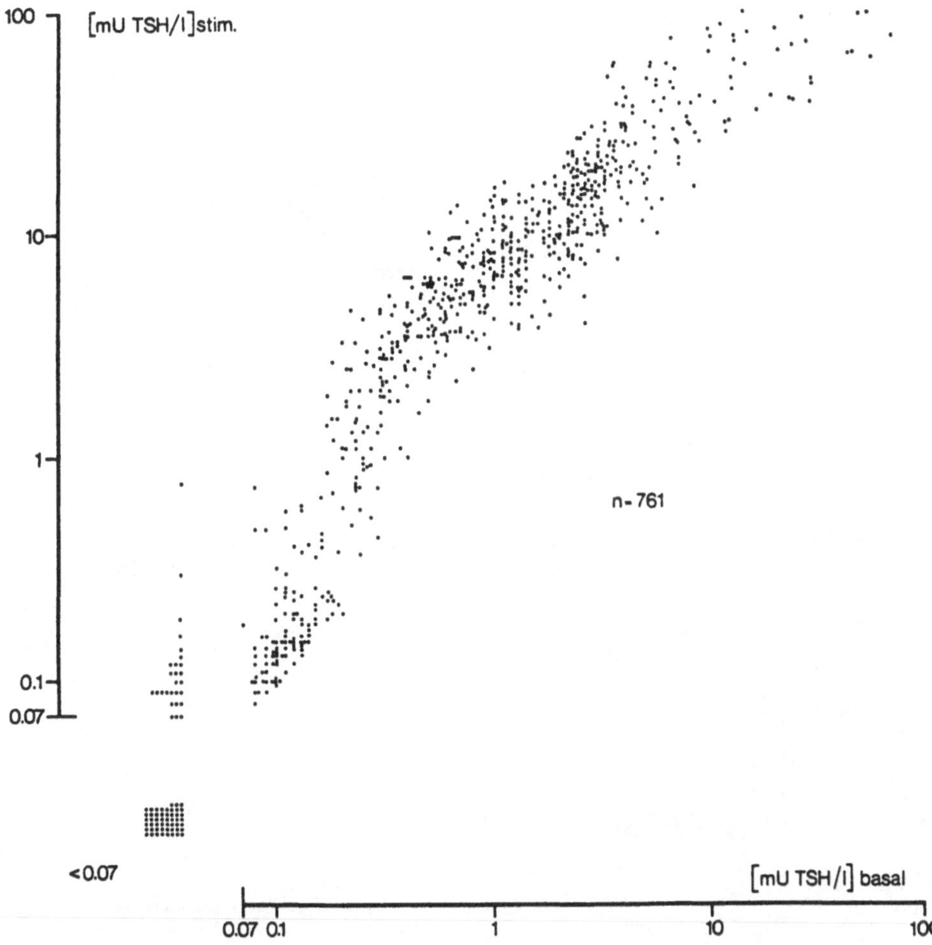

Fig. 1 Relationship of basal and corresponding TRH-induced TSH serum concentrations upon supersensitive TSH determination in non-selected patients from a radioimmunological-radiochemical laboratory.

The mean standard deviation for TRH-induced TSH was calculated to be ln Sy = 0.46787. This enables calculation from the mean curve and equation I of the ranges ± S. D. and ± 2 S. D. as also shown in figure 2. Only 30 (4.5%) pairs of TSH levels were found to be outside of the + 2 S. D. range, 2 pairs of which just being outside the ± 3 S. D. range.

The turning points of the mean curve derived from the correlation polynoma (equation I) are discribed in table 1 as well as the ± 2 Sy ranges as calculated via ln Sy and the graphically obtained ± 2 Sx ranges.

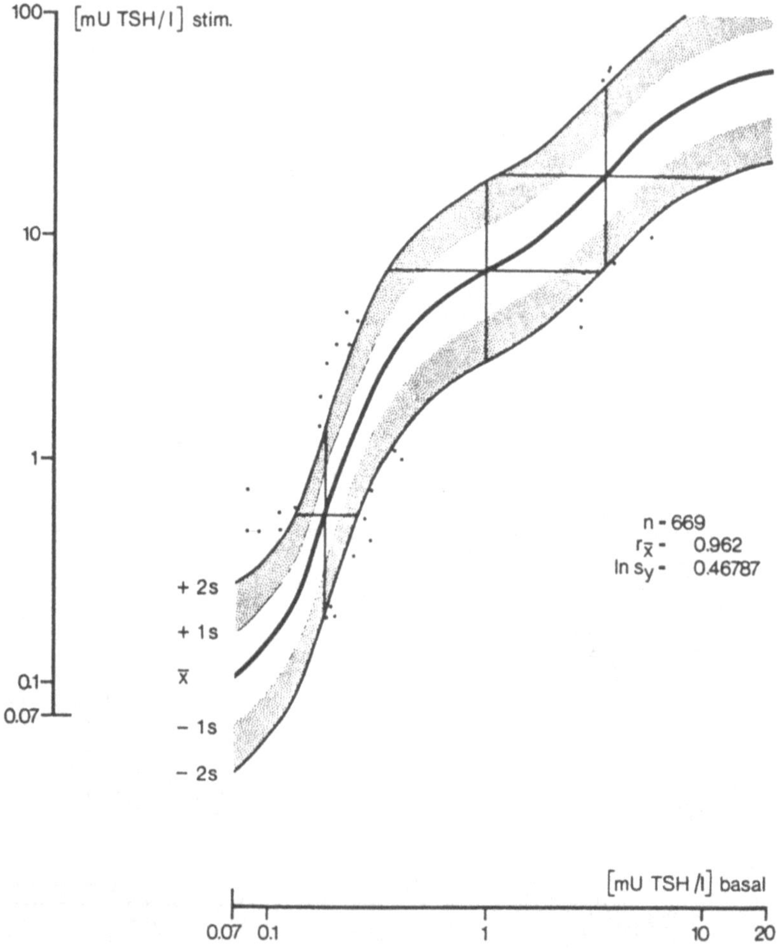

Fig. 2 Polynomial function with the mean curve and the respective reference ranges concerning the correlation between basal and TRH-induced TSH.

Table 1 Definition of turning points of the polynomial function from figure 2 describing the correlation between basal and TRH induced TSH concentrations

	$\bar{x}$ [mU TSH/l] (± 2 SD-range)	$\bar{y}$ [mU TSH/l] (± 2 SD-range)
W_1	0.18 (0.12 – 0.25)	0.52 (0.2 – 1.4)
W_2	0.96 (0.33 – 3.0)	7.05 (2.8 – 18)
W_3	3.4 (1.2 – 15)	19.8 (8.0 – 54)

As shown in figure 2 the mean curve was found to be significantly steeper close to turning point 1 in comparison to turning point 2. Therefore, alternatively a differentiated linear x-y correlation was studied. Such linear correlation was found for the basal TSH range 0.07 – 0.32 mU/l (close to ± 2 S.D. range of turning point 1 according to table 1) as expressed in equation II:

$$\ln y = 2.53522 \ln x + 3.79084 \qquad \text{(II)}$$
$$(r = 0.858,\ Sy = 0.58939)$$

An analogous linear relationship for TRH tests with basal TSH levels between 0.33 and 3.00 mU/l (2 S.D. range of turning point 2) is described by equation III:

$$\ln y = 0.73833 \ln x + 1.97661 \qquad \text{(III)}$$
$$(r = 0.761,\ \ln Sy = 0.39606)$$

As depicted in figure 3 the slopes of the two linear curves according to equations II and III differ by a factor of 3.4. Their intercept corresponds to a basal TSH level of 0.34 and to a TRH-induced TSH level of 3.1 mU/l.

In comparison to these limited range linear correlations one continuously covering the whole range of basal TSH concentrations from 0.07 – 20 mU/l (n = 669) was calculated as expressed in equation IV:

$$\ln y = 1.16727 \ln x + 1.71612 \qquad \text{(IV)}$$
$$(r = 0.908,\ \ln Sy = 0.65372)$$

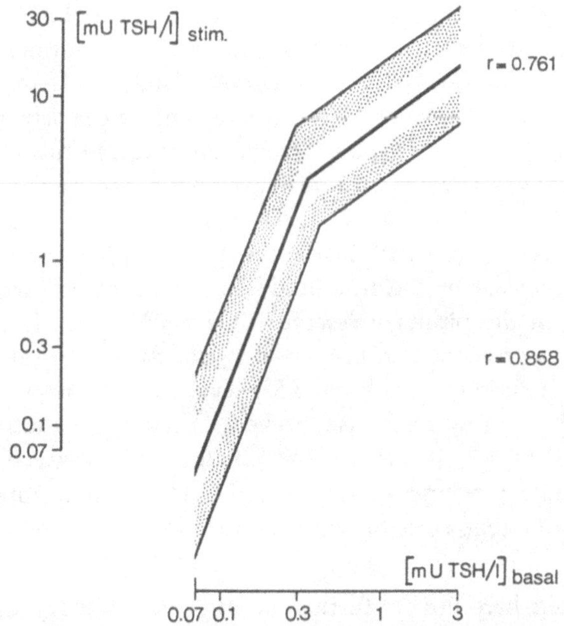

Fig. 3 Linear correlations of basal and TRH-induced TSH limited to the subnormal and normal range for basal TSH.

As can be seen this coefficient of correlation comes close to that from the correlation polynoma (fig. 2), however, the mean standard deviation being much larger.

Discussion

Our results demonstrate a correlation between basal and TRH-stimulated serum TSH concentrations which can be described by a 6th degree polynoma extending earlier findings of Seidel [14] and, thus, correcting the original assumption of a rather linear, yet not very close correlation [3, 6, 11]. Due to lower sensitivity, specificity and precision of the formerly used assay, a research assay, the subnormal range of basal TSH levels could not be included into such calculation because of absent normal distribution [14).

The availability of new supersensitive TSH IRMAs enabled our new calculations presented here. The appearance of the deducted correlation curve is that of two superimposed titration curves with a total of three turning points within the range studied (fig. 2). Interestingly, these turning points happen to be located in the range of subnormal, normal and hypernormal basal TSH concentrations with the respective TRH-induced correlates. The impact of these findings upon pituitary-thyroid regulation are already clearly demonstrable upon computation of limited range linear correlations concerning the basal TSH ranges of 0.07 – 0.32 and 0.33 – 3.00 mU/l (fig. 3). It becomes obvious that in the subnormal basal TSH range the slope of the linear correlation curve is much different and markedly higher compared to that for the normal range. This is consistent with the view of fine regulation of pituitary-thyroid interrelationship. In this context it may be pathophysiologically important that once thyroid function turns toward hyperthyroidism or thyroid suppression, which is obviously a continuous process without a defined cut-off, relatively small changes in basal TSH concentration cause a rather significant decrease in TRH-induced TSH concentration which is equivalent to a reduction in the pituitary reserve. This mechanism of thyroid regulation may be viewed as protection from thyroid dysfunction. The same can be observed in the region of supranormal basal TSH levels which, however, has not been computed linearily. In the latter case, however, there is no continuous increase in TRH-induced TSH in response to rather small changes in basal TSH, because of the limited pituitary reserve to secrete TSH. This system obviously represents kind of a buffer system agreeing with the titration curves mentioned above.

Thus, our studies presented here enable further insight into pituitary thyroid regulation. Furthermore, relevant diagnostic conclusions may be deducted, especially by looking at the findings concerning the "gray zone" between normal and suppressed basal TSH levels. Generally, the diagnostic use of Δ TSH appears to be no longer correct in face of an absent linear but existing polynomial correlation between basal and TRH-induced TSH levels.

A detectable increase in TSH concentration within the subnormal TRH test excludes hyperthyroidism. Therefore, the TRH test results used up to now have to be redefined if supersensitive TSH determination is used. Furthermore, suppressed, that is non-detectable basal TSH, which in rare instances may be associated with a slight, yet significant, increase in TRH-induced TSH (fig. 1) may be unsuitable to confirm complete TSH-suppressive treatment in all of the cases, particularly applying to thyroid carcinoma therapy. Thus, the TRH test should be continued to be performed in the above mentioned "gray zone" for security reasons. However, a normal basal TSH concentration per se excludes the presence of hyperthyroidism. In this case there is no need for a TRH test. These considerations and suggestions are only valid upon use of one of the supersensitive TSH assays clearly discriminating between normal and suppressed basal TSH levels being separated from each other by a "gray zone".

References

[1] Alexander, W. D., D. J. Kerr, M. Ferguson: First-line test of thyroid function, Lancet **II** (1984) 647.

[2] Allen, R. K., D. Watson: Thyrotropin as the initial screening test for thyroid disease. Clin. Chem. **30** (1984) 502–503.

[3] Beckers, C., A. Maskens, C. Cornette: Thyrotropin response to synthetic thyrotropin releasing hormone in normal subjects and in patients with non-toxic goiter. Europ. J. Clin. Invest. 2 (1972) 220.

[4] Böttger, I., H. W. Pabst: Time for a new concept in thyroid in vitro diagnostics. Nuklearmedizin (1984) 655–659.

[5] Böttger, I., H. W. Pabst, R. Senekowitsch, et al.: Performance of two new solid-phase ligand assays for TSH using monoclonal antibodies. Nucl. Med. Common. **6** (1985) 195–207.

[6] Kochupillai, N., M. G. Deo, M. G. Karmaker, et al.: Pituitary-thyroid axis in Himalayan endemic goitre, Lancet **I** (1973) 1021–1024.

[7] Mahlstedt, J., A. Hotze: Experience with an ultrasensitive immunoradiometric assay. Nuc. Compact **16** (1985) 72–76.

[8] Mewissen, B., R. Hehrmann: Kann ein hochsensitiver Radioimmunoassay für TSH den TRH-Test ersetzen? Akt. Endokr. Stoffw. **6** (1985) 1–6.

[9] Pfannenstiel, P., N. Panitz: Erste Erfahrungen mit einem hochsensitiven immunometrischen TSH-Assay zur Diagnostik von Schilddrüsenerkrankungen. Der Nuklearmediziner **8** (1985) 185–189.

[10] Rattle, S. J., D. R. Purnell, P. I. M. Williams, et al.: New separation method for monoclonal immunoradiometric assays and its application to assays for thyrotropin and human choriogonadotropin. Clin. Chem. **30** (1984) 1457–1461.

[11] Sawin, C. T., J. M. Hershman: The TSH response to thyrotropin-releasing hormone (TRH) in young adult men: Intra-individual variation and relation to basal serum TSH and thyroid hormones. J. Clin. Endocrinol. Metab. **42** (1976) 809–816.

[12] Seidel, Ch., D. Ziegelitz, H.-J. Correns: Zur klinischen Eingruppierung supprimierter und niedrig-normaler TSH-Spiegel bei Euthyreose. Nuc. Compact **12** (1981) 2–7.

[13] Seidel, Ch., D. Ziegelitz, K. Sydow, et al.: TSH-Basiswerte in der Diagnostik von Schilddrüsenerkrankungen. Dt. Gesundheitswesen **34** (1979) 2029–2038.

[14] Seidel, Ch., D. Ziegelitz, A. Weber, et al.: Zum klinischen Stellenwert eines empfindlichen TSH-RIA. Endokrinilogie **80** (1982) 181–193.

[15] Wide, L., P. A. Dahlberg: Quality requirements of basal S-TSH assays in predicting an S-TSH response to TRH. Scand. J. Clin. Lab. Invest. **40**, Suppl. 155 (1980) 101–110.

Clinical value of blunted TSH-response

P. Lind, G. Klima, P. Költringer, O. Eber, G. Bienhaus, Ch. Seidel

Introduction

In 3130 patients of our hospital TSH values were established prior and after TRH stimulation by means of an ultrasensitive immunoradiometric assay.

In the course of this investigation we used as stimulant
- in 1201 patients 200 μg TRH intravenously, and
- in 700 patients 400 μg TRH, while
- in 1229 patients a peroral dosage of 40 mg TRH

were administered.

Following stimulation blood sampling was done 30 minutes after intravenous injection, but 3 hours following oral administration.

Results

In the following diagrams basal TSH values were plotted separately according to the corresponding dosages against the respective TSH response values (fig. 1, 2). In both these diagrams – in double logarithmic plotting – the graphs show the response values covering a range of 0.07 – to 20 μU/ml basal TSH.

Figure 1 describes the stimulation following 200 μg TRH intravenously, while in figure 2 we see the response values following peroral stimulation. Since a linear plotting of basal TSH as against response values does not demonstrate clearly the correlation between both these parameters, we established mean value curves for each individual group by means of a polynomial calculation (fig. 3, 4).

When comparing the curves in figure 3 and 4 (mean value curves and the + and −2 s ranges) the graph showing TSH response after 200 μg TRH stimulation differs greatly as against the other two groups (e. g. the response curve after oral TRH stimulation). In all three curves we see a point of inflection a 0.18 to 0.25 μU/ml basal TSH.

The curve representing TSH response following 200 μg TRH shows two further inflection points a 1.05 and 3.2 μU/ml respectively.

Thyrotropin

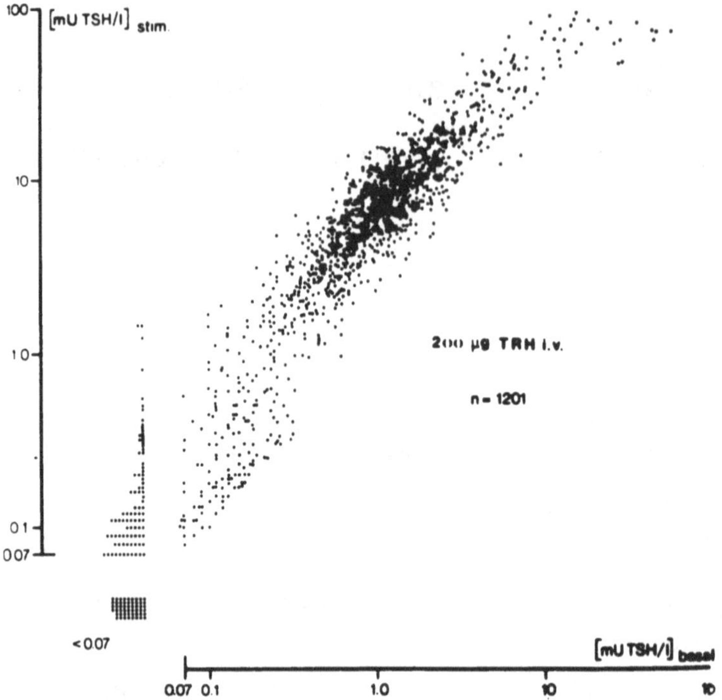

Fig. 1 TSH response values (n = 1201) after 200 µg TRH i.v. covering a basal TSH range of 0.07 – 20 mU/l (double logarithmic plotting).

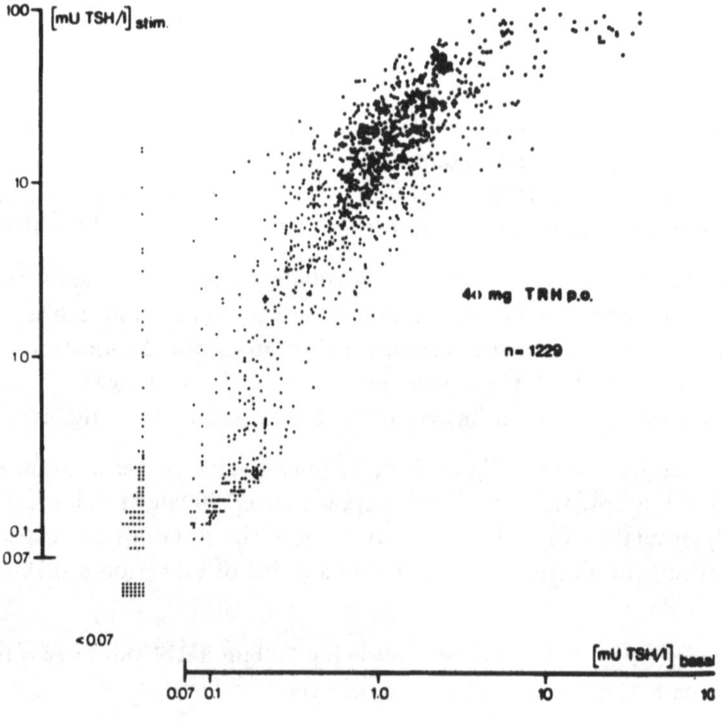

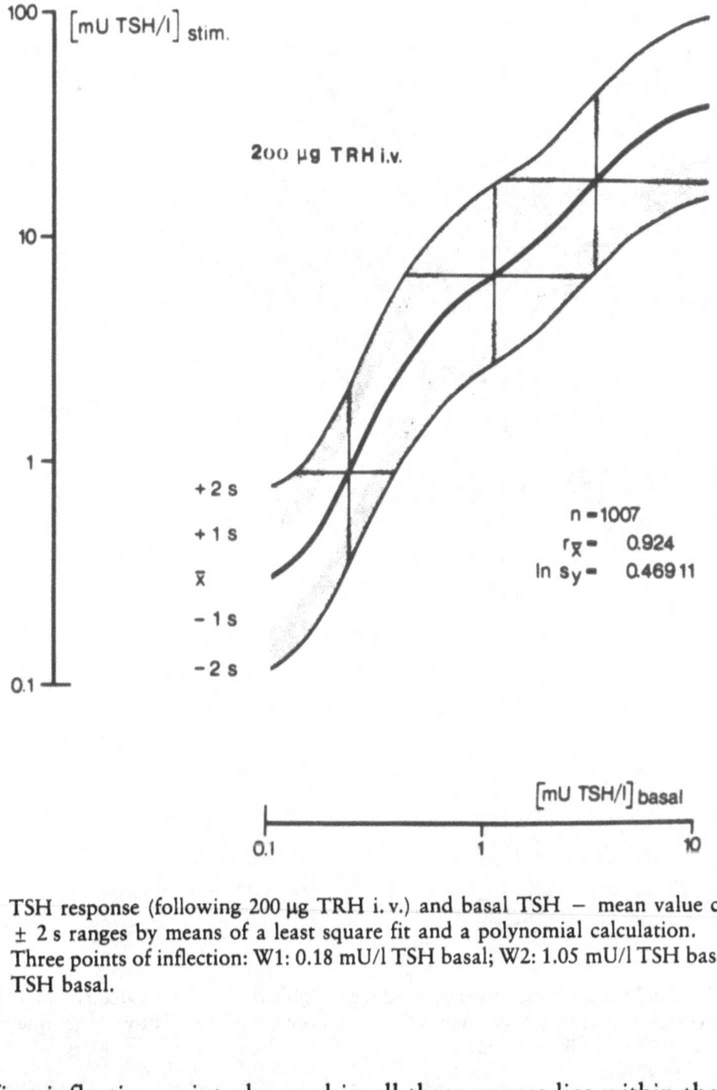

Fig. 3 TSH response (following 200 µg TRH i. v.) and basal TSH – mean value curve, ± 1 s and ± 2 s ranges by means of a least square fit and a polynomial calculation.
Three points of inflection: W1: 0.18 mU/l TSH basal; W2: 1.05 mU/l TSH basal; W3: 3.2 mU/l TSH basal.

The first inflection point observed in all three curves lies within the range of the so called "blunted TSH response", while the second inflection point is located within the mean value range of euthyroid subjects, moreover, the third point of inflection is situated near the transition of hypothyroidism. The situation of these inflection points suggests that by means of stimulation below maximum of 200 µg TRH i. v. we can best demonstrate the subtle correlation between basal and response values in the diagram.

Fig. 2 TSH response values (n = 1229) after oral TRH administration (40 mg) covering a basal TSH range of 0.07 – 20 mU/l (double logarithmic plotting).

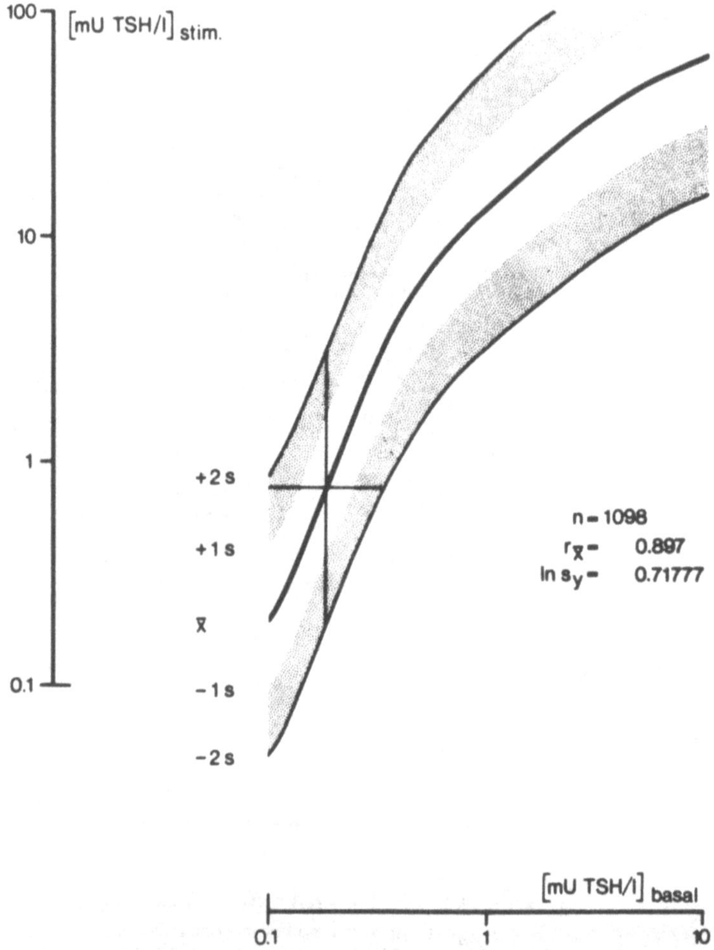

Fig. 4 Basal TSH and TSH response (following 40 mg TRH p. o.) – mean value curve, ± 1 s and ± 2 s ranges by means of a least square fit and a polynomial calculation. Only one point of inflection at 0.25 mU/l basal TSH.

Figure 5 demonstrates the calculated polynomial mean curves according to the three different administrations of TRH.

In figure 6 and 7 we see the two standard deviation ranges of response values of all three groups with the distinct deviation of the + 2 s ranges corresponding to the TRH stimulation doses.

In this connection we see a basal value of 0.2 μU/ml corresponding to a + 2 s – response value of 1.6 μU/ml following 200 μg TRH i. v., while after 400 μg TRH i. v. this value amounts to 3.2 μU/ml and 4.0 μU/ml in case of peroral stimulation.

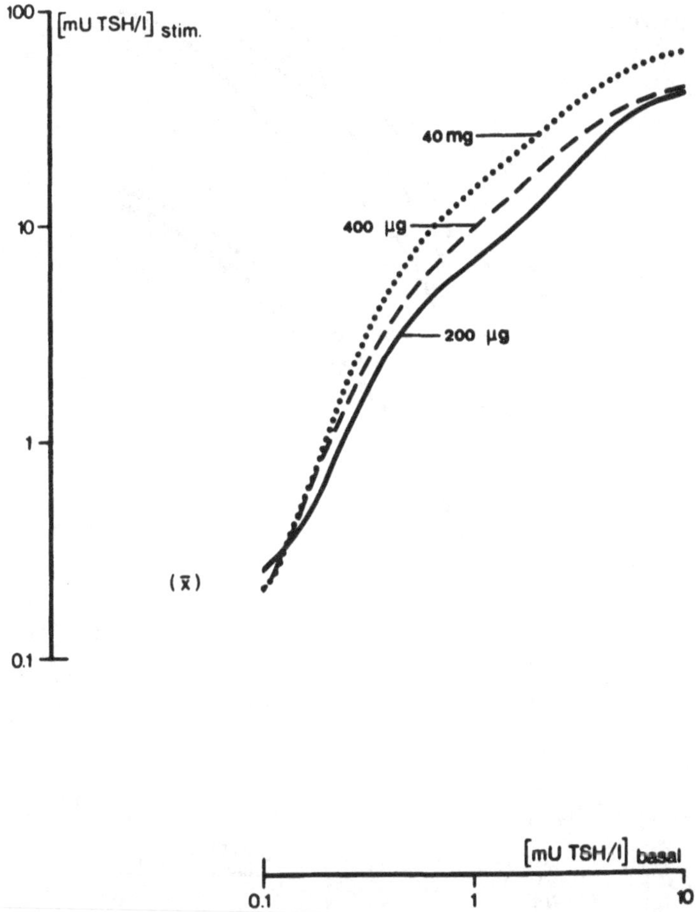

Fig. 5 Mean value curves – basal TSH against TSH response following different TRH dosages: ——— 200 µg i. v. – – – 400 µg TRH i. v., ... 40 mg TRH p. o.

The −2 s standard deviation curves (fig. 8) differ only slightly in their course and are even identical in a range below 2.5 µU/ml TSH response. Values below this response have been summarized up to now in the group of the so called "blunted TRH test".

The response values of the latter – namely below 2.5 µU/ml – gained by means of ultrasensitive TSH assays make us doubt as to the uniformity of the underlying material. This doubt caused us to introduce a clinical evaluation of this group: 357 patients showing a TSH response below 2.5 µU/ml were divided into three classes according to

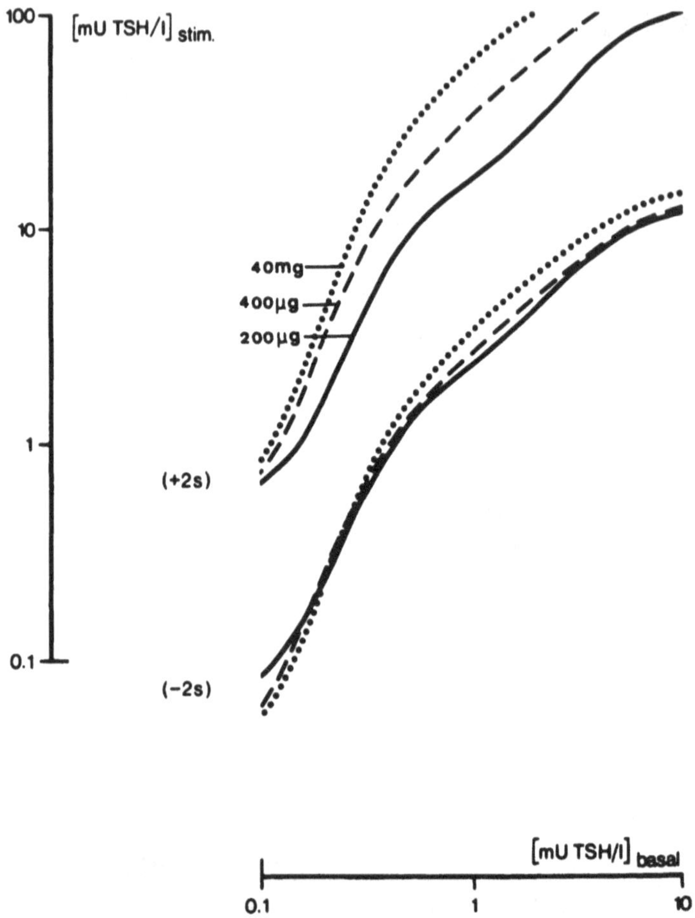

Fig. 6 The two standard deviation ranges (±) – basal TSH against TSH response – following different TRH dosages: ——— 200 µg TRH i. v., – – – 400 µg TRH i. v., ... 40 mg TRH p. o.

- clinical parameters as body weight, heart rate, blood pressure and individual complaints such as heat intolerance, tremor, perspiration and following
- peripheral thyroid hormone levels:

A Hyperthyroidism
B Clinical borderline cases
C Euthyroidism, subdivided into

group 0 = without clinical cause
group 1 = due to autonomous tissue

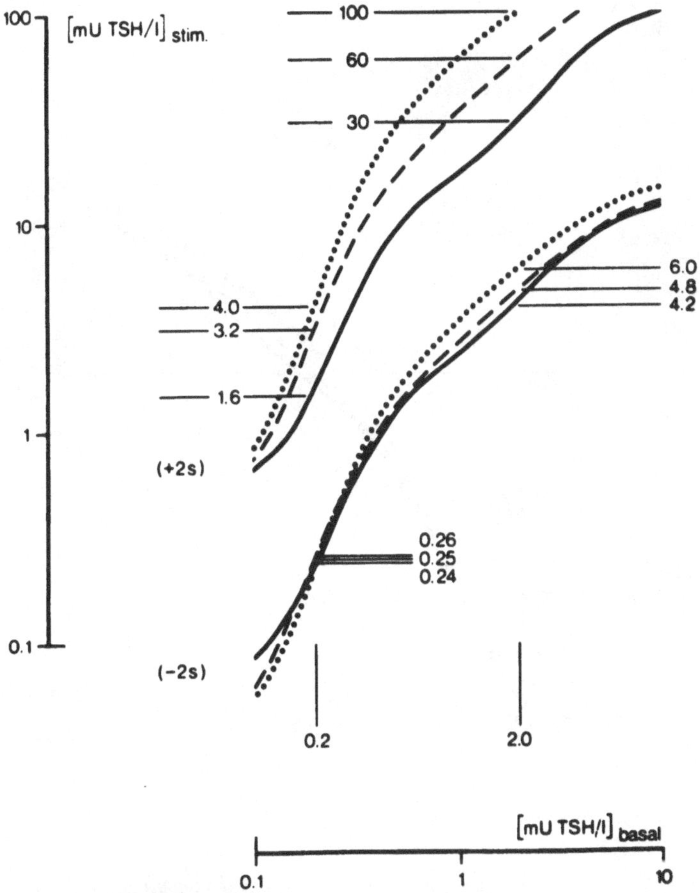

Fig. 7 BasalTSH values (e.g. 0.2 mU/l and 2 mU/l) and their + and – two standard deviation values according to their different TRH stimulation dosages.

group 2 = due to post radioiodine therapy
group 3 = due to surgery after hyperthyroidism
group 4 = due to suppression of hormone substitution therapy

Moreover, the same 357 patients (tab. 1) were classified again in
class α with a response below 0.5 μU/ml, and in
class β with a response of 0.5 up to 2.5 μU/ml

Class α (fig. 9) with a response below 0.5 μU/ml shows
26% of clinically and laboratory overt hyperthyroidism,
12% of clinical borderline cases with euthyroid peripheral thyroid hormone levels and finally
62% showing clinical and peripheral euthyroidism

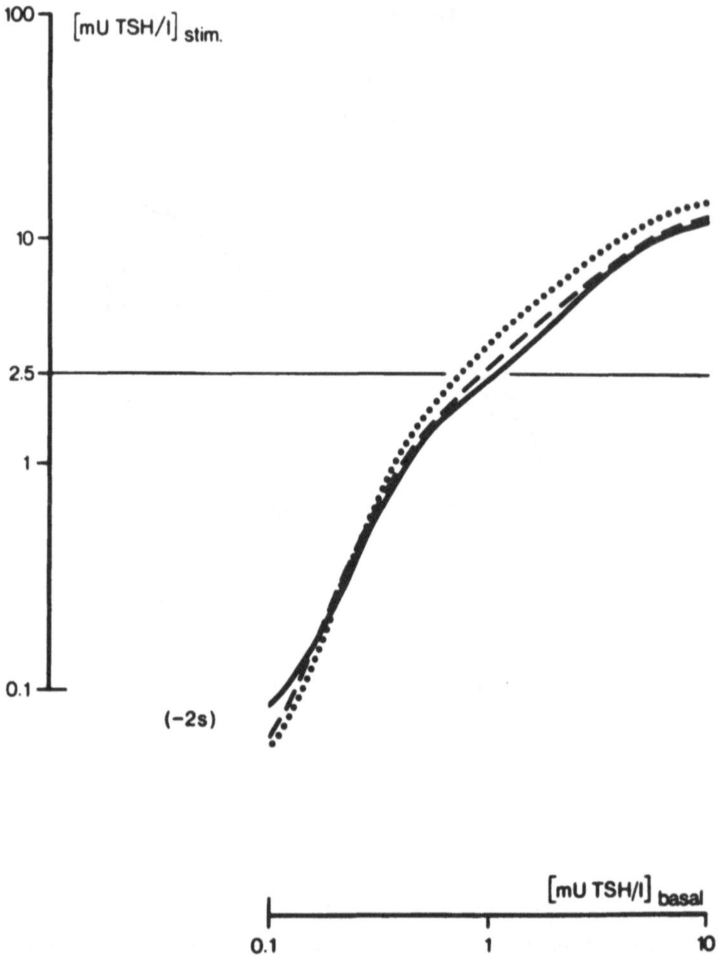

Fig. 8 The course of the −2 s deviation ranges following different TRH stimulation dosages: ——— 200 μg TRH i. v., – – – 400 μg TRH i. v., …… 40 mg TRH p. o.

In class β (fig. 10) response between 0.5 and 2.5 μU/ml
not overt clinical hyperthyroidism was observed, while
12% were clinical borderline cases, and
88% were clinical and laboratory euthyroid

However, when excluding patients under thyroid hormone treatment we observed in class α (fig. 11)
54% clinically overt hyperthyroidism,
24% clinical borderline cases and
22% euthyroid subjects

Table 1 Classification of the 357 patients in class α (TSH response < 0.5 mU/l) and class β (TSH response 0.5 – 2.5 mU/l) according to their clinical functional status

	TSH response < 0.5 μU/ml (α)	TSH response 0.5 – 2.5 μU/ml (β)
A	44	–
B	20	22
C		
0	–	20
1	10	16
2	7	9
3	1	–
4	89	119
	171	186

A = Hyperthyroidism; B = Borderline cases; C = Euthyroidism

Fig. 9

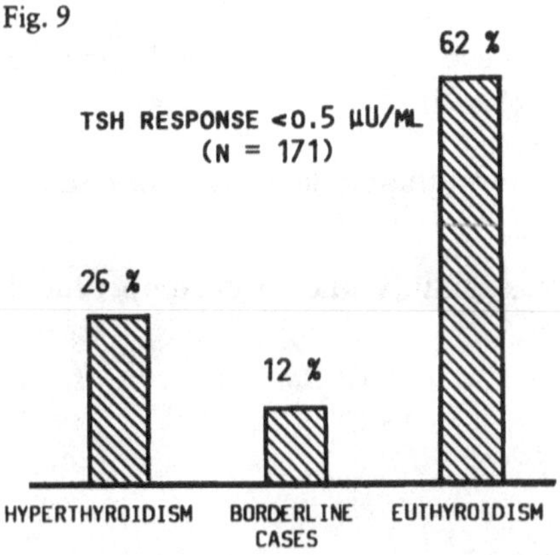

Fig. 10

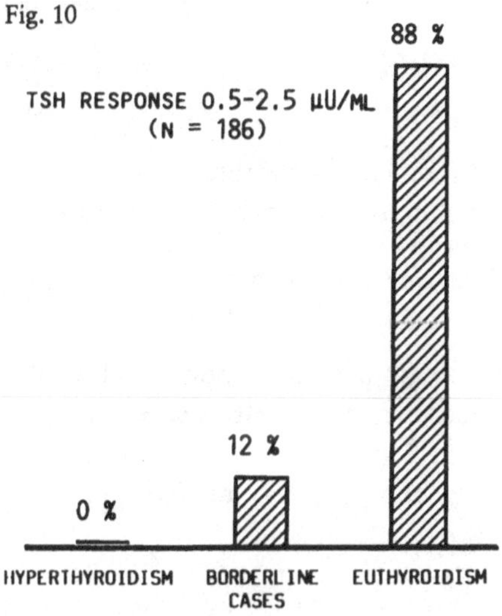

Fig. 9 Percentage of hyperthyroidism, borderline cases and euthyroidism in class α (n = 171 – including patients with thyroid hormone replacement therapy).

Fig. 10 Percentage of hyperthyroidism, borderline cases and euthyroidism in class β (n = 186 – including patients with thyroid hormone replacement therapy).

In class β (fig. 12) there were
two thirds of the patients clinically euthyroid and
one third clinical borderline cases

Fig. 11

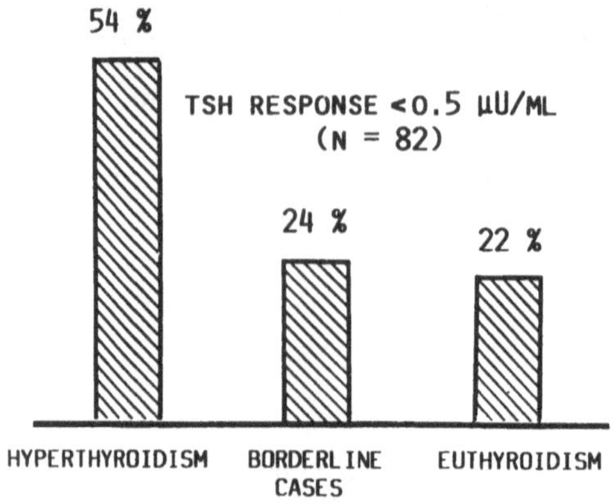

Fig. 12

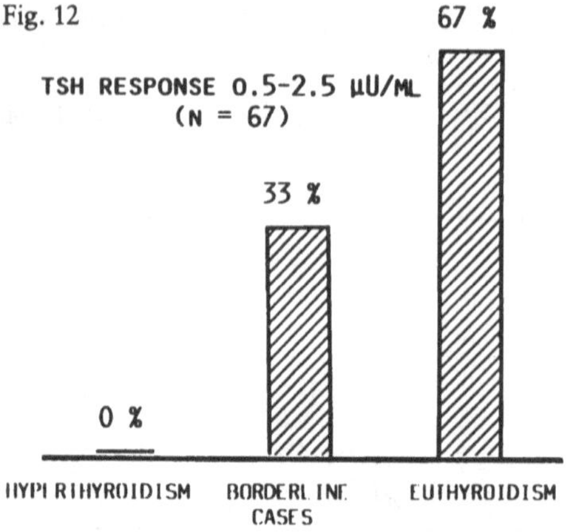

Fig. 11 Percentage of hyperthyroidism, borderline cases and euthyroidism in class α (n = 82 – excluding patients with thyroid hormone treatment).

Fig. 12 Percentage of hyperthyroidism, borderline cases and euthyroidism in class β (n = 67 – excluding patients with thyroid hormone treatment).

Of clinical borderline cases the term "preclinical hyperthyroidism" may be attributed only to 24% in class α and 33% in class β.

The question arises as to the clinical syndroms underlying such pre-clinical hyperthyroidism (tab. 2, 3):

Class α, with a response below 0.5 µU/ml was mainly due to decompensated adenomas and multifocal autonomies, while in
Class β (with a response of 0.5 to 2.5 µU/ml) almost half the patients suffered from compensated autonomous adenoma

Table 2 Clinical syndromes (scintigraphic diagnosis) as a cause of borderline cases in class α (TSH response < 0.5 mU/ml)

Borderline cases (24%)	
45%	Solitary hot nodule ("decompensated")
45%	Multinodular goiter with autonomy
0%	Solitary hot nodule ("compensated")
10%	Disseminated thyroid autonomy
0%	Graves' Disease
0%	Subacute thyroiditis (de Quervain)

Table 3 Clinical syndromes (scintigraphic diagnosis) as a cause of borderline cases in class β (TSH response 0.5 – 2.5 mU/l)

Borderline cases (33%)	
23%	Solitary hot nodule ("decompensated")
14%	Multinodular goiter with autonomy
41%	Solitary hot nodule ("compensated")
14%	Disseminated thyroid autonomy
0%	Graves' Disease
8%	Subacute thyroiditis (de Quervain)

The following conclusions may be drawn:

I a) A TRH dosage of 200 μg intravenously demonstrates best the relation between basal TSH and TSH response.

b) The course of TSH response following 200 μg TRH intravenously differs greatly in its functional transitory ranges as against euthyroidism and enables us to understand better the thyroid pituitary interaction.

c) Diagnostic accuracy in judging thyroidal function is far greater when applying TRH tests, especially in the basal range between 0.1 and 0.4 μU/ml.

II a) The so called "blunted TRH-test" comprises a heterogenous material and should not be identified with preclinical hyperthyroidism.

b) 22% of patients with a TRH response below 0.5 showed no symptomes of overt hyperthyroidism.

c) A TSH response above 0.5 μU/ml invariably excludes overt hyperthyroidism.

Sensitive TSH test in clinical routine: possibility of prediction of response to TRH from baseline TSH concentrations

H. Köhn, B. Tham, B. König, B. Wonder, P. Kahn, A. Mostbeck

Introduction

So far, thyrotropin measurements lacked the sensitivity to distinguish between hyper- and euthyroids, since detection limits were generally not lower than approximately 1 μU/ml. Consequently, for correct assessment of equivocal TSH levels additional TRH tests measuring the response of thyrotropin to thyroliberin had to be performed.

Recently, immunoradiometric assays using monoclonal antibodies for very sensitive measurement of thyrotropin with a detection limit lower than 0.05 μU/ml became available. We investigated the potential of very sensitive thyrotropin measurement for assessment of different states of the thyroid in clinical routine as well as the ability to reliably predict the thyrotropin response to thyroliberin from baseline TSH values, thus possibly reducing the need for performing TRH stimulation tests.

Material and methods

In 260 patients without previous history of thyroidal disease or therapy, thyroid function was assessed by standard clinical criteria, scans, serum T4, FT4, T3, TSH measurements and in most cases also by TRH tests.

Very sensitive measurement of TSH was performed using a commercially available one-step sandwich immunoradiometric assay (RIA gnost TSH coated tube, Behringwerke AG) with a lower detection limit of 0.03 μU/ml (according to the manufacturer's specification).

In order to assess the potential of predicting the TSH response to thyroliberin from baseline thyrotropin levels, data of 774 TRH tests were examined. 657 of these tests were performed at the Wilhelminenspital and 117 tests at the Hanuschkrankenhaus. Since the results of the TRH tests from both institutes demonstrated a similar significant correlation between baseline TSH values and delta TSH after thyroliberin stimulation, data from both institutes were merged.

Thyrotropin

Statistical analysis of thyrotropin concentrations in patients with different state of the thyroid was performed by means of a non parametric test (U-test, Mann-Whitney).

Results

Assessment of thyroidal function by baseline thyrotropin

In euthyroids, both baseline TSH and delta TSH after thyroliberin stimulation had a log normal distribution (figs. 1, 2). Euthyroid range for baseline thyrotropin (n = 208) was 0.28 – 2.74 μU/ml (median: 0.87 μU/ml) and for delta TSH (n = 192) 2.05 – 16.79 μU/ml (median: 5.99 μU/ml).

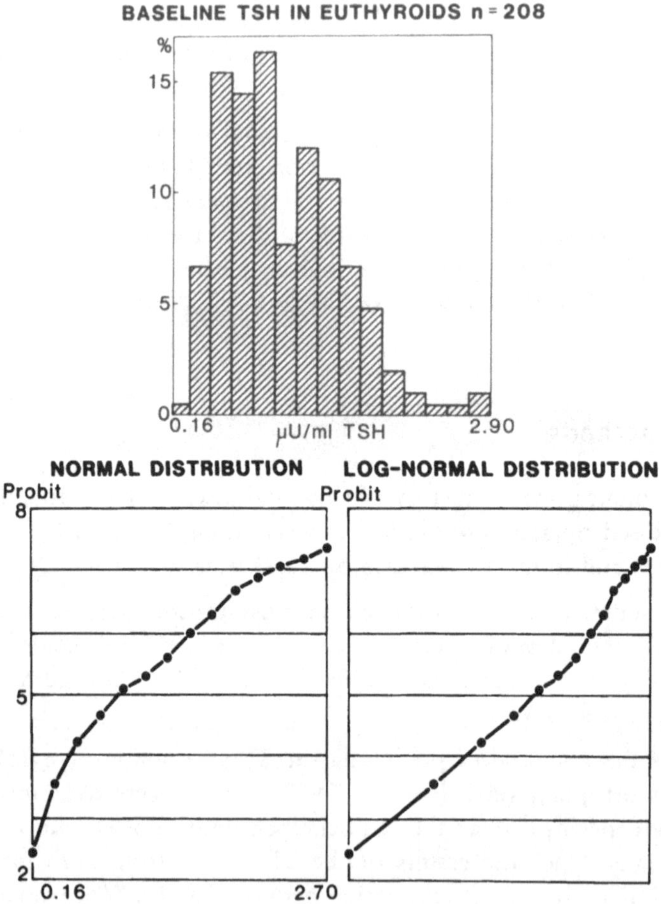

Fig. 1 Log normal distribution of baseline thyrotropin in euthyroids.

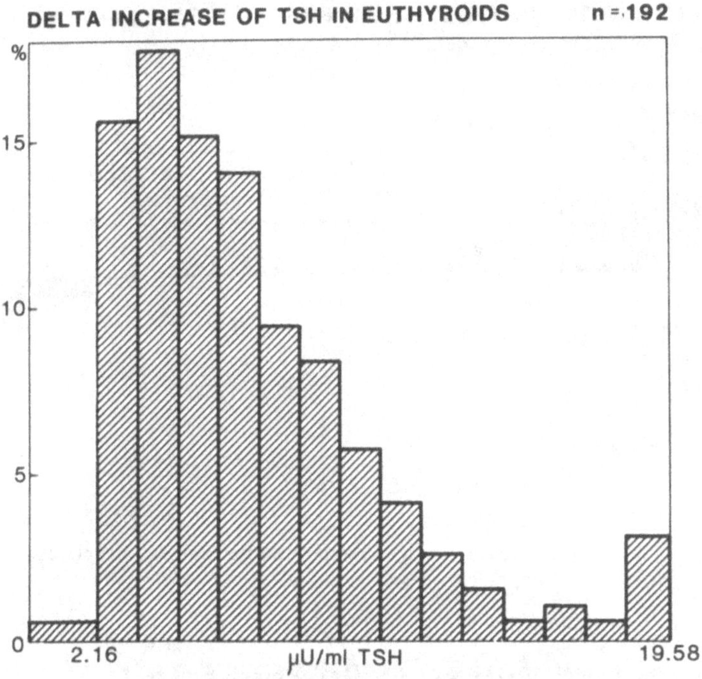

Fig. 2 Log normal distribution of delta TSH in euthyroids.

Hyperthyroid range for thyrotropin was 0.005 – 0.43 µU/ml (median: 0.05 µU/ml) and for delta TSH 0 – 0.22 µU/ml (median: 0.011 µU/ml) (n = 31).

In hypothyroids (n = 21), the mean of thyrotropin was 41.3 µU/ml (range 5.5 – 78.5 µU/ml) and of delta TSH 29.3 µU/ml (range 8.5 – 42.0 µU/ml) (tab. 1).

Thyrotropin in euthyroids differed significantly from hyper- or hypothyroids ($p < 0.001$).

Table 1 Ranges of baseline thyrotropin and of delta TSH after stimulation in eu-, hyper- and hypothyroid patients

	Baseline			ΔTSH		
	n	median	95%-confidence limits	n	median	95%-confidence limits
Euthyroids	208	0.87	0.28 – 2.74	192	5.99	2.05 – 16.79
Hyperthyroids	31	0.05	0.005 – 0.43	31	0.011	0 – 0.22
		$\bar{x}$	range		$\bar{x}$	range
Hypothyroids	21	41.3	5.5 – 78.5	21	29.3	8.5 – 42

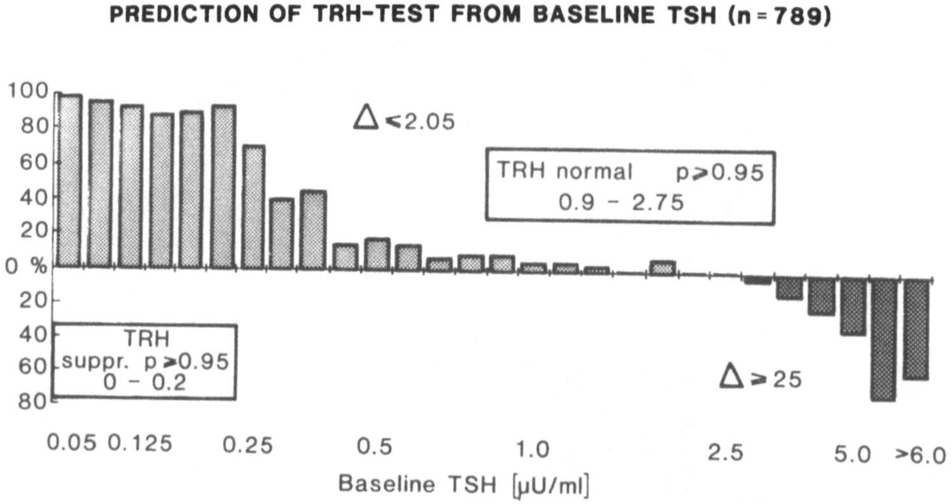

Fig. 3 Prediction of thyrotropin response to thyroliberin from baseline thyrotropin concentrations.

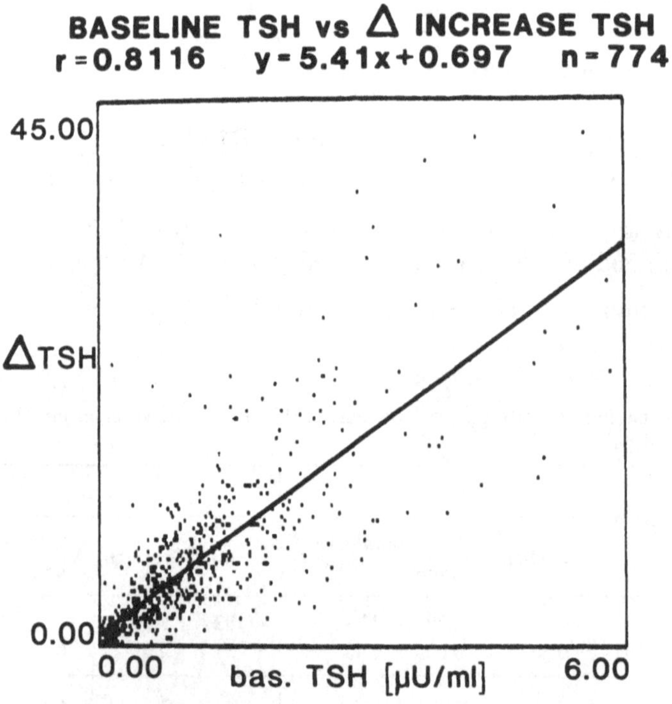

Fig. 4 Correlation between baseline thyrotropin and delta TSH after thyroliberin stimulation ($n = 774$, $r = 0.81$, $p < 0.001$).

Prediction of thyrotropin response to thyroliberin from baseline TSH

As shown in figure 3, a suppressed thyroliberin test (delta TSH < 2.05 µU/ml) was found with 95% probability in patients with baseline thyrotropin less than 0.2 µU/ml.

A baseline TSH of 0.9 – 2.75 µU/ml had a 95% probability of a normal TRH test (delta TSH > 2.05 µU/ml < 25 µU/ml). Baseline thyrotropin greater than 3.0 µU/ml was always related to latent or primary hypothyroidism, but in only 46% of these patients a delta TSH greater than 25 µU/ml was found. Using thyrotropin as the primary diagnostic tool, more than 50% of thyroliberin tests could have been spared in these patients.

Baseline thyrotropin concentrations correlated highly significant with delta TSH after thyroliberin stimulation ($r = 0.81$, $p < 0.001$, $n = 774$) (fig. 4).

Discussion

Very sensitive measurement of thyrotropin by immunoradiometric assays using monoclonal antibodies with a detection limit lower than 0.05 µU/ml enables discrimination between hyper- and euthyroid patients in most cases without the need of performing time consuming thyroliberin tests.

Baseline thyrotropin concentrations found in euthyroid patients ranged from 0.27 – 2.75 µU/ml being in good agreement with the literature. Mahlstedt et al. [1] reported an euthyroid range of 0.2 – 3.0 µU/ml and Wood et al. [2] of 0.26 – 2.8 µU/ml.

While Joseph [3] described a Gaussian distribution of thyrotropin in euthyroids with a range of 0.1 – 2.5 µU/ml, in our patients the distribution was log normal.

A similar lower limit of 2.0 µU/ml of the delta TSH after TRH stimulation was used by Mahlstedt et al. [1] as criterion of a normal thyroliberin test, while the upper limit of 12.0 µU/ml was somewhat lower than that of 16.8 µU/ml found in our euthyroid patients. Nevertheless, for predicting the TSH response to TRH we found an upper limit of the delta TSH of 25 µU/ml more useful.

Reliable prediction of the thyrotropin response to thyroliberin was possible in certain ranges of baseline thyrotropin concentrations. Baseline TSH values < 0.2 µU/ml will have a 95% probability of a suppressed TRH test (delta TSH < 2.05 µU/ml) and baseline TSH levels between 0.9 – 2.75 µU/ml a 95% probability of a normal TRH test (delta TSH > 2.05 < 25 µU/ml).

A similar strong relationship between baseline thyrotropin and TSH response to TRH has been reported by Joseph [3] and Mahlstedt et al. [1]. These authors found suppressed TRH tests in patients with baseline thyrotropin concentrations

< 0.1 μU/ml and Mahlstedt et al. [1] found normal TRH tests in patients with baseline thyrotropin > 0.6 μU/ml as compared to 0.9 μU/ml in our study.

Baseline thyrotropin concentrations greater than 3.0 μU/ml were always related to latent or primary hypothyroidism and seemed to be a more reliable diagnostic tool in these patients than the thyroliberin test, since a delta TSH after TRH greater than 25 μU/ml was found in only 46%. In case of longer lasting or more severe hypothyroidism there is probably already maximum stimulation of the pituitary so that thyroliberin cannot cause an exaggerated response.

Our results suggest that very sensitive measurement of baseline thyrotropin has great diagnostic potential for discriminating euthyroids from hyper- or hypothyroid patients and that for certain ranges of baseline thyrotropin no significant improvenment can be expected by performing additional thyroliberin tests.

References

[1] Mahlstedt, J. A. Hotze: Erste Erfahrungen mit einem ultrasensitiven immunoradiometrischen TSH-Assay. Nuc. Compact **16** (1985) 72–76.

[2] Wood, W. G., D. Waller, U. Hantke: An evaluation of six solid-phase thyrotropin (TSH) kits. J. Clin. Chem. Clin. Biochem. **23** (1985) 461–471.

[3] Joseph, K.: Erstdiagnostik und Verlaufskontrolle bei Schilddrüsenfunktionsstörungen mit der immunoradiometrischen TSH Bestimmung. Nuc. Compact **16** (1985) 240–254.

TSH measured with sensitive RIA method in euthyroid goiter patients

Z. Kusic, H. Prpic, Lj. Lukinac, S. Spaventi, I. Simonovic

Introduction

There has been general tendency to atribute sporadic euthyroid goiter to increased TSH stimulation, following different factors which potentially decreased the levels of thyroid hormones. This hypothesis provides the physiological basis for treatment of goiter with thyroid hormones. In majority of patients with sporadic euthyroid goiter TSH concentration is, however, not increased [1, 11, 16, 17]. This phenomenon could be caused by many factors: increased sensitivity of iodine-depleted thyroid to the normal level of TSH [2], periodic elevations of TSH [20], greater nocturnal surge of TSH secretion in goitrous patients [9], altered antigenecity of TSH in goitrous patients [23] and insensitivity of standard RIA tests which are unable to determine small changes in TSH concentrations still in normal range.

The objective of the present study was to determine the possible change of serum TSH concentration in patients with sporadic euthyroid goiter using a sensitive "in house" method.

Subjects and methods

Sixty-four patients with sporadic non-toxic goiter were investigated: 1. 32 patients with diffuse goiter (29 women and 3 men aged 19 – 64 yr) 2. 32 patients with nodular goiter (27 women and 5 men aged 21 – 79 yr). Control group consisted of 19 women and 13 men aged 21 – 52 yr.

Goiter size and nodularity were estimated by palpation, ^{99m}Tc or ^{123}I scan or by ultrasound. Group of patients with nodular goiter included only those with solitary nonfunctional nodule. Duration of goiter was not determined. Patients who had previous thyroidectomy or thyroid hormone therapy were excluded from the study. All patients were euthyroid according to clinical and laboratory results. Patients with thyroiditis, which was confirmed by cytologic examination or determination of thyroglobulin autoantibodies, were excluded. Controls were euthyroid subjects, without goiter and history of thyroid disorders.

Thyrotropin

Sensitive "in house" TSH RIA method was performed as follows: TSH standards (MR 80/558) in concentrations of 0.06 mU/l, 0.12 mU/l, 0.24 mU/L, 0.48 mU/L, 0.96 mU/l, 1.92 mU/l, 3.84 mU/l, 7.69 mU/l and 15.37 mU/l were dissolved in TSH free serum. TSH antiserum (M 168/2 from prof Butt, Edinburgh) was used in final titre of 1 : 300 000 in 50 mmol/l phosphate buffer, pH 7.3 (10 mmol/l EDTA, 3.08 mmol/l NaN_3, 77 mmol/l NaCl, 2 g/l BSA, 5 ml/l tween-20). Label ^{125}I-TSH was prepared by the modification of Chloramine-T method using L-cysteine instead of sodium metabisulfite; the total activity was 5000 cpm per tube. Sheep anti rabbit IgG in titre of 1 : 50 was prepared in the same phosphate buffer. The first incubation, without label, was carried out for 72 hours, and the second incubation, with ^{125}I-TSH, lasted 24 hours. The last incubation period of 5 hours, with the second antibodies, was stopped by addition of PEG-6000 (90 g/l). After centrifugation the bound fraction was counted in gamma counter.

Determinations of total T_3 and T_4 were performed by "in house" RIA methods using commercial antisera (T_3/LuzernaChem, T_4/Biodata) and relevant standards dissolved in hormone free serum. As the precipitation agent PEG-4000 was used.

Statistical analysis was performed using Student's t test except for TSH where due to the nonparametric distribution of values the Mann-Whitney test was employed.

Results

Patients with goiter had normal levels of T_3, T_4 and TSH that were not significantly different from control values (fig. 1). The same was with T_3/T_4

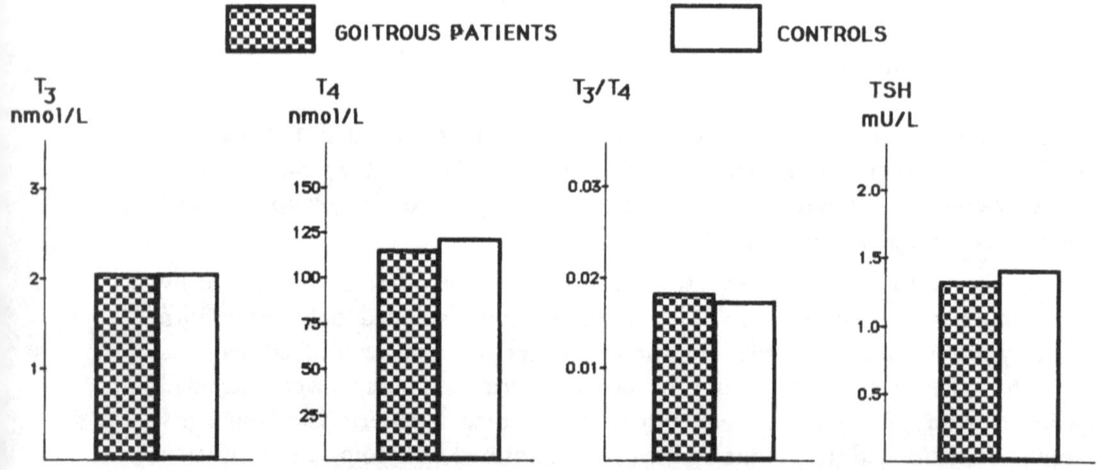

Fig. 1 Comparison of mean T_3, T_4, T_3/T_4 and median TSH values in group of goitrous patients and controls.

ratio. It was not possible to demonstrate a significant difference between any parametar of the groups of patients with diffuse or nodular goiter and control group either (tab. 1). Also, there was no difference between the two groups of patients.

Table 1 Hormone values in goitrous patients and control subjects

	Diffuse goiter	Nodular goiter	Controls
n	32	32	32
T_3 nmol/l			
mean	1.9	2.1	2.0
± 2 SD	1.1 – 2.7	1.3 – 2.8	1.2 – 2.8
T_4 nmol/l			
mean	115	111	119
± 2 SD	69 – 161	68 – 159	77 – 161
T_3/T_4			
mean	0.0173	0.019	0.0173
± 2 SD	0.0095 – 0.0251	0.0096 – 0.0284	0.0099 – 0.0247
TSH mU/l			
median	1.44	1.22	1.4
range	0.06 – 7.2	0.06 – 3.95	0.19 – 4.2

Discussion

Despite of many investigations the cause of sporadic euthyroid goiter is not clear. The heterogenecity of the disease entity "non-toxic" goiter may complicate the interpretation of results. There were undoubtedly several different causes for the development of goiter in majority of studies. Besides diffuse goiter different size and duration they often included nodular goiter with autonomous nodules and large proportion of patients with chronic thyroiditis. It would appear that any population defined as "idiopathic" goiter would contain a larger proportion of patients with Hashimoto's thyroiditis, as a primary etiology. In our study this was avoided by determining thyroid autoantibodies or by cytologic examination. Our group of nodular patients consisted only of patients with solitary nonfunctional nodules. Multinodular goiters often contain autonomous nodules which could cause blunted TSH response to TRH or lower levels of TSH measured with sensitive method. A good correlation was found between TRH test and TSH measured with sensitive method [13].

Several studies showed no difference in TSH levels between goitrous and normal subjects [1, 11, 16, 17]. Young et al. [25] found, however, elevated TSH in 42% of patients and Dige-Petersen et al. [4] in 26% of the patients. In the study of Young et al. [25] there was significantly higher TSH concentration in patients with goiter known to be present less than 1 year, compared to goiter of longer than 1 year duration. This finding is explained by authors with new "steady state" in which TSH levels fall either as a result of an increase in the mass of abnormally functioning tissue or an increased sensitivity to TSH. Duration of goiter was not recorded in our study, however, such data are usually not reliable. Hypothesis that TSH might be elevated only early in the course of goiter development could be proved in longitudinal studies. Pezzino et al. [16] found significantly greater T_3/T_4 ratio in serum of goitrous patients which is believed to reflect hypoiodination of thyroglobulin [8]. In this study we did not find statistically significant difference of T_3, T_4 and T_3/T_4 between the groups of goiter patients and the control group. There was no difference between the two groups of goiter patients, either. Changes in TSH concentration in goiter patients could not be proved even with sensitive TSH RIA method which enables differentiation between low concentration in hyperthyroid and euthyroid subjects [12]. Rothenbuchner and Yamada found larger increase of TSH in response to TRH in patients with euthyroid goiter [17, 24]. They concluded that TSH has an important participary role in the maintenance of goiter. Several investigations indicated that the transition from diffuse to nodular goiter is associated with a significant reduction in plasma TSH levels, which may reflect development of autonomy [4, 22, 25]. A blunted TSH response to TRH has been recorded in a considerable proportion of patients with euthyroid nodular goiter, even if patients with autonomously functioning adenoma were excluded [7, 10, 15]. It appears that autonomously functioning tissue may not be confined only to nodules and can be manifested as microscopic areas [14].

There are concepts that TSH is not involved in the pathogenesis of sporadic goiter and responsible factors are growth-stimulating immunoglobulins or small amounts of conventional thyroid-stimulating immunoglobulins [3, 21]. There is an increasing number of evidence for the existence of growth-stimulating immunoglobulins in the serum of majority of patients with euthyroid goiter [5, 6, 18, 19]. These immunoglobulins seem to promote primarily the multiplication of epithelial cells rather than to stimulate their function. These findings support the concept that the majority of patients with sporadic non-toxic goiter have a variant of thyroid autoimmune disease separate from lymphocytic thyroiditis. This is particularly evident for goiters growing in spite of thyroxine therapy and for goiters associated with supressed TSH response to TRH. It is, however, rather unlikely that growth-stimulating immunoglobulins are the sole and only cause of sporadic non-toxic goiter.

Although the role of TSH is undoubtedly important in the endemic goiter development, the obtained results suggest that at least the maintenance of goiter in our regions is not dependent upon a raised level of serum TSH.

Abstract

The role of thyrotropin in the development and maintenance of sporadic non-toxic goiter is still not clear. In spite of normal concentration in majority of patients, therapy with thyroid hormones is often successful. One of offered explanations for this phenomenon is relative insensitivity of standard RIA tests which are unable to determine small changes in TSH concentrations.

We determined TSH concentration with sensitive TSH "in house" method in 64 euthyroid goiter patients and 32 controls. Goiter patients were divided in two groups: 32 patients with diffuse goiter and 32 patients with solitary nonfunctional nodule. In all patients T_3 and T_4 concentrations were determined and scans with ^{99m}Tc or ^{123}I were performed. In goiter patients citology or histology examinations of nodules were done or titre of thyroglobulin antibodies were determined. Patients with autonomous nodules, hyperthyroidism, hypothyroidism and thyroiditis were excluded from the study.

There was no statistically significant difference of T_3, T_4, TSH and T_3/T_4 between the groups of patients and the control group. Also, there was no difference between the two groups of goiter patients.

Changes in TSH concentration in goiter patients could not be proved even with sensitive TSH RIA method.

References

[1] Beckers, C., C. Cornette: TSH Production Rate in Nontoxic Goiter. J. Clin. Endocrinol. 32 (1971) 852–854.

[2] Bray, G. A.: Increased Sensitivity of the Thyroid in Iodine-Depleted Rats to the Goitrogenic Effects of Thyrotropin. J. Clin. Invest. 47 (1968) 1640–1647.

[3] Brown, R. S., S. L. Pohl, et al.: Do Thyroid-Stimulating Immunoglobulins cause Non-toxic Multinodular Goiter. Lancet I (1978) 904–906.

[4] Dige-Petersen, H., L. Hummer: Serum Thyrotropin Concentrations Under Basal Conditions and after Stimulation with Thyrotropin-Releasing Hormone in Idiopathic Non-toxic Goiter. J. Clin. Endocrinol. Metab. 44 (1977) 1115–1120.

[5] Doniach, D.: Les immunoglobulines stimulantes de croissance (TGI) peuvent-elles expliquer certains goitres sporadiques euthyroidiens? Ann. Endocrinol. (Paris) 43 (1982) 534–547.

[6] Drexhage, H. A.: Immunoglobulins Affecting Thyroid Growth. Thyroid Today 4 (1985) 1–5.

[7] Emrich, D., M. Bahre: Autonomy in Euthyroid Goiter: Maladaption to Iodine Deficiency. Clin. Endocrinol. (Oxf.) 8 (1977) 257–265.

[8] Greer, M. A.: Factors Regulating Triiodothyronine (T3) and Thyroxine (T4) in Blood. Mayo Clin. Proc. **47** (1972) 944–952.

[9] Ingbar, S. H., K. A. Woeber: The Thyroid Gland. In: Textbook of Endocrinology, p. 117. W. B. Sounders Comp., Philadelphia–London–Toronto 1981.

[10] Kirkegaard, C., J. Faber, et al.: Intravenous and Peroral TRH Stimulation in Sporadic Atoxic Goitre. Acta Endocrinol. (Copenh.) **85** (1977) 508–514.

[11] Kusic, Z.: Thyroid Hormones and Thyrotropin in Patients with Euthyroid Nodular Goiter. Acta Med. Iugos. **33** (1979) 321–329.

[12] Lukinac, Lj., A. Kurtz: RIA Method for Determination of h-TSH in Human Serum. Radiol. Iugosl. **15** (1981) 507–511.

[13] Lukinac, Lj., Z. Kusic: Very Sensitive RIA TSH Method as a substitution for TRH test? Eur. J. Nucl. Med. **9** (1983) A 28.

[14] Miller, J. M., M. A. Block: Functional Autonomy in Multinodular Goiter. J. Am. Med. Assoc. **214** (1970) 535–539.

[15] Morgans, M. E.: Sporadic Non-toxic Goitre: An Investigation of the Hypothalamic-Pituitary-Thyroid Axis. Clin. Endocrinol. **8** (1977) 101–108.

[16] Pezzino, V., R. Vigneri, et al.: Increased Serum Thyroglobulin Levels in Patients with Nontoxic Goiter. J. Clin. Endocrinol. Metab. **46** (1978) 653–657.

[17] Rothenbuchner, G., D. A. Koutras, et al.: The Effect of Thyrotropin-Releasing Hormone on Serum TSH, T_4, and T_3 Levels in Endemic and Sporadic Nontoxic Goitre. Horm. Metab. Res. **6** (1974) 501–506.

[18] Schumml, P. M., K. Badenhoop, et al.: Significance of Thyroid-Growth-Stimulating Immunoglobulins in the Development of Euthyroid sporadic Goiter. Ann. Endocrinol. (Paris) **45** (1984) 86.

[19] Smyth, P. P. A., D. Neylan, et al.: Association of Thyroid-Stimulating Immunoglobulins and Thyrotropin-Releasing Hormone Responsiveness in Women with Euthyroid Goiter. J. Clin. Endocrinol. Metab. **57** (1983) 1001–1006.

[20] Stanbury, J. B., Chiu-an Wang: Nontoxic Goiter. Thyroid Today **3** (1981) 1–5.

[21] Studer, H.: Pathogenesis of Goiter: A Unifying Hypothesis. Thyroid Today **4** (1984) 1–7.

[22] Toft, A. D., W. J. Irvine, et al.: A Comparison of Plasma TSH Levels in Patients with Diffuse and Nodular Non-Toxic Goiter. J. Clin. Endocrinol. **42** (1976) 973–976.

[23] Vanhaelst, L., M. Bonnyns, et al.: Pituitary TSH in Normal Subjects and in Patients with Asymptomatic Atrophic Thyroiditis: Evidence for its Immunological Heterogenity. J. Clin. Endocrinol. Metab. **41** (1975) 115–119.

[24] Yamada, T., M. Naka, et al.: Age-related alterations of pituitary-thyroid function in normal female subjects and in female patients with simple goitre. Acta Endocrinol. (Copenh.) **107** (1984) 346–351.

[25] Young, R. L., W. C. Harvey, et al.: Thyroid-Stimulating Hormone Levels in Idiopathic Euthyroid Goiter. J. Clin. Endocrinol. Metab. **41** (1975) 21–26.

Application of a sensitive immunoradiometric assay (IRMA) for TSH in the diagnosis and follow-up thyroid disorders

R. G. Bretzel, G. Siedenberg, E. Skribelka, H. Schatz, K. Federlin

Introduction

Currently, the TRH-test (thyreotrophin-releasing-hormone) seems to be the only reliable method to differentiate between hypo, hyper and euthyroidism in the primary diagnosis of thyroid function [1, 2]. In addition, the efficacy of a thyroid suppressive treatment by L-thyroxine, as used in various thyroid diseases, is examined by the TRH-test [3]. But this test includes an in vitro challenge of the patient by thyreotrophin and it may occassionally exert some side effects. The test is time consuming because at least two blood samples need to be drawn at different times. Finally, it is an expensive test.

Recently, highly sensitive immunoradiometric assays (IRMA) for TSH have been developed and are commercially avialable now, which make use of monoclonal antibodies against TSH and which may detect much smaller concentrations of TSH. In this study, we examined whether a single determination of the basal TSH value with the help of these "ultrasensitive" TSH-IRMA's is capable of replacing the TRH-test in the primary diagnosis of thyroid function and in the control of a thyroid-suppressive therapy. Finally, we evaluated the clinical relevance of TRH-test results with low basal and/or subnormal TSH responses ("Borderline Cases").

Subjects and methods

The studies were performed in more than 500 outpatients and ward patients of our department of Internal Medicine and Endocrinology. Patients had simple goiter, nodular goiter, thyroiditis or had undergone resections of goiter or thyroid cancer. Patients without overt thyroid disease in whom the thyroid function had to be examined were also included. TRH-tests were done using the nasal application route (TRH-Relefact, Hoechst, Frankfurt), the second serum sample being drawn after 30 minutes. Measurement of TSH serum concentration was done using an automatic routine radioimminoassay with a lower limit of detection of

Thyrotropin

0.50 mU/l (ARIA II, Becton-Dickinson, Heidelberg). In addition, TSH concentration was determined by means of "ultrasensitive" assays with a lower limit of detection of at least 0.05 mU/l (TSH-IRMAclon, Henning, Berlin; RIA-gnost hTSH-coated-tube, Behring, Marburg; hTSH-EIA, Abbott, Wiesbaden). Finally, other relevant parameters such as TT4, TT3, and T3U were also determined in an automatic routine radioimmunoassay (ARIA II, Becton-Dickinson, Heidelberg).

Results

Sensitivity of an immunoradiometric assay (IRMA) in comparison to a radioimmunoassay (RIA) for TSH

We have determined TSH levels in 311 non-selected consecutively collected serum samples from outpatients with a fully automatic conventional TSH-RIA (ARIA II) and with a TSH-IRMA (TSH-IRMAclon). Only 162 serum samples (52%) were found to be within the detection range of the RIA, whereas TSH levels could be measured in 277 samples (89%) using the IRMA. Of the 149 serum samples showing suppressed values (less than 0.5 mU/l) in the TSH-RIA, only 40 samples showed "truly" suppressed (less than 0.1 mU/l) TSH levels after re-evaluation with the TSH-IRMA. The remaining 109 samples had TSH levels above this limit. In 49 of these 109 cases, levels greater than 0.5 mU/l were observed. At least in the latter cases, representing one third of the patients in question, the more sensitive TSH-IRMA would provide the exclusion of hyperthyroidism.

Comparing two different TSH-IRMA methods both using monoclonal antibodies (IRMAclon and RIA-gnost hTSH-coated-tube) we found practically identical results in the range of TSH values above 0.2 – 0.3 mU/l based on determinations of 397 serum samples. However, at TSH concentrations below 0.2 – 0.3 mU/l, a few discrepancies were observed.

In 279 cases the TSH concentration was also determined with a new enzymometric immunoassay (hTSH-EIA) also using monoclonal antibodies against TSH. We also found a good correlation of the values when compared to that determined by an IRMA (IRMAclon) with a few discrepancies in the range of TSH concentrations below about 0.3 mU/l (fig. 1). These and the above mentioned discrepancies occurred with roughly equal frequency and with different serum samples in all sensitive assays, thus probably reflecting non-specific matrix binding effects or interassay variations in this very low concentration range.

Primary diagnosis of thyroid function

Thyroid function was determined in 100 non-treated patients using a nasal TRH-test. It was investigated whether the TSH basal value determined with a sensitive

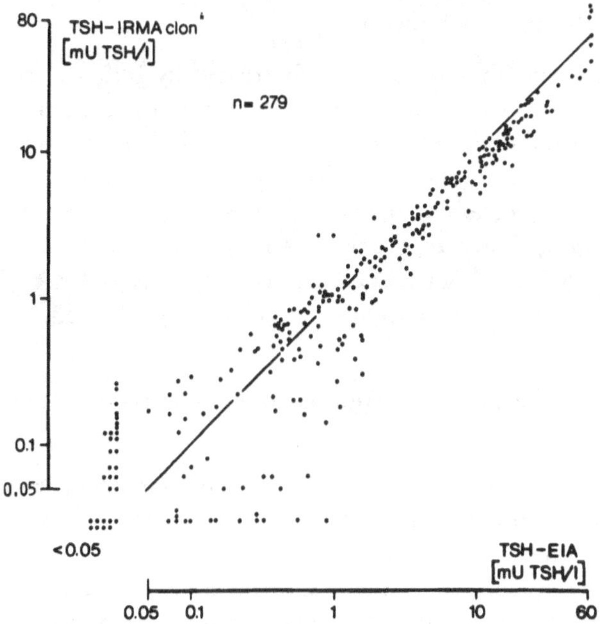

Fig. 1 TSH serum concentrations determined in 279 serum samples using two different ultrasensitive TSH-assays. TSH-IRMAclon (Henning, Berlin); TSH-EIA (Abbott, Wiesbaden); theoretical line of equivalence is depicted.

IRMA could predict the result of a TRH-test. We found a predictive value of 94% for basal TSH values in the range of less than 0.1 mU/l ("0") and 100% for values between 0.30 – 2.40 mU/l (tab. 1). In 84% of the cases with a basal TSH concentration above 2.40 mU/l a TRH-test which followed revealed a hypothyroid state ("pos." i. e. exaggerated TSH response). Basal values between 0.10 – 0.30 mU/l seem to reflect hyperthyroidism or borderline cases with a negative or an impaired TSH response (see also the last chapter).

Table 1 Predicative value of a TSH basal serum value determined with an ultrasensitive IRMA for a TRH-test with follows

IRMA-basal (mU/l)	TRH-test	Predicative value	No. of cases	
"0"	neg.	94%	15/16	1 x N
0.10 – 0.30	neg./low	83%	10/12	2 x N
0.30 – 2.40	normal	100%	40/40	
► 2.40	pos.	88%	28/32	4 x N

N = normal TRH-test.

The control of a thyroid-suppressive therapy

Thirty-five out of 120 patients thyreosuppressively treated by L-thyroxine (29%) showed a basal serum TSH concentration of more than 0.50 mU/l when analysed by the automatic routine radioimmunoassay (ARIA II). These cases were considered as being under poor control and the L-thyroxine dose was adjusted. In the remaining 85 cases the TSH secretion appeared to be sufficiently suppressed. 56 patients of that group (66%), however, proved to still have a basal TSH secretion with concentrations up to 3 mU/l when evaluated by a sensitive IRMA (IRMAclon). In that cases the dosage of L-thyroxine had also to be adjusted.

Evaluation of an impaired basal or/and stimulated TSH secretion ("Borderline Cases")

We evaluated TRH-tests in 163 non-selected patients of our department with different thyroid diseases or thyroid function disorders using an "ultrasensitive" TSH-IRMA (TSH-IRMAclon) (fig. 2). 103 cases showed a normal or an exaggerated TSH response. The remaining 66 patients showed either a basal serum TSH concentration of less than 0.1 mU/l and/or a delta-TSH (TSH response to TRH) below 2.5 mU/l. This group reflects cases which would be normally classified as "hyperthyroidism" or "maximally TRH-suppression" or "negative TRH-test"

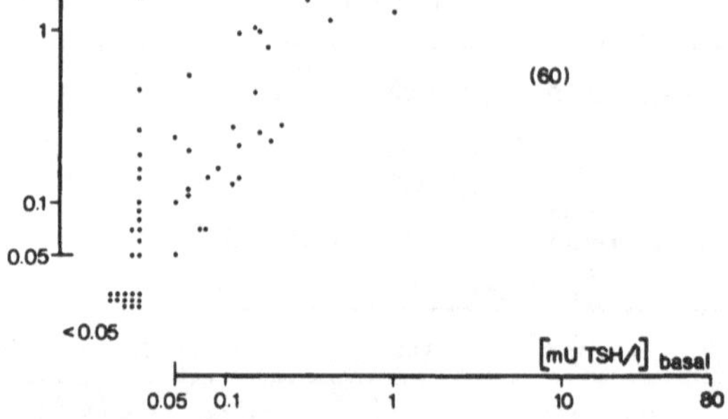

Fig. 2 Results of TRH-tests performed in 163 patients with various thyroid diseases and thyroid function disorders. The x-axis represents the basal TSH concentration, the y-axis the TSH concentration 30 minutes following nasal TRH challenge. Each point represents the result of one distinct patient. TSH concentration determined using the TSH-IRMAclon (Henning, Berlin).

according to the old definition of a delta-TSH below 2.5 mU/l or to the new definition of a basal TSH value below 0.1 mU/l determined in a sensitive assay.

Then, we further evaluated these 66 cases for the underlying diagnosis and the clinical status (fig. 3). The most interesting subgroup consisted of cases with suppressed basal TSH values but a normal TRH-response as shown in 6 patients: One patient with a thyroid cancer treated by L-thyroxine, three patients with clinically euthyroid benign thyroid disease under L-thyroxine, one patient with an autonomic thyroid nodule currently in euthyroidism, and one female with hypothalamic amenorrhoea. At least in these cases the determination of the basal serum TSH concentration would misclassify the thyroid function. Only the TRH-test enables reliable differentiation. Another subground consisted of 25 cases who showed a basal TSH value below 0.1 mU/l and a TRH-response of less than 0.1 mU/l (fig. 3) including 6 patients with true clinically overt hyperthyroidism

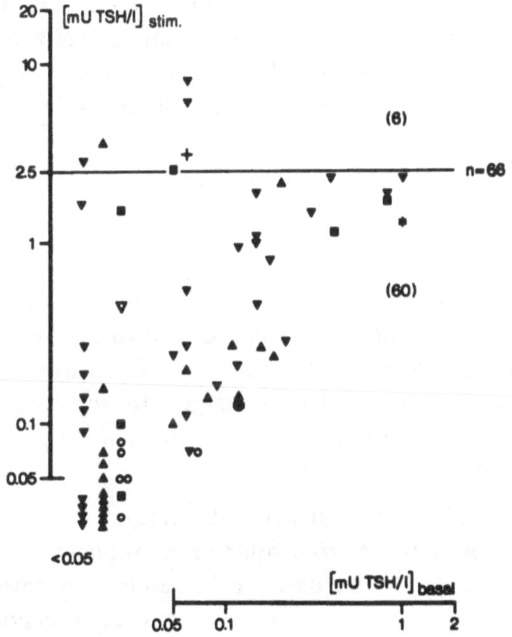

Fig. 3 Results of impaired basal or/and stimulated TSH serum levels (so-called borderline cases): TSH basal of less than 0.1 mU/l and/or a delta-TSH following TRH below 2.5 mU/l.

▲ thyroid cancer, treated by L-thyroxine
▼ clinically euthyroid benign thyroid disease, treated by L-thyroxine
■ autonomic thyroid nodule, clinically euthyroid
✱ Addisons disease
+ hypothalamic amenorrhoea
● Euthyroidism, non-classified disease
▽ clinically overt hyperthyroidism, treated by methimazol and L-thyroxine
○ clinically overt hyperthyroidism, non-treated

and 17 patients under apparently optimal thyreosuppressive treatment. In these cases, the basal TSH value correctly predicts the TRH-test result. Two non-treated patients proved to have autonomic nodules in clinically euthyroidism probably indicating "latent hyperthyroidism".

Another subgroup of 14 patients showed basal TSH concentrations of less than 0.1 mU/l and a subnormal delta-TSH (0.1 – 2.5 mU/l) in the TRH-test (fig. 3). It consisted of 13 patients under L-thyroxine given for various reasons and one patient with an autonomic nodule in clinically euthyroidism. At least in the latter case, determination of only the basal TSH concentration would misinterprete the actual thyroid function.

Finally, a large subgroup of 21 patients showed a basal TSH value greater than 0.1 mU/l but a subnormal TSH response (delta 0.1 – 2.5 mU/l). These was a total of 17 patients under L-thyroxine, 2 patients with autonomic thyroid tissue, 1 patient with Addison's disease, and 1 patient with a still non-classified diagnosis in clinically euthyroidism. In all these cases determination of basal serum TSH values would interprete the thyroid function as euthyroidism respectively non-suppressed TSH secretion. But, actually there is only a subnormal TSH response (delta TSH less than 2.5 mU/l) whose clinical relevance needs to be further evaluated in each case.

Discussion and Conclusion

Determination of serum TSH concentrations by means of sensitive immunoradiometric or enzyme-linked assays using monoclonal antibodies against TSH proved to be superior to a routine radioimmunoassay. No relevant differences were seen comparing various sensitive assays in a wide detection range. Minor discrepancies occurred in the very low concentration range (less than about 0.3 mU/l). This confirms and extends recent findings of own studies [4].

The use of these sensitive methods in the primary diagnosis of non-treated patients enables the differentiation of the thyroid function in about 90 to 100% of the cases depending on the range of the basal TSH serum concentration. Nearly all misinterpreted cases were patients with autonomic thyroid nodules. Therefore, measuring the basal TSH serum level using these sensitive methods (IRMA, EIA) seems to be a sufficiently reliable screening test to replace the TRH-test. Basal TSH serum values between 0.10 and 0.30 mU/l though still require a TRH-test, which was already recently found by other investigators [5, 6, 7]. A TRH-test was sometimes also recommended for another "borderline zone" between the euthyroid and hyperthyroid range [5].

For studies in patients under thyroid-suppressive treatment we recommended the determination of the basal TSH concentration by means of the new sensitive methods as reliable too [4, 8]. From the studies shown here, we conclude that this holds true in about 80% of the cases. Interestingly, all of these cases had basal TSH concentrations above 1 mU/l and in this situation the TRH-test seems to be avoidable also in treated patients. In the remaining cases a TRH-test is still required.

To summarize, these new sensitive methods proved to be a useful tool to replace the TRH-test in most of the clinical situations. However, in borderline cases – i.e. non-treated cases with a basal serum TSH concentration between 0.10 – 0.30 mU/l and probably all patients under L-thyroxine having a basal TSH concentration of less than 1 mU/l – we would still recommend the performance of a TRH-test.

References

[1] Scriba, P. A., W. Börner, D. Emrich, et al.: Endokrinologie-Informationen **9** (1985) 65.
[2] Hesch, R.-D.: Klin. Wochenschr. **62** (1984) 1059.
[3] Hesch, R.-D., K. LeBlanc, A. von zur Mühlen: Dtsch. Med. Wochenschr. **106** (1981) 146.
[4] Bretzel, R. G., G. Siedenberg, E. Skribelka, et al.: Schilddrüse 85, Homburg/Saar (im Druck).
[5] Mewissen, B., R. Hehrmann: Akt. Endokr. Stoffw. **6** (1985) 1.
[6] Joseph, K.: Diagnose und Labor **35** (1985) 133.
[7] Mahlstedt, J., A. Hotze: Nuc. Compact **16** (1985) 72.
[8] Bretzel, R. G., K. Federling: Klin. Wochenschr. **63**, Suppl. 4 (1985) 203.

Significance of TRH test in strumectomized patients for life-long thyroid hormone treatment

H. Fritzsche, E. Hillbrand, H. Hugl, M. Kargl, P. Weiß

Introduction

Life-long treatment of patients after strumectomy with thyroid hormones for prevention of recurrent goiter was generally accepted because of a considerable lower incidence of recurrent goiter [14]. With the more precise diagnosis of thyroid function by the TRH-test several authors reported normal TT3 and TT4, but an increased response of TSH to TRH (preclinical hypothyroidism) in 50 – 70% of bilateral subtotal strumectomized patients 4 – 8 weeks after operation [1 – 3, 10, 16]. These results supported the hypothesis, that recurrent goiter growth is stimulated by increased TSH-secretion. In consequence patients after strumectomy were selected by TRH-test for longlife treatment. However no prospective studies about the significance of increased TSH-secretion for recurrent goiter growth were published in the literature [11].

Recent research of goiter genesis demonstrated development of nodular goiter (therefore also recurrent goiter) by autonomous or stimulated growth of heterogenetic follicular cells]9, 12]. TSH is discussed as a growth stimulating factor in animal experiments but no dose dependent action was described. If an abnormal TRH-test would indicate risk of recurrent goiter, up to 50% of strumectomized patients should develop recurrent goiter. But in fact these figures have never been reported in literature. Additionally from clinical experience we know strumectomized patients up to 60 years after operation without any hormone prophylaxis with normal remnants and preclinical hypothyroidism.

Therefore we examined thyroid function in three patient groups 4 – 6 weeks, 6 – 15 years and 16 – 64 years after strumectomy and compared the results of Δ TSH between patients with normal remnants or recurrent goiter.

Patients and methods

The study was performed in 457 strumectomized patients. The different patient groups, sex, range and median of age at operation and median of time interval since strumectomy are listed in table 1. All patients were off therapy since a

Thyrotropin

minimum of 4 weeks and showed normal TT_3 and TT_4. In addition to the clinical investigations technetium scintiscans and sonography were performed in all patients. Normal thyroid remnants were defined by a normal scintiscan and by a homogenous echogenicity in the sonography with a total volume less than 20 ml (mean thyroid volumen + 3 SD of healthy individuals).

Serum total T_3 (n. v.: 80 – 220 ng/dl), serum total T_4 (n. v.: 3.4 – 13.0 µg/dl) and TSH were determined by radioimmunoassay. Δ TSH (n. v.: 2.5 – 25 µU/ml) was calculated from TSH 30 minutes after 200 µg/TRH (400 µg in patients > 70 years) minus TSH-basal.

For statistical analysis the U-test (Mann, Whitney) for unpaired samples and the Wilcoxon-Test for paired samples were used ad a significance level of $\alpha = 0.01$.

Results

Patients with normal remnants and patients with recurrent goiter do not show any statistical significant difference of age at operation and of years since strumectomy within the groups 4 – 6 weeks, 6 – 15 years and 16 – 64 years after operation and are comparable for this study (tab. 1).

In the course of years (tab. 2) TT_4 shows a statistical significant increase from $\tilde{x} = 6.0$ µg/dl and $\tilde{x} = 6.7$ µg/dl in patients with normal remnants and recurrent goiter 4 – 6 weeks after surgery to $\tilde{x} = 7.3$ µg/dl 6 – 15 years and $\tilde{x} = 7.3$ and $\tilde{x} = 7.6$ µg/dl respectively 16 – 64 years after operation.

Within the three groups only patients 16 – 64 years after operation show a statistical significant difference of TT_4. TT_3 is equal within and between the patient groups.

Table 1 Sex, range and median of age at operation and median of time interval since strumectomy of patients with normal remnants and recurrent goiter

Time interval since thyrectomy	Normal remnants				Nodules/recurrent goiter			
	N	M/W (%)	age at op. range median	years since thyrectomy median	N	M/W (%)	age at op. range median	years since thyrectomy median
4 – 6 weeks	171	15/85	16 – 75 47	0	56	25/75	27 – 72 48	0
6 – 15 years	26	8/92	22 – 56 34	11	42	15/85	19 – 64 34	12
16 – 64 years	46	15/85	16 – 64 30	24	116	10/90	16 – 63 28	28

Table 2 Range and median of TT_4 and TT_3 in strumectomized patients with normal remnants or recurrent goiter at different time intervals since operation

Time interval since thyrectomy	Normal remnants			Nodules/recurrent goiter		
	N	TT_4 (μg/dl) range, median	TT_3 (ng/dl) range, median	N	TT_4 (μg/dl) range, median	TT_3 (ng/dl) range, median
4 – 6 weeks	171	4.5 – 13.0 6.0	80 – 220 115	56	4.5 – 13.0 6.7	80 – 220 124
6 – 15 years	26	4.6 – 12.0 7.3	85 – 212 130	42	5.3 – 12.0 7.3	81 – 207 130
16 – 64 years	46	4.5 – 11.5 7.3	80 – 217 121	116	4.5 – 13.0 7.6	80 – 208 125

Table 3 Range and median of ΔTSH and incidence of ΔTSH > 25 μU/ml in strumectomized patients with normal remnants and recurrent goiter at different time intervals since operation

Time interval since thyrectomy	Normal remnants			Nodules/recurrent goiter		
	N	ΔTSH, range, median (μU/ml)	% ΔTSH > 25 μU/ml	N	ΔTSH, range, median (μU/ml)	% ΔTSH > 25 μU/ml
4 – 6 weeks	171	1.0 – 80 26.2	53	56	1.4 – 73.9 21.1	44
6 – 15 years	26	6.9 – 71.4 16.4	19	42	0 – 72.2 16.7	14
16 – 64 years	46	1.7 – 65.8 16.0	19	116	0 – 73.2 9.9	13

Patients with normal thyroid remnants show a Δ TSH of $\tilde{x}$ = 26.2 μU/ml 4 – 6 weeks after surgery and a statistical significant lower Δ TSH 6 – 15 years and 16 – 64 years after operation (tab. 3). Also patients with recurrent goiter show a statistical significant lower Δ TSH years after surgery. In patients with recurrent goiter 16 – 64 years after operation Δ TSH of $\tilde{x}$ = 9.9 μU/ml is statistical significant lower than Δ TSH $\tilde{x}$ = 16.7 in patients with recurrent goiter 6 – 15 years after operation and also statistical significant lower than Δ TSH $\tilde{x}$ = 16.0 in patients with normal remnants 16 – 64 years after operation. Preclinical hypothyroidism (Δ TSH > 25 μU/ml) was observed in 53% of patients with normal remnants and in 44% of patients with nodules in the remnants 4 – 6 weeks after strumectomy. 6 – 15 years and 16 – 64 years after operation the incidence of Δ TSH > 25 μU/ml is statistical significant lower. But within and between the patient groups 6 – 15 and 16 – 64 years after operation there is no statistical significant differnce of incidence of preclinical hypothyroidism.

Because previous hormone treatment in some patients may have influenced our results we compared incidence of Δ TSH > 25 μU/ml in patients with normal remnants and recurrent goiter according to previous hormone treatment (tab. 4).

Table 4 Incidence of ΔTSH > 25 μU/ml, range and median of years since strumectomy in patients with normal remnants and recurrent goiter without and with consequent hormone treatment

Hormone prophylaxis	Normal remnants			Nodules/recurrent goiter		
	N	years after op. range, median	% ΔTSH > 25 μU/ml	N	years after op. range, median	% ΔTSH > 25 μU/ml
no hormone prophylaxis	38	7 – 42 24	15	90	6 – 65 30	15
consequent hormone prophylaxis	19	6 – 26 16	16	19	7 – 34 16	16

Strumectomized patients with normal remnants or recurrent goiter without any hormone treatment 7 – 42 and 6 – 65 years after operation respectivley show a similiar incidence of Δ TSH > 25 μU/ml of 15%. Patients with normal remnants or recurrent goiter and with a consequent hormone treatment for 6 – 34 years both show an incidence of Δ TSH > 25 μU/ml of 16% when off therapy. There is no statistical significant difference.

Discussion

Preclinical hypothyroidism observed in 50 – 70% of patients after bilateral subtotal strumectomy several weeks and month after operation was thought to be the pathogenesis of recurrent goiter growth [1 – 3, 10, 16]. But the real action of increased TSH-secretion in recurrent goiter growth has never been proved by a prospective randomized study [11]. Additionally there are no reports about incidence of preclinical hypothyroidism in patients several years after operation.

Our results show a statistical significant lower incidence of Δ TSH > 25 μU/ml in strumectomized patients 6 – 15 years and 16 – 64 years after operation (tab. 3). The lower but statistically not significant differnt incidence of preclinical hypothyroidism in patients with recurrent goiter may be the result of autonomous functioning thyroid tissue left at operation or slowly growing in the years following surgery as documented by significant lower Δ TSH $\tilde{x}$ = 9.9 μU/ml and significant higher TT_4 $\tilde{x}$ = 7.6 μg/dl in the patient group with recurrent goiter 16 – 64 years after operation.

There is no statistical significant difference of the incidence of Δ TSH > 25 μU/ml between the patient groups 6 – 15 years after surgery actually known as period with the peak of recurrent goiter incidence [13] and 16 – 64 years after operation.

In the course of years thyroid function tends to normalize in strumectomized patients with normal remnants and recurrent goiter similarly as indicated by the incidence of preclinical hypothyroidism 50 – 70% several weeks after operation and only 13 – 19% more than 6 years later.

There is no difference of incidence of preclinical hypothyroidism in patients with normal remnants and recurrent goiter more than 6 years after strumectomy without any or with consequent hormone treatment. Therefore from these results the pathogenetic action of TSH as growth stimulating factor appears to be doubtful.

The data suggest rather an independence of recurrent goiter growth and increased Δ TSH. The growth stimulating effect of increased TSH on nodular goiter also observed in animal experiments [12] may act as a permissive factor in strumectomized patients, where adenomas or heterogenetic follicules sensitive to TSH stimulation have been left at operation. Such remnant adenomas can be found in up to 30% of recent strumectomized patients by ultrasound [6].

Additional measurement of serum-thyroglobulin (TG) seems to be useful in the detection of recurrent goiter growth. High TG-levels indicate goiter growth [4, 7, 8] and are described in recurrent goiter [15] and sometimes also in normal remnants [5].

From our results we conclude that TRH-test is useful for diagnosis of preclinical hypothyroidism with regard to further treatment, but not sufficient for selection of strumectomized patients for a life-long hormone prophylaxis.

Conclusion

Preclinical hypothyroidism with a high incidence of 50 – 70% in patients after bilateral strumectomy was reported in literature and thought to be the pathogenetic factor of recurrent goiter. In consequence strumectomized patients were selected by TRH-test for a life-long hormone treatment. Comparing different patient groups with normal remnants and recurrent goiter incidence of Δ TSH > 25 μU/ml is statistically significantly lower with 19 and 14% respectively 6 – 15 years after strumectomy and 19% and 13% 16 – 64 years after operation. There is no statistically significant difference of preclinical hypothyroidism incidence in patients with normal remnants or recurrent goiter without or with consequent hormone treatment more than 6 years since strumectomy.

These results suggest independence of preclinical hypothyroidism and recurrent goiter growth. Increased TSH may act as a permissive factor in strumectomized patients with nodules or heterogenetic follicules in the remnants, which can be detected by ultrasound or by serum TG-measurement. Therefore TRH-test is only useful for diagnosis of preclinical hypothyroidism with regard to treatment but not sufficient for selection of risk patients of recurrent goiter.

References

[1] Arlt, B., A. Arlt, W. Brinkmann, et al.: Untersuchungen zur thyreotropen Partialfunktion des HVL nach Schilddrüsenoperation. Med. Welt **31** (1980) 550.

[2] Bonelli, E., J. Brändle, H. Fritzsche, et al.: Die Kontrolle der Schilddrüsenfunktion nach Strumaresektion als Basis der Rezidivprophylaxe. Acta Chir. Austr. **16**, Suppl. 51 (1983).

[3] Börner, W., A. Weber, E. Moll, et al.: Spontanverlauf der Schilddrüsenfunktion nach Resektion euthyreoter Strumen, p. 442. Nuklearmedizin, 17. Intern. Jahrestagung der Gesellschaft für Nuklearmedizin, Innsbruck 1979. F. K. Schattauer Verlag, Stuttgart – New York 1980.

[4] Bürgi, U., F. Gebel, H. Gerber: Die diagnostische Bedeutung der Thyreoglobulinbestimmung im Blut. Schweiz. Med. Wochenschr. **114** (1984) 365.

[5] Fritzsche, H., E. Brändle, P. Weiss: Thyreoglobulin als Parameter für die Indikation zur Rezidivprophylaxe. Schilddrüse 1985. Georg Thieme Verlag, Stuttgart – New York (in press).

[6] Fritzsche, H., M. Kargl, E. Blum, et al.: Morphologische und funktionelle Ergebnisse der Strumaresektion unter Berücksichtigung der präoperativen Sonographie. Schilddrüse 1985. Georg Thieme Verlag Stuttgart – New York (in press).

[7] Gärtner, R., A. Hainzinger, K. Korn, et al.: Evidence for Autonomous Thyroglobulin Release from Euthyroid and Hyperthyroid Nodular Goiter – Thyroglobulin, a Possible Helpful Parameter in Diagnosis of Non-malignant Thyroid Desorders. Klin. Wochenschr. **61** (1983) 737.

[8] Gebel, F., F. Ramelli, U. Bürgi, et al.: The Site of Leakage of Intrafollicular Thyroglobulin into the Blood Stream in Simple Human Goiter. J. Clin. Endocrinol. Metab. **57** (1983) 915.

[9] Gerber, H., H. J. Peter, F. Ramelli, et al.: Autonomie und Heterogenität der Follikel in der euthyreoten und hyperthyreoten menschlichen Knotenstruma: Die Lösung alter Rätsel? Schweiz. Med. Wochenschr. **1178** (1983) 113.

[10] Hüfner, M., R. Wahl, B. Müller, et al.: Das Verhalten der thyreotropen Hypophysenfunktion nach Operation euthyreoter Strumen und autonomer Adenome. Endokrinologie **75** (1980) 35.

[11] Köbberling, J.: Pathogenese des Strumarezidivs nach Strumaresektion. Schilddrüse 1983, pp. 204 – 209. Georg Thieme Verlag Stuttgart – New York 1985.

[12] Peter, H. J., H. Gerber, H. Studer, et al.: Pathogenesis of Heterogeneity in Human Multinodular Goiter. J. Clin. Invest. **76** (1985) 1992.

[13] Steiner, H.: Das Strumarezidiv. Springer-Verlag, Wien 1960.

[14] Steiner, H.: Rezidivprophylaxe nach Schilddrüsenoperationen. Wien. Med. Wochenschr. **161** (1977) 127.

[15] Steurer, Th., Chr. Reiners: Serum-Thyreoglobulin (hTG) nach Operation blander Strumen. Akt. Endokrinol. Stoffw. 3 (1982) 126.

[16] Wahl, R., Ch. Hornstein, M. Grussendorf, et al.: Ansätze zu einer differenzierten Rezidivprophylaxe nach Strumaoperation, p. 161. Langenbecks Arch. Chir. Suppl: Chirurgisches Forum 78 für experimentelle und klinische Forschung, 1978.

Diagnostic significance of basal TSH-concentrations (TSH-IRMA)

A. Passath, G. Leb, H. Warnkroß

With the introduction of immunoradiometric TSH-assays it has become possible to establish the effect of thyroid hormone excess or deficiency upon the pituitary cells by means of serum TSH determinations without the necessity of TRH-stimulation [3].

Up to now the TRH test, applying TSH-RIA has been accepted as the sole functional parameter to differentiate between euthyroidism and hyperthyroidism. The sensitivity of the TSH-RIA method was insufficient in the lower ranges to determine TSH suppression by means of a single basal value.

TSH measurement using the IRMA-method, however, is highly sensitive so that TSH concentration may be precisely established even below 0.1 mU/l [4, 6]. Since a close linear relation between basal TSH (bTSH) and TRH-stimulated TSH-concentrations (sTSH) was found, it was suggested to describe pituitary-thyroid regulation by means of a single basal TSH serum value [1, 5].

Yet, it is not generally accepted that a linear relation exists between bTSH and sTSH [2]. In this connection it may be stated, that endocrine organs are subject to complicated regulation – and feedback mechanisms and hormonal effects upon these – e. g. thyroid hormone upon the pituitary – are governed by different mechanisms than those affecting other body cells.

Non-detectable TSH-concentrations prior and after TRH-stimulation rather frequently occur in hypermetabolism. However, in spite of thyroid hormone excess in the pituitary gland (i. e. "pituitary hormone excess") there may be a state of eumetabolism of the entire organism.

In low bTSH concentrations the sTSH values can not be accurately anticipated. The reason is that identical bTSH concentrations may at one time be associated with reduced (blunted) TSH-stimulation following TRH ("relative pituitary hormone excess") while at another with normal TRH stimulation ("euthyroid regulation").

Increased basal TSH levels indicating a thyroid hormone deficiency in the pituitary gland (i. e. "pituitary hormone deficiency") are not always associated with a general hypometabolism. On the other hand TSH stimulation following

Thyrotropin

TRH is not so pronounced in case of hypothyroid bTSH values as may occur with normal bTSH levels.

Thus the functional interdependence between bTSH and sTSH may not be believed to follow a linear relationship and must not be considered from an isolated pituitary aspect. A theoretical regression line would have to pass approximately the zero point (bTSH and sTSH beeing zero) flattening out in the hypothyroid range. In plotting such a regression line a potency function would give the best fit.

Results

Interrelation of sTSH and bTSH levels for determining diagnostic value of basal TSH-concentrations:
TRH-tests in non-selected thyroid patients including out-patients and in-patients partely with severe ailments were evaluated. In about 10% of TRH-tests (n = 1039) bTSH values ranged below 0.1 mU/l, while 6% of bTSH values exceeded 4 mU/l and were within the hypothyroid range. Thyroid hormone levels and clinical classification as to thyroid function were disregarded. The regression line based on logarithmic transformated TSH data approximately represented the expected tendency (fig. 1). All TSH values (RIA gnost hTSH c.t. – Behring Institut) were utilized for calculating the regression equation. The course of the regression line does not fully correspond to the mean sTSH values within the respective bTSH ranges of 0.2 – 0.8 and 1.8 – 4 mU/l.

Yet, for the majority of basal TSH concentrations a relatively precise assessment of stimulated TSH values may be given as follows:

1. Basal TSH-concentrations <0.1 mU/l (fig. 2): in 96% of cases there was no, or blunted TSH stimulation following TRH but only in 4% Delta-TSH was > 2.5 mU/l.
2. Basal TSH-concentrations ranging from 0.1 to 0.4 mU/l: in 30 – 60% normal TSH stimulation following TRH was recorded (Delta-TSH > 2.5 mU/l), the percentage of blunted stimulation decreases with extent of bTSH-concentrations.
3. Basal TSH-concentrations of 0.4 – 4 mU/l: with 96 – 100% accuracy a normal TRH test is to be expected, sTSH values rise according to bTSH in an approximately linear relation.
4. Basal TSH-concentrations between 1.7 – 4 mU/l: with increasing bTSH, stimulated TSH values exceeding 25 mU/l are observed more frequently.
5. Basal TSH-concentrations ranging above 4 mU/l may be considered as hypothyroid.

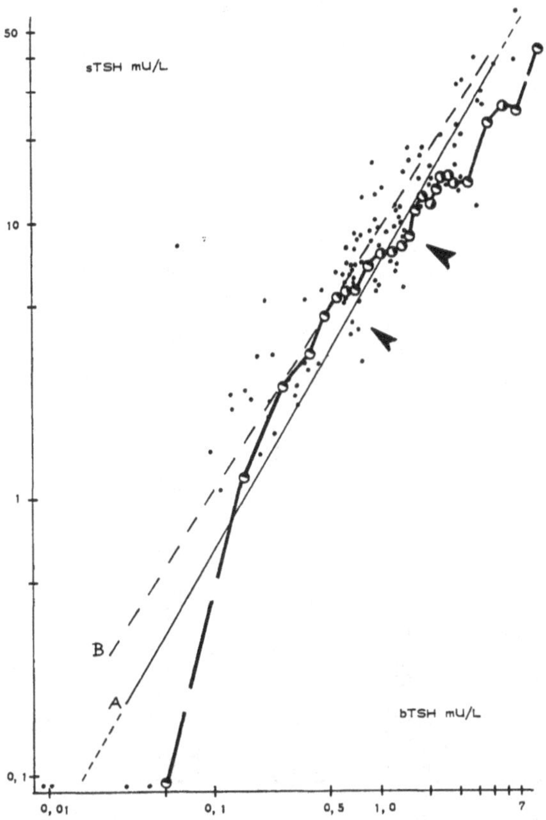

Fig. 1 1039 TRH-tests: Correlation between bTSH and sTSH (potency function).
r = 0.94 $\bar{y} = 0.96\ x^{0.82}$

——— regression line (A)

◐ mean sTSH-data (logarithmic transformed) in the corresponding bTSH range

114 TRH-tests from subjects with euthyroidism
r = 0.97 $\bar{y} = 0.95\ x^{0.97}$

– – – – regression line (B)

● TSH-data

The question arises in which way these ranges may be indicative in thyroid diagnostics.

TRH tests of a series of clearly defined euthyroid patients were evaluated in order to establish the relation between bTSH and sTSH within the euthyroid range. 114 thyroid patients with clinically determined euthyroidism and with normal T_4 and T_3 parameters were selected. In this series there were normal-sized thyroid glands as well as diffuse and nodular goitres with cold, warm and hot nodules including patients with strumectomy and on thyroid hormone therapy.

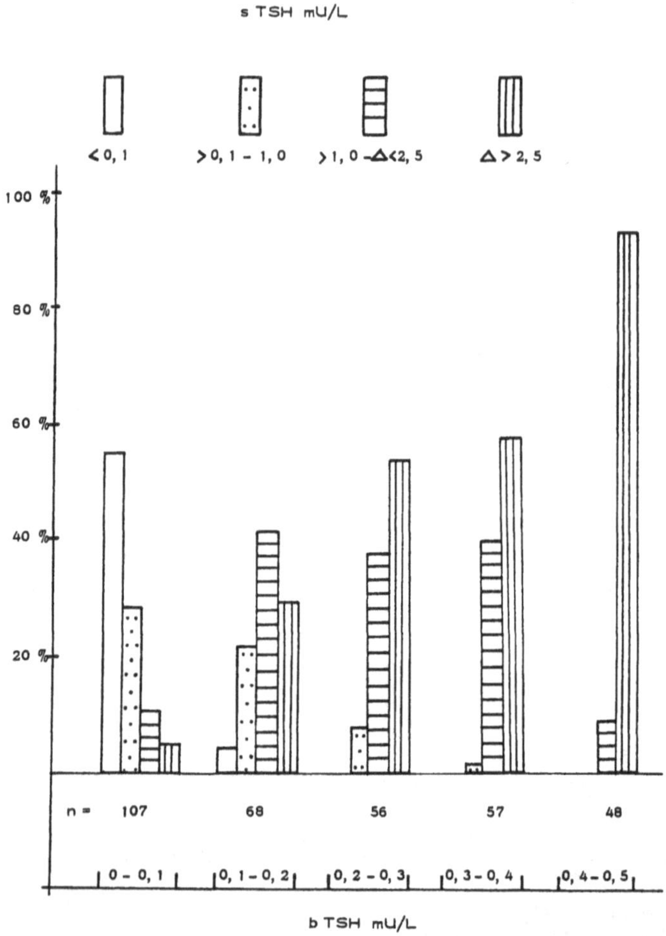

Fig. 2 Percentage distribution of sTSH-data in different bTSH ranges (bTSH 0 – 0.5 mU/L).

sTSH < 0.1 — sTSH > 0.1 – < 1.0

sTSH > 1.0, Delta-TSH < 2.5 — Delta-TSH > 2.5 mU/L

The regression line thus calculated shows the same incline but is better correlated to the mean sTSH values in the bTSH ranges between 0.2 and 1 mU/l than the regression line described before (fig. 1). In other words the predictability of sTSH on basis of bTSH values is very limited regarding the border range of 0.1 – 0.3 mU/l. In this euthyroid series we found normal TRH-tests in more than 95% when bTSH-concentrations was above 0.3 mU/l.

Discussion

In comparison to TSH-RIA assays the sensitivity in the lower concentration range could be greatly improved by using the TSH-IRMA-method. Whereas TSH-RIA allowed to evaluate TRH-tests only qualitatively (positive or negative), when using IRMA-assays also a quantitative assessment is possible ("absolute or relative pituitary hormone excess or deficiency").

The pattern of this potency function showing the interdependence of sTSH and bTSH-concentrations allows to predict with great probability pituitary-thyroid regulation in the following ranges:

With bTSH-concentrations below 0.1 mU/l there is a probability of more than 96% of any existing either "absolute or relative pituitary hormone excess" so that TRH-tests will not be required [3 – 5]. To establish the degree of any systemic hypermetabolism it is however necessary to determine thyroid hormone levels in serum.

In case these show no elevation, a bTSH value below 0.1 mU/l indicates merely a disturbed pituitary-thyroid regulation or TSH suppression by thyroid hormones with high pituitary thyroid-hormone content, respectively. Two examples will illustrate this: Under thyrostatic medication, bTSH values below 0.1 mU/l, will indicate a still existing pituitary thyroid-hormone excess and in the course of thyroid hormone therapy would proof the desirable suppressive effect. In both cases there is no evidence of any systemic hypermetabolism when thyroid hormone levels are normal or high normal.

With basal TSH values ranging from 0.3/0.4 to 4 mU/l an adequate TSH stimulation following TSH may be anticipated with almost 100% certainty. In these bTSH findings neither a TRH-test nor thyroid hormone measurements are required [3]. Consequently, this bTSH range yields evidence for euthyroid regulation in the individual subject.

However, no exact predictions are possible with basal TSH-concentrations between 0.1 and 0.3/0.4 mU/l. In this case ther may be either a "relative pituitary hormone excess" or a normal pituitary-thyroid regulation. Within this range it may be stated that ouvert systemic hyperthyroidism is unlikely in most cases and therefore thyroid hormone determinations will be superfluous. TRH-test, however, is still necessary for quantitative evaluation to distinguish normal TSH stimulation and low responders (blunted stimulation) [5].

There may be exceptions e.g.: Under thyroid hormone therapy the desired substitution effect is achieved when bTSH values are within this range. Under thyrostatic therapy such values indicate that an adequate pituitary regulation be lacking. In older patients and those with severe ailments a low response to TRH seems difficult to interpret so that further investigations and follow ups will be essential.

With bTSH values ranging from 1.7 to 4 mU/l a "relative pituitary hormone deficiency" can only be defined by TRH-test in individual cases.

Summary

In conclusion, it may be stated that the application of sensitive TSH-IRMA assays represents a great advance in thyroid diagnostics since within clearly defined bTSH ranges (below 0.1 and between 0.4 – 4 mU/l) the extent of TSH stimulation following TRH may be predicted with great accuracy thus enabling a simple and precise determination of thyroid function.

References

[1] Bayer, M. F., J. P. Kriss, I. R. McDougall: Clinical experience with sensitive Thyrotropin measurements: Diagnostic and therapeutic implications. J. Nuc. Med. **26** (1985) 1248 – 1256.

[2] Böttger, I. G., H. W. Pabst, G. Bienhaus, et al.: TSH tesponse to TRH as a function of basal TSH – new aspects in pituitary-thyroid regulation. International Symposium on Thyrotropin, April 17 – 18, 1986, Graz/Austria (in press).

[3] Joseph, K.: Schilddrüsenerstdiagnostik: TSH immunradiometrisch. Diagnose und Labor **35** (1985) 133 – 149.

[4] Klingler, W., P. Ball: Die Bestimmung des Thyreotropin (TSH) im Serum mit einer sensitiven immunradiometrischen Methode. Ärztl. Lab. **31** (1985) 219 – 223.

[5] Martino, E., G. Bambini, L. Bartalena, et al.: Human serum Thyrotrophin measurement by ultrasensitive immunoradiometric assay as a first-line test in the evaluation of thyroid function. Clin. Endocrinol. **24** (1986) 141 – 148.

[6] Wood, W. G., D. Waller, U. Hantke: An evaluation of six solid-phase Thyrotropin (TSH) kits. J. Clin. Chem. Clin. Biochem. **23** (1985) 461 – 471.

Impaired conversion of thyroxine to triiodothyronine causing elevated concentrations of thyroxine and TSH in an euthyroid patient

H. Vierhapper, W. Waldhäusl

Methods

To determine concentrations of total thyroxine (TT4, normal range: 5.0 – 11.2 µg/dl), thyroid function index (TFI, normal range 0.86 – 1.13), total triiodothyronine (TT3, normal range: 0.9 – 1.75 ng/ml), reverse triiodothyronine (rT3, normal range: 0.09 – 0.35 ng/ml), thyrotropin (TSH, normal range: < 4 µU/ml, following stimulation by 400 µg TRH: < 20 µU/ml) and thyroxine binding globulin (TBG, normal range 13 – 26 mg/l) the following commercially available radioimmunoassays were used: TT4, TFI: Bio-Rad, Richmond, CA, USA; TT3, rT3: Serono Co., Freiburg, FRG; TBG: Behringwerke, Marburg/Lahn, FRG; TSH: Byk-Mallinckrodt, Dietzenbach-Steinberg, FRG (TSH-Standard: MRC 68/38). The intra- and interassay coefficient of variation of all radioimmunoassays was smaller than 10%.

Case report

This 60 year old female patient was first referred to the thyroid outpatient department for suspected hyperthyroidism. The patient's clinical symptoms (e. g.: tachycardia, weight loss of 15 kg) were in accordance with that diagnosis. A diffuse goiter (clinical stage III) was palpated and confirmed by 99 mTc thyroid scintigraphy. Serum concentration of TT4 and TT3 where 20 µg/dl and 6.4 ng/ml, respectively and TFI was 1.65. Concentrations of TSH were not determined at this point. Following normalization of serum concentrations of TT4 and of clinical symptoms by initial therapy with methimazole partial thyroidectomy was performed. During the following two years the patient underwent craniotomy for the removal of a neurinoma of the acoustic nerve. Furthermore total hysterectomy was performed due to a myomatous uterus. Possibly due to the ensuing treatment with conjugated estrogens the patient then presented elevated serum concentrations of TT4, whereas TFI remained normal. Subsequently estrogen therapy was discontinued. One year later the patient appeared clinically euthyroid

Thyrotropin

but presented elevated serum concentrations of TT4, TFI and TSH (basal and stimulated). Identical concentrations of TT4 were seen in one serum sample both with and without ethanol extraction prior to radioimmunoassay, thus excluding the presence of endogenous antibodies directed against TT4. Concentrations of TT3 were in the low-normal range, whereas concentrations of rT3 were slightly elevated (tab. 1). Concentration of TBG was normal (19.3 mg/l). X-ray examination and CT-scanning of the sella region were normal as were physical examination and the result of routine screening of kidney and liver function.

The patient was then given T3 (Trijodthyronin, Sanabo, Wien, Austria) perorally at doses of 25 µg b. i. d., 25 µg t. i. d. and 25 µg q. i. d. for three days each (tab. 1) resulting in supraphysiological concentrations of TT3 and a reversible suppression of TT4, TFI, rT3 and TSH. When p. o. T4 (Thyrex, Sanabo; 100 µg/day) was given instead of T3, concentrations of TT4 and TFI remained elevated above the normal range. Finally the patient was placed on a maintenance therapy with T3 (25 µg/day) resulting in normal serum concentrations of both, TT4 and TT3 as well as a normal responsiveness of TSH to TRH.

Table 1 Serum concentrations of thyroid hormones and TSH (before (b) and 20 minutes after (a) stimulation by 400 µg TRH) in a clinically euthyroid patient prior to and during treatment with p.o. triiodothyronine or thyroxine

Therapy		TT_4 (µg/dl)	FTI	TT_3 (ng/ml)	FT_3 (ng/ml)	TSH (µU/ml) (b)	TSH (µU/ml) (a)
off therapy	($\bar{x}$, n = 3)	15.2	1.27	0.95	0.36	4.2	23.0
50 µg T_3/day	(day 3)	13.4	1.26	1.25	0.29	3.2	–
75 µg T_3/day	(day 3)	12.3	1.13	1.80	0.29	2.4	–
100 µg T_3/day	(day 3)	9.9	1.09	4.50	0.30	2.2	3.0
off therapy	(day 42)	15.9	1.21	1.30	–	3.8	23.0
100 µg T_4/day	(day 7)	20.5	1.21	1.30	–	4.4	19.0
25 µg T_3/day	(day 100)	10.2	–	1.10	–	2.9	13.0
normal range		5.0 – 11.2	0.86 – 1.12	0.90 – 1.75	0.09 – 0.35	< 4.0	< 20.0

Discussion

At present, three different clinical conditions have to be considered when an explanation for elevated serum concentrations of TSH is sought in man: Firstly, the removal of physiological feedback inhibition in primary hypothyroidism results in increased concentrations of TSH in the presence of subnormal thyroid hormone production; secondly, elevated concentrations of TSH are encountered together with increased production of T4 and T3 in patients with secondary hyperthyroidism with or without radiologically apparent TSH-producing pituitary adenomas [1]; and thirdly, inappropriately high concentrations of TSH in the presence of supranormal concentrations of thyroid hormones may indicate pheripheral resistance to thyroid hormone action [2, 3].

The patient described in this report does not fit into any of these three groups: As opposed to the combination of subnormal levels of TT3 and low-normal concentrations of TT4 frequently encountered in mild primary hypothyroidism [4] she presented hyperthyroxinemia together with low-normal concentrations of TT3.

If, on the other hand, hyperthyrotropinemia was the primary cause of the results obtained at the follow-up of our patient one would then expect increased serum concentrations of TSH and both, of T3 and T4 [1, 5]. The same consideration applies to and consequently excludes resistance to thyroid hormones in our patient [3]. A supranormal concentration of T3 was indeed documented when the patient was first seen. Unfortunately, TSH was not determined at this point and although the available evidence indicates that the patient then suffered from primary hyperthyroidism the presence of hyperthyrotropinema cannot, in retrospect, be excluded with certainty. However, once initial hyperthyroidism had been successfully treated by subtotal thyroidectomy TT3 in our patient remained in the low-normal range and there was neither clinical evidence of recurrent hyperthyroidism nor any radiological evidence of a pituitary adenoma.

The demonstration of identical concentrations of TT4 prior to and after ethanol extraction excluded the presence of endogenous T4-binding antibodies in our patient. It should also be noted that TFI paralleled the concentrations of TT4. Since the method employed for the determination of TFI corrects for the presence of abnormal T4-binding proteins [6], euthyroid thyroxine excess due to an abnormal binding protein with higher affinity to T4 than to T3 [7] may be excluded.

The concentrations of TT3 and rT3 seen in the patient described in this report resemble the metabolic situation frequently encountered in severe non-thyroidal illness [8, 9], where a decrease in the extrathyroidal conversion of T4 to T3 results in subnormal concentrations of T3 and in elevated serum concentrations of its metabolically inactive homologue, rT3. However, in contrast to her counterparts suffering from nonthyroidal diseases [6] our patient exhibited hyperthyroxinemia and an enhanced response of TSH to TRH and thus does not alltogether fit into the frame of the so-called 'Euthyroid sick syndrome'.

To explain the results presented in our report we propose that a primary deficit in T3, presumably due to a decreased deiodination of T4 in peripheral tissues caused a rise in pituitary TSH subsequently resulting in increased thyroidal production of T4 thus increasing substrate supply to peripheral monodeiodinases and eventually resulting in lownormal concentrations of TT3. The fact that chronic pituitary stimulation may induce hyperplasia of the thyrotroph [10] provides the rationale for low-dose, long-term T3-substitution therapy in our patient. In conclusion it appears that future differential diagnoses of euthyroid hyperthyroxinemia should include the possibility of an impaired conversion of T4 to T3 in association with a compensatory rise in TSH secretion.

Abstract

Thyroid function was studied in a 60 year old female patient 2 years after partial thyroidectomy had been performed for hyperthyroidism. Serum concentration of TT4 and TSH were elevated, whereas the serum concentrations of TT3 and TBG were within the normal range. Within two weeks increasing doses of peroral T3 suppressed serum concentrations of TT4 and TSH into the normal range. Physiological concentrations of TT4, TT3 and TSH were subsequently maintained during long-term administration of 25 μg T3 p. o/day. We propose that the possibility of an impaired conversion of T4 to T3 associated with a compensatory rise in TSH secretion has to be considered in the differential diagnosis of euthyroid hyperthyroxinemia.

References

[1] Waldhäusl, W., P. Bratusch-Marrain, P. Nowotny, et al.: Secondary hyperthyroidism due to thyrotropin hypersecretion: Study of pituitary tumor morphology and thyrotropin chemistry and release. J. Clin. Endocrinol. Metab. **49** (1979) 879 – 887.

[2] Refetoff, S., L. T. De Wind, L. J. De Groot: Familial syndrome combining deaf-mutism, stippled epiphyses, goiter and abnormally high PBI: Possible target organ refractoriness to thyroid hormone. J. Clin. Endocrinol. Metab. **27** (1967) 279 – 294.

[3] Gheri, R. C., R. Bianchi, G. Mariani, et al.: A new case of familial partial generalized resistance to thyroid hormones: Study of 3,5,3'-triiodothyronine (T3) binding to lymphocyte and skin fibroblast nuclei and in vivo conversion of thyroxine to T3. J. Clin. Endocrinol. Metab. **58** (1984) 563 – 569.

[4] Ingbar, S. H., K. A. Woeber: The thyroid gland. In: Textbook of Endocrinology (R. H. Williams, eds.), p. 215. W. B. Saunders, Philadelphia – London – Toronto 1981.

[5] Rösler, A., Y. Litvin, C. Hage, et al.: Familial hyperthyroidism due to inappropriate thyrotropin secretion successfully treated with triiodothyronine. J. Clin. Endocrinol. Metab. **54** (1982) 76 – 82.

[6] Vierhapper, H., A. Laggner, W. Waldhäusl, et al.: Impaired secretion of TSH in critically ill patients with 'low T4-syndrome'. Acta Endocrinol. (Kbh) **101** (1982) 542 – 549.

[7] Stockigt, J. R., D. J. Topliss, J. W. Barlow, et al.: Familial euthyroid thyroxine excess: An appropriate response to abnormal thyroxine binding associated with albumin. J. Clin. Endocrinol. Metab. **53** (1981) 353 – 359.

[8] Chopra, I. J., D. H. Solomon, U. Chopra, et al.: Alterations in circulating thyroid hormones and thyrotropin in hepatic cirrhosis: Evidence for euthyroidism despite subnormal serum triiodothyroine. J. Clin. Endocrinol. Metab. **39** (1974) 501–511.
[9] Cavalieri, R. R., B. Rapoport: Impaired peripheral conversion of thyroxine to triiodothyronine. Annu. Rev. Med. **28** (1977) 57–65.
[10] Tachmann, M. L., G. P. Guthrie: Hypothyroidism: Diversity of presentation. Endorinol. Rev. 5 (1984) 456–465.

TSH-levels after operation of autonomously functioning thyroid tissue-enucleation versus resection of solitary nodules

G. Wolf, A. Passath, W. Langsteger

Introduction

The heterogenous presentation of autonomously functioning thyroid tissue (AFFT) and the better knowledge on pathogenesis of hot and cold follicles has had a major influence on surgical tactics in recent years. Bilateral subtotal resection, leaving small remnants, has ceased to be standard procedure for AFTT. Several studies showed the dependance of postoperative thyroid function on the quality and quantity of the remnants. Uni- or multifocal appearance of the autonomous disease has led to development of selective or supraselective operative methods, i. e. enucleation of solitary nodules. This means a minor surgical trauma, a shorter and safter procedure and lower risk of specific complications. As according to Studer [6], cohorts of potentially autonomous follicles can be found around scintigraphically detectable nodes, we designed this study to investigate wether these methods lead to a higher rate of postoperative endocrine disfunction or recurrent goitrous enlargement.

Patients and methods

We analysed our patients from the period 1981 – 1984 retrospectively. A total of 125 patients was examined, which means 14.1% from all thyroid operations. T3, T4 basal and stimulated TSH were determined before operation, 6 and 12 months postoperatively. Double stratification resulted in 4 groups:

I: Multinodular autonomous goitre, standard bilateral resection.

II: Multinodular autonomous goitre, selective enucleation of autonomous adenomas.

III: Solitary nodules, (single adenomas), bilateral resection.

IV: Solitary nodules, selective enucleation of adenoma.

Thyrotropin

Choice between either methods was made by scintigram, intraoperative palpation and, recently, mostly by ultrasound examination. A total of 55% were found hyperthyroid with elevated T4 and T3-levels. One quarter of the singular nodes proved to be "compensated", three quarters to suppress all the surrounding tissue. Depending on postoperative TRH-test patients were set on thyroid hormone substitution.

Results (figs. 1 a – c, 2 a – c)

In group I (n = 45) mean bTSH rose from 0.6 mU/l to 3.6 after 6 and 4.1 mU/l after 12 months, mean dTSH from 4.3 to 16.8. After six months a 24.5%-rate of subclinical hypothyroidism, indicated by elevated bTSH, was found. 12 months postoperatively still in 17.7%. These cases excluded, mean bTSH was 1.9 mU/l and 1.8 mU/l. No re-operations due to recurrent goitre had to be performed, nevertheless there was an inadequate tissue reduction in one case and discrete recurrent thyroid growth in ten cases leading to scintigraphically measureable enlargement. They were called „morphological" recurrencies. It led to higher suppression dose in 5 cases and could be left untreated in 6. In this group a 4.4%-rate of subclinical hyperthyroidism (all out of primarily hyperfunctioning cases) was found, leading to re-intervention (1 operation, 1 radio-iodine).

Group II represents only a few cases (n = 11), because selective enucleation of multiple adenomas is hardly to achieve. It resulted in 1 hypothyroid case but no functional or morphological recurrence. Mean TSH-levels were lower (n. s.) compared to group I.

When solitary nodes had to resected (group III; n = 36) due to goitrous enlargement or technical problems, only a rate as high as 11% of postoperative hypothyroidism could be achieved, changing to 2.7% after one year. As far as functional restitution is concerned, none of the 19 hyperthyroid or decompensated [27] patients showed hyperthyroid recurrence. Mean bTSH was 3.72 mU/l after 6 months and fell to 1.6 mU/l after one year, dTSH was mean 15.3 and 16.8.

In 33 cases of all AFTT patients there was one singular node in an otherwise unaffected gland. This was the indication for selective enucleation of the adenoma. Mean bTSH was here 1.3 mU/l after 6 and 12 months, dTSH 10.5 and 4.5. Elevated bTSH was only found in one case after 6 months. 4 patients who were first treated by enucleation had to be excluded from this group. They stayed hyperthyroid with AFTT remnants but these could be discovered retrospectively as unremoved nodules or enlarged thyroids at first operation becoming hyperthyroid. After adequate treatment none of our patients presented with functional disregulation.

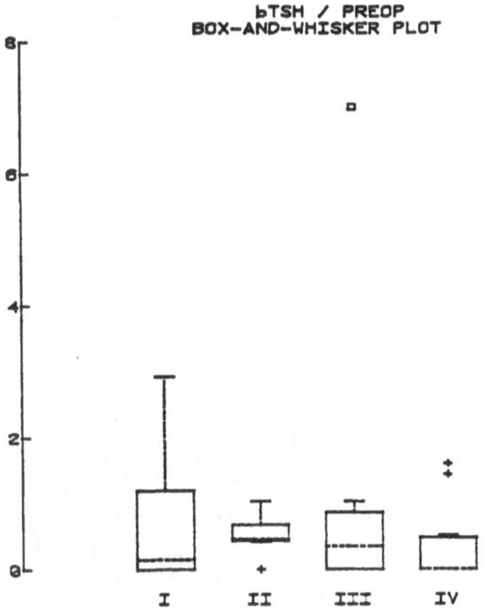

a

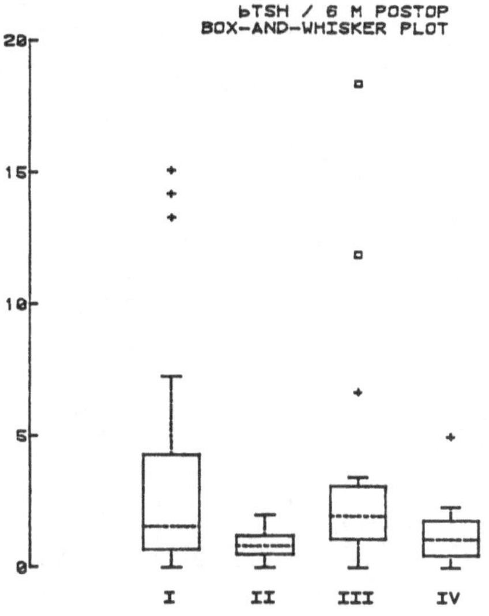

b

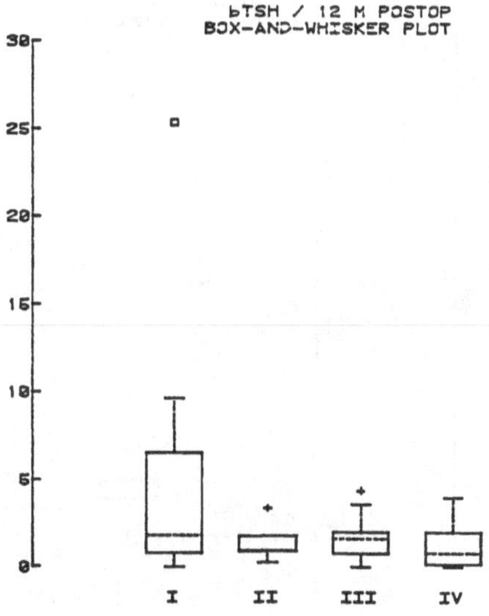

c

Fig. 1 a – c bTSH-levels preoperatively, 6 and 12 months postoperatively.

Regarding all AFTT patients together, hyperthyroidism was persistent in one case, possible due to inadequate treatment, and recurrent in 2 (i.e. 1.6%). Hypothyroidism is evident in 16.6% of the primarily euthyroid and 9.2% of the hyperthyroid patients after 6 months and still in 4.8% after one year. Most cases are represented in the resection groups.

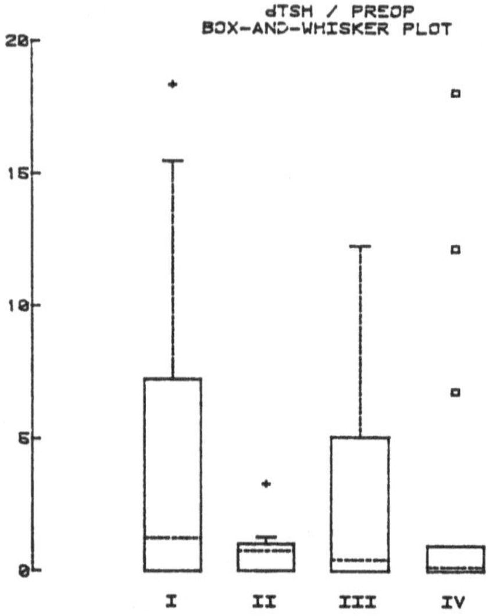

a

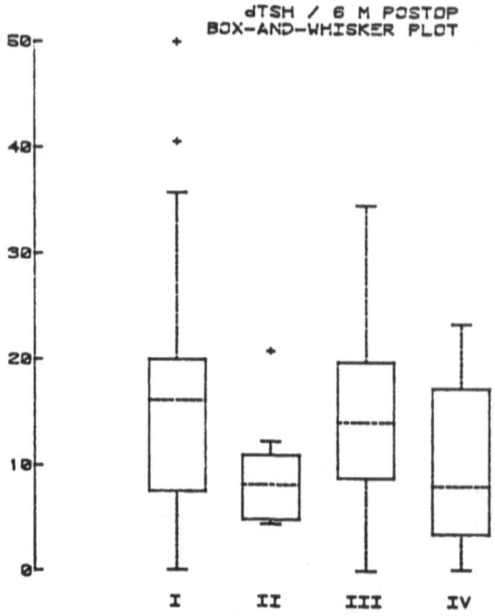

b

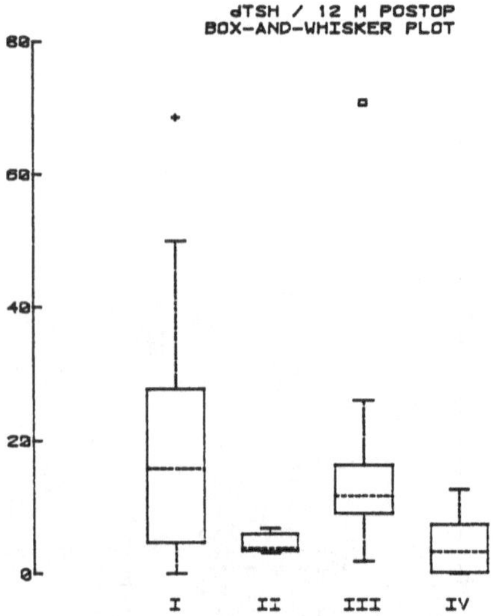

c

Fig. 2 a – c dTSH-levels preoperatively, 6 and 12 months postoperatively.

Discussion

In areas with an iodine replete diet, AFTT accounts for only 0.5 – 6% of thyroid operations [1, 3, 4]. In our endemic goitre area it accounts for 14.1% which is lower than the reports by Ladurner [5] form a more alpine region of Austria but in good correlation with the reports by Röher (17.2%) [3] from an endemic area in the FRG. In contrast to several other experiences [3, 4] our patients did not show increasing clinical features (thyroid parameters, clinical symptoms) correlated with goitre size or with number of autonomous lesions. Moreover, the most impressing medical history was presented by patients with single nodes in glands of normal size. There is a striking preponderance on female patients [24 : 1), mean age was 43.2 ± 10.3 years, hyperthyroidism was well distributed, but more common in younger patients, which differs again to other reports [4].

The extent of surgery has changed in recent years. Formerly standard bilateral resection was performed for every kind of thyroid disorder. The goal of the now preferred selective methods (enucleation, unilateral resection) is to leave at least one macroscopially normal thyroid lobe or as much as normal tissue possible. Wahl was able to show [7] that after selective surgery for autonomous goitre T3/T4 concentrations increased and basal and stimulated TSH decreased on iodine substitution. If there is adequate reduction of autonomous tissue, there is no risk from normal iodine intake which seems rather to protect against ongoing development of functional autonomy.

Both "selective" groups showed good results concerning elevated or upper-normal dTSH (fig. 3). Enucleation seems to be the minor trauma on the gland, as the missing postoperative hypothyroidism might indicate. Leaving remnants

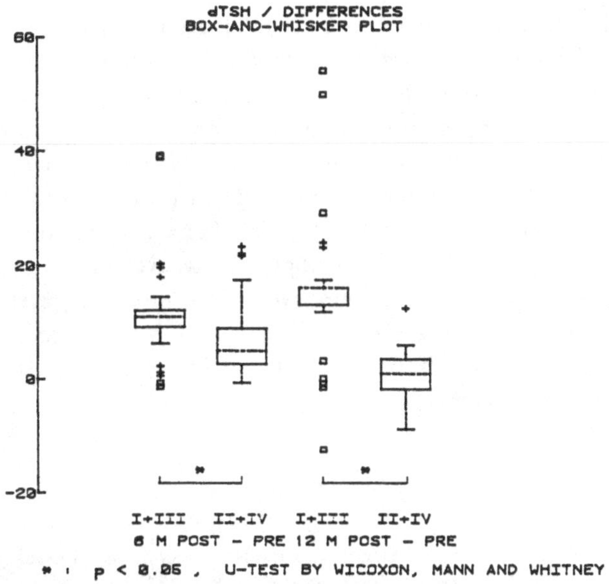

Fig. 3 dTSH-levels in the resection groups (I, III) and the enucleation groups (II, IV) at 6 and 12 months compared with preoperative values.

comparably to normal in size and quality in multinodular glands will hardly be achieved by enucleation. In an older review [8] from a period were enucleation was widely performed, we found an 11%-rate of undiagnosed and unremoved nodules. At this time in 20% the preoperative diagnosis (singular adenoma) had to be revised intraoperatively. Recently, with the obligate use of preoperative ultrasound, scintigraphically invisible nodes can be accurately predicted in 95%, thus leading to more resection cases. Under this trategy no recurrence due to inadequate operation occured.

Bilateral resection led to elevated bTSH and dTSH in 8% of the primarily hyperthyroid patients and in 9.6% of the euthyroid. As patients with resection had thyroxine medication regularly there was not therapeutic consequence of this sublinical hypothyroidism except elevation of substitution in one third of the cases. The 4.8%-rate of hyperfunction has to be taken into account, these were all patients with enlarged remnants. Our frequency is in good correlation with the dates by Röher [3] but higher than those of Berchtold [2].

Intensified specialisation has led to an 1.8%-rate of specific complications in thyroid surgery (all operations) and none of these were observed in enucleation cases.

Conclusion

Our results indicate that also removement of affected thyroid tissue is able to have the same functional results compared with standard resection, mean bTSH-levels revealed a lower rate of sublinical hypothyroidism. We prefer selective operation, which is a minor surgical trauma, a short and safe procedure. The goal has to be an adequate reduction of tissue to "normal" gland size, which seems to be sufficient, even leaving potential autonomous follicles around. This is an mayor technical problem in multinodular goitre. Here enucleation bears a high risk of adenomas to go undedected intraoperatively. Resection is recommended, as well as for concomitant goitre. Selective treatment can be safely done

- if all nodules (hot and cold) can be removed. This makes preoperative desirable but has also to lead to intraoperative inspection of the entire thyroid;
- if there is not goitrous enlargement.

References

[1] Belfiore, A., L. Sava, F. Runello, et al.: Solitary Autonomously Functioning Thyroid Nodules and Iodine Deficiency. J. Clin. Endocrinol. Metab. 55 (1983) 283–287.

[2] Berchtold, R., H. Studer, J. Teuscher: Operationsstrategie bei Schilddrüsenautonomie und Basedow-Hyperthyreose. Langenbecks Arch. Chir. 366 (1985) 51–54.

[3] Goretzky, P. E., R. Wahl, O. Branscheid, et al.: Indication for Operation of Patients with Autonomously Functioning Thyroid Tissue in Endemic Goiter Areas. World J. Surg. 9 (1985) 149–155.

[4] Hamburger, J. I.: Evolution of Toxicity in Solitary Nontoxic Autonomously Functioning Thyroid Nodules. J. Clin. Endocrinol. Metab. 50 (1980) 1089–1093.

[5] Ladurner, D., K. Hufler: Hyperthyreoter Knotenkropf. In: Chir. Endokrinologie (H. D. Röher, R. Wahl, eds.). Thieme, Stuttgart–New York 1983.

[6] Peter, H. J., H. Studer, R. Forster, et al.: The Pathogenesis of "Hot" and "Cold" Follicles in Multinodular Goiters. J. Clin. Endocrinol. Metab. 55 (1982) 941–946.

[7] Wahl, R. A., K. Joseph, E. Bögner, et al.: Thyroid Function after Surgery for Autonomous and Non-Autonomous Nodular Endemic Goitre-Effect of Iodine-Substitution. Klin. Wochenschr. 63 (1985) 812–820.

[8] Wolf, G., D. Kronberger, J. Smolle: Rezidive beim autonomen Adenom? Acta Chir. Austr. Suppl. 43 (1982) 185.

Serum TSH determination by IRMA-mat-TSH assay in patients with functioning thyroid nodules

J. Földes, J. Csillag, P. Lakatos, G. Tarján

In hyperthyroidism TSH secretion is suppressed and serum TSH level is lower than normal. Previous commercial assays applying RIA method to determine serum TSH concentration were insensitive to differenciate hyperthyroidism from euthyroidism. The aim of the present study was to detect serum TSH level by a TSH-IRMA assay in patients with functioning thyroid adenoma of various severity and to answer the question whether the TRH stimulation test can be replaced by a sensitive serum basal TSH determination. Serum basal TSH level was measured by IRMA-mat-TSH (Mallinckrodt) kits (normal range: 0.3 – 3.8 mU/l).

The investigated female subjects with untreated functioning thyroid adenoma (age: 18 – 56 years) were subdivided into 4 groups.

Group I (n = 9). Subjects with a single functional nodule without suppressing perinodular parenchyma; euthyroid clinical state with normal serum FT_4 and FT_3 level and a positive TRH-test.

Group II (n = 7). Scanning shows a "hot" thyroid nodule, but subjects are still clinically euthyroid with normal FT_4 and FT_3 levels and a positive TRH-test.

Group III (n = 9). A "hot" nodule is demonstrated; patients are clinically euthyroid; serum FT_4 and FT_3 values are within the normal range, but TSH response is absent to TRH stimulation (i. e. preclinical hyperthyroidism).

Group IV (n = 18). Toxic nodular goiter; patients are hyperthyroid, FT_4 and/ or FT_3 level is elevated, TRH-test is negative.

Beside these patients 20 untreated healthy female subjects served as controls.

Table 1 demonstrates that in groups I=III serum FT_4 and FT_3 levels are within the normal range, though a stepwise increase of their value is observed. In group III (preclin. hyperthyroidism) the mean serum FT_3 level is already significantly higher than in the control group, however, its value is still within the normal range. In euthyroid perinodular parenchyma (group I) the increment of serum TSH level after a TRH stimulation test is the same as in the controls. Some euthyroid patients having a "hot" thyroid nodule still respond to the TRH loading test (group II), however, the Δ TSH after the administration of TRH is

Thyrotropin

Table 1 Serum-free thyroxine, -free triiodothyronine and ΔTSH after a TRH-stimulation test in patients with functioning thyroid adenomas

	FT_4 pmol/l	FT_3 pmol/l	TRH-load ΔTSH mU/l
Controls (20)	16.8 ± 2.0	6.9 ± 1.2	10.8 ± 4.0
Group I (9)	17.0 ± 1.9	7.3 ± 1.2	10.4 ± 4.3
Group II (7)	17.6 ± 2.3	7.5 ± 1.3	5.3 ± 1.7***
Group III (9)	18.2 ± 2.5	8.2 ± 1.4*	0.3 ± 0.2***
Group IV (18)	34.1 ± 2.9***	18.6 ± 4.3***	0.2 ± 0.1***
Means ± S.D.	* $p < 0.05$	*** $p < 0.001$	

Table 2 Serum TSH level in TRH-test positive and negative patients with functioning thyroid adenomas

	Se.	TSH-IRMA	mU/l
Functional thyroid nodule	<0.1	0.1 – 0.3	0.3 – 3.8
TRH positive n = 16	–	9	7
TRH negative n = 27	26	1	–

significantly less compared with the controls. In the preclinical hyperthyroid and in the toxic nodular goiter groups (groups III – IV) TSH response was absent following TRH stimulation.

Figure 1 shows that among the 20 control subjects only 1 had a serum TSH level less than 0.3 mU/l. In cases of functioning thyroid nodules without suppressed perinodular tissue in 7 out of the 9 patients (group I) serum basal TSH concentration was normal, however, in 2 subjects its value was found in the intermediate

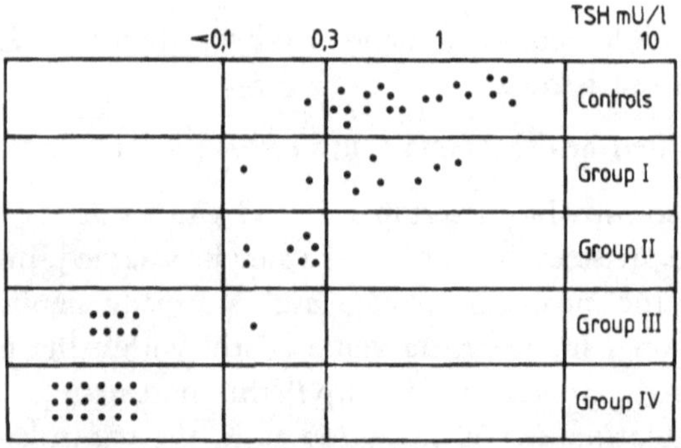

Fig. 1 Serum TSH-IRMA level in patients with functioning thyroid adenomas of various severity (see text).

zone (range: 0.1 – 0.3 mU/l). These findings are in agreement with the previous data of Izembart et al. [2].

As demonstrated recently by Lerro et al. [3] in some clinically euthyroid patients with "hot" nodules serum thyroid hormone level is normal and an increase of TSH level is encountered after TRH administration. We investigated 7 such patients (group II) and in all of them serum TSH concentration was found in the intermediate zone (0.1 – 0.3 mU/l). A regular follow up of these subjects in recommended.

In preclinical hyperthyroidism (group III), in clinically euthyroid patients with a single thyroid "hot" nodule, where an absent TSH response to TRH is found despite normal serum free thyroid hormone concentration, serum basal TSH level was lower than 0.1 mU/l in all but one of the 9 cases. And at last in the toxic nodular goiter group (group IV) serum basal TSH level was unequivocally less than 0.1 mU/l. This finding is corresponding to the previous data of Pfannenstiel [5, 6], Caldwell et al. [1] and Martino et al. [4] that an undetectable serum TSH level discriminates hyperthyroidism from euthyroidism.

Classifying the patients with functioning thyroid adenomas into groups with positive and negative TRH-test results, table 2 shows that among the 27 patients with absent TSH response to TRH the serum basal TSH level was less than 0.1 mU/l in 26 cases; on the other hand in the 16 subjects with a positive TRH test 9 had a serum TSH level in the intermediate zone, while in 7 patients TSH concentration was normal.

Our results point to the following conclusions:

1. In a group of subjects an autonomous non-toxic nodular goiter may evolve gradually – through a preclinical hyperthyroid state – into toxic nodular goiter. This transition of the clinical state is sensitively reflected by a successive decrease of serum basal TSH level determined by a sensitive IRMA method.

2. A serum basal TSH level lower than 0.1 mU/l might replace the TRH stimulation test. However, in cases of borderline TSH values the performance of a TRH stimulation test and the determination of serum thyroid hormone level is recommended to differentiate euthyroidism from hyperthyroidism.

References

[1] Caldwell, G., S. M. Grow, V. M. Sweeting, et al.: Lancet *I* (1985) 1117 – 1119.
[2] Izembartt,M., M. Heshamati, A. Chevalier, et al.: Nuc. Compact **16** (1985) 441 – 443.
[3] Lerro, S., M. Losa, M. T. Trisorio, et al.: Clin. Endocrinol. (Oxf.) **23** (1985) 373 – 378.
[4] Martino, E., G. Bambini, L. Bartalena, et al.: Clin. Endocrinol. (Oxf.) **24** (1986) 141 – 148.
[5] Pfannenstiel, P., N. Panitz: In: Freie Schilddrüsenhormone in der Klinischen Diagnostik (O. Eber, W. Langsteger, eds.), pp. 159 – 189. Köln 1985.
[6] Pfannenstiel, P.: Nuc. Compact **16** (1985) 396 – 398.

High sensitivity TSH in assessing thyroid function of patients

G. Gallone, O. Testori, L. Mongardi, V. De Filippis

Introduction

Abnormalities of thyroid hormones binding can be quantitative or qualitative. The most common are the deficit and the excess of thyroxine binding globulin (TBG). They can be congenital or acquired. In our region, the incidence of TBG congenital deficits is 1/2400 newborn [8]. Moreover, pregnancy, hepatopathy and many drugs can determine transient or permanent alterations of TBG plasmatic levels [5, 10]. Polymorphic electrophoretic variants of TBG and albumin that can alter hormone binding have been described. Cases of familiar hyperthyroxinaemia due to abnormal T4 binding by albumin or by TBPA have also been found [2, 4, 6, 9]. Non physiological antithyroid hormones antibodies were demonstrated in patients affected by thyroidal and non-thyroidal illnesses. Such immunoglobulins can act as hormone carriers and interfere with the binding capacity of the system [11, 15]. In all situations so far described, the determination of total thyroid hormones (TT3 and TT4) provides unreliable information about the gland function. Many methods have been proposed to overcome this difficulty, namely: The determination of percent T3 uptake, TBG and free fractions of thyroid hormones. These tests represent a good improvement for the assessment of the thyroid function. Nevertheless, the determination of free fractions carried out with different methods can give unreliable results [1, 7, 8, 9, 14].

Therefore, the final decision about the real thyroidal functional status of some patients must be reached with the help of clinical findings and through the TRH test.

Recently, the measurement of blood TSH by monoclonal antibodies (TSH IRMA) has proved to be a useful tool in order to discriminate between normal and hyperthyroid subjects [3, 12, 13].

During the last two years, we have encountered 47 subjects with thyroid hormones binding proteins abnormalities, mainly TBG excess and deficiency.

TSH IRMA has provided an effective "first-line" parameter to rule out a false hyperthyroidism (TBG excess) or a false hypothyroidism (TBG deficit) suspected on the basis of the total hormones, and to correct some misleading results of

Thyrotropin

free hormones determination (supranormal FT3 or FT4 in euthyroid subjects with TBG deficit).

Materials and methods

Most of the subjects are in- and out-patients of the Endocrine Division of the Mauriziano Hospital of Turin (Italy). TBG abnormalities have been found in 46 patients. One patient is reported with antiT3 antibodies.

For the determination of blood thyroid hormones and carrier proteins the following commercial kits have been employed: T3 and T4 Amerlex RIA kits (solid phase antibody), Lisophase method Sclavo for free T3 (FT3) and free T4 (FT4), TSH Biodata Maiaclone IRMA, Corning TBG Immophase (125I). Anti-T3 antibodies have been detected by radioimmunoprecipitation.

Results

Results are summarized in tables 1, 2 and 3.

Comments

Patients with TBG excess (tab. 1)

In subjects 1–31, TT3 and/or TT4 are in the hyperthyroid range. However, TSH IRMA was alsways detectable, as in normal subjects, assessing a normal thyroid function.

On the contrary, in patients 32 and 33 the hyperthyroid status is confirmed by the TSH values.

Patient 34 is an example of preclinical hyperthyroidism.

TBG was above normal range in all subjects.

The clinical findings and the values of FT3 and of FT4 confirmed the informations given by TSH, both in normal and hyperthyroid subjects.

Patients 35 and 36 are examples of hypothyroidism with TBG excess. In such cases TSH IRMA does not offer any better information than TSH RIA.

Patients with TBG deficit (tab. 2)

In subjects 1–9, TT3 and TT4 were in the hypothyroid range but the values of TSH IRMA were in the normal range. TBG level was always subnormal, as in

Table 1 Patients with TBG excess

Patients	Age	Sex	TT3 ng/dl	TT4 ug/dl	TSH mU/l	TBG mg/l	FT3 pg/ml	FT4 pg/ml
Min			51	4.2	0.2	12.0	2.8	6.6
Max			160	11.0	6.5	30.0	5.6	14.0
1. A.G.	47	F	163	14.0	2.9	33.4	2.8	7.6
2. B.A.	37	F	120	12.0	1.6	38.2	–	–
3. C.P.	64	F	270	12.3	2.6	43.2	4.4	7.5
4. C.V.	53	F	187	12.9	2.4	33.6	4.1	10.2
5. C.S.	58	F	211	15.0	2.4	50.2	2.7	7.5
6. C.R.	66	F	212	11.4	1.1	33.3	3.7	8.3
7. C.P.	58	F	201	16.6	5.7	69.6	2.9	11.0
8. D.F.	26	F	163	9.9	1.6	54.2	3.1	6.5
9. F.R.	–	F	170	12.0	1.1	35.2	3.3	8.0
10. F.A.	–	F	146	13.1	0.7	32.9	–	–
11. G.E.	26	F	149	13.9	2.4	35.7	4.4	11.1
12. G.A.	–	F	175	12.5	4.4	31.5	3.2	7.5
13. G.I.	69	F	146	14.9	1.5	55.7	2.9	8.6
14. G.L.	–	F	156	15.9	1.1	36.8	3.7	12.4
15. G.G.	–	F	135	12.2	1.7	38.3	3.1	8.3
16. P.J.	68	F	212	13.4	1.6	69.1	2.8	11.7
17. P.O.	–	F	160	9.5	0.2	37.2	3.1	6.8
18. P.R.	75	F	181	14.6	1.8	60.2	2.3	6.7
19. T.A.	60	F	218	14.2	3.4	64.8	3.2	10.2
20. M.S.	61	F	180	13.1	2.7	36.8	4.5	10.8
21. G.L.	38	F	127	14.9	3.1	45.7	2.4	11.7
22. C.A.	66	F	192	13.1	2.5	65.0	3.1	6.3
23. P.C.	–	F	161	17.2	2.0	72.5	2.3	7.0
24. D.N.B.	–	F	145	12.4	2.4	40.6	2.6	8.1
25. M.P.	31	F	167	15.2	2.7	62.2	3.0	7.3
26. M.M.	–	F	173	17.9	1.5	69.8	2.4	8.4
27. L.M.	–	F	166	13.5	1.7	70.2	2.5	7.0
28. C.M.	–	F	154	14.2	6.4	60.0	2.9	7.2
29. C.A.	25	F	184	11.5	3.0	55.2	3.6	6.6
30. C.P.	57	F	160	12.2	2.5	42.9	3.5	9.1
31. B.D.	62	M	158	13.1	1.8	45.6	3.4	8.8
Mean			172	13.5	2.3	49.0	3.2	8.5
S.D.			30	1.9	1.3	13.7	0.6	1.8
32. P.G.	29	F	448	29.2	0.0	86.6	15.8	34.9
33. T.E.	25	F	432	10.1	0.0	32.2	10.7	10.1
34. D.M.R.	–	F	200	20.1	0.0	39.3	4.4	13.3
35. D.R.	72	F	84	10.4	11.4	53.1	2.4	8.6
36. T.L.	–	F	169	8.5	10.4	81.0	1.9	3.2

partial deficit of this carrier protein. Furthermore, in 3 of these subjects (1 – 7 – 9) the values of FT3 were above the normal range. The normal blood TSH ruled out the diagnosis of hyperthyroidism.

Patient 10 had practically undetectable blood TBG and low TT3 and TT4. A value of zero of TSH IRMA was compatible with the diagnosis of hyperthyroidism which was confirmed by the results of the FT3 and FT4 determination and by the history of excessive intake of LT4.

Table 2 Patients with TBG deficit

Patients	Age	Sex	TT3 ng/dl	TT4 ug/dl	TSH mU/l	TBG mg/l	FT3 pg/ml	FT4 pg/ml
Min			51	4.2	0.2	12.0	2.8	6.6
Max			160	11.0	6.5	30.0	5.6	14.0
1. B.M.	28	M	46	2.3	1.7	2.1	6.4	13.3
2. B.B.	51	M	77	5.5	1.4	9.7	5.3	13.1
3. C.A.	81	M	55	6.9	4.3	8.5	4.2	11.4
4. D.L.	–	M	21	2.7	4.4	6.3	2.0	7.4
5. P.A.	54	M	59	3.8	2.8	8.4	3.3	8.3
6. Q.O.	56	M	47	0.9	3.7	0.8	–	–
7. S.S.	5	M	66	3.4	1.9	7.7	6.7	10.7
8. P.B.	57	F	49	3.4	4.9	6.4	4.0	8.4
9. P.E.	43	F	71	3.3	3.2	6.6	5.9	9.4
Mean			54	3.6	3.1	6.3	4.7	10.2
S.D.			16	1.6	1.2	2.8	1.5	2.1
10. Z.E.	–	M	61	4.8	0.0	0.1	8.2	38.8

Patient with antiT3 autoantibodies (tab. 3)

In this patient TT_3 suggested the possibility of hyperthyroidism, that was dried by the normal TSH value and by FT3. The demonstration of antiT3 autoantibodies allowed us to explain the cause of high TT3.

Table 3 Patient with antiT3 autoantibodies

Patient	Age	Sex	TT3 ng/dl	TT4 ug/dl	TSH mU/l	FT3 pg/ml	FT_4 pg/ml	AbT3 %
Min			51	4.2	0.2	2.8	6.6	
Max			160	11.0	6.5	5.6	14.0	
L.A.	30	M	192	9.8	3.1	3.6	10.6	59

Conclusions

In many laboratories the determination of TT3, TT4 and TSH is routinely employed for the assessment of thyroid functional status. In the majority of the cases such system gives satisfactory informations. However, in the presence of abnormalities of the carrier proteins, the results of TT3 and TT4 do not allow a right diagnosis. The determination of TSH by RIA methods does not allow a discrimination between normal and hyperthyroid subjects. The availability of ultrasensitive TSH IRMA allows to overcome the latter difficulty.

Our results prove the possibility of assessing the real thyroid functional status by using TT3, TT4 and TSH IRMA also in presence of abnormalities of binding proteins.

The determination of TBG and other carrier proteins may explain the cause of "abnormal" TT3 and TT4 values. The measurement of FT3 and FT4 gives additional informations on the real thyroid functional status.

References

[1] Beck-Peccoz, P., et al.: In: Terze Giornate Italiane della Tiroide, Abs. 26. Turin, Italy, November 1985.
[2] Bernstein, R. S., et al.: Endocrinology **86** (1970) 383.
[3] Caldwell, G., et al.: Lancet **8348** (1985) 1117.
[4] Daiger, S. P., et al.: Am. J. Hum. Gen. **33** (1981) 640.
[5] DeGroot, L.: The Thyroid and its Deseases, p. 181. Wiley Medical, New York 1984.
[6] Dick, M., et al.: Clin. Chim. Acta **116** (1981) 361.
[7] Ferdeghini, M., et al.: In: Terze Giornate Italiane della Tiroide, Abs. 27. Turin, Italy, November 1985.
[8] Gallone, G., et al.: In: Aspetti Critici delle Metodiche RIA, p. 449. Turin, Italy, January 1984.
[9] Hennemann, G., et al.: In: Free Hormones in Blood (A. Albertini, R. P. Ekins, eds.), p. 203. Elsevier Biomedica Press, Amsterdam – Oxford – New York 1982.
[10] Ingbar, S. H., et al.: In: Principles of Internal Medicine (T. R. Harrison, ed.), p. 1697. McGraw Hill Book, New York 1980.
[11] Merlin, P., et al.: In: Advances in Thyroid Hormones (A. Carpi, ed.), p. 27. ETS, Pisa 1982.
[12] Pinchera, A., et al.: In: Cost/Benefit and Predictive value of Radioimmunoassay (A. Albertini, R. P. Ekins, R. S. Galen, eds.), p. 151. Elsevier Science Publishers B. V., New York – Oxford – Shannon 1984.
[13] Seth, J., et al.: Br. Med. J. **891** (A) (1985) 1334.
[14] Stocking, J. R., et al.: In: Free Hormones in Blood (A. Albertini, R. P. Ekins, eds.), p. 223. Elsevier Biomedical Press, Amsterdam – Oxford – New York 1982.
[15] Trimarchi, F., et al.: J. Endocrinol. Invest. **6** (1983) 203.

V The thyroid TSH receptor and TSH receptor antibodies

The subunit structure of the TSH receptor

B. Rees Smith, J. Furmaniak, F. A. Hashim, E. Davies Jones,
R. D. Howells, Y. Nakajima

Introduction

The TSH receptor is an integral membrane glyco-protein which forms a binding site for TSH on the outside surface of thyroid follicular cells. The binding of TSH to the receptor causes the hormone-receptor complex to interact with the regulatory subunits of adenylate cyclase. This interaction takes place in the lipid bilayer or at the cytoplasmic surface of the cell membrane and results in production of increased amounts of cyclic AMP which mediate most, if not all, of the actions of the hormone. In Graves' disease, a relatively common autoimmune disorder, autoantibodies to the TSH receptor are formed. They bind to the receptor in such a way as to mimic the effects of TSH and this results in the development of hyperthyroidism [22, 23].

This short review considers the properties of the receptor and the nature of its interaction with TSH and TSH receptor antibodies.

Photoaffinity labelling of the TSH receptor

The TSH receptor is present on the cell surface in very small amounts (in the region of 10^3 sites per cell; [23]) and consequently special techniques are often required to study the receptor. One of the most powerful techniques currently available for studying trace amounts of cell surface receptors is affinity labelling [14]. In the case of the TSH receptor, we have found TSH coupled to photoactive crosslinking reagents to be particularly useful [5]. These studies have indicated that both subunits of TSH form part of the hormone's receptor binding site [5].

Analysis by SDS-PAGE of porcine TSH receptors crosslinked to 125-I labelled TSH have shown that the receptor contains 2 subunits linked by a disulphide bridge. One of the subunits (A; mol. wt. 50 k) is water soluble and forms the binding site for TSH on the outside surface of the cell membrane. The other (B) subunit (mol. wt. 30 k) penetrates the lipid bilayer [15, 16]. The non-covalent bonds between the A and B subunits of the porcine or human TSH receptor are readily dissociated at neutral pH in the presence of 50 mM NaCl. Consequently,

Thyrotropin

when thyroid membranes are reduced under these conditions, the TSH receptor A subunit is released. The release is much less in the absence of NaCl indicating that the non-covalent interactions between A and B subunits are markedly dependant on the ionic environment. The binding of TSH to its receptor is also markedly influenced by ionic strength and this phenomenon may be related to the effects of salt on the non-covalent interactions between the A and B subunits.

The TSH receptor A subunit can be released from thyroid membrane preparations whether or not the A subunit has been crosslinked to TSH [10]. The free A subunit will bind TSH and TSH receptor antibodies indicating that both thyroid stimulators bind to the same receptor subunit [10, 11]. Furthermore, immunoprecipitation and gel filtration studies have shown that the binding of TSH and the receptor antibodies to the TSH receptor is mutually exclusive [21]. In addition, monovalent Fab fragments of TSH receptor antibodies compete effectively with TSH in receptor binding studies and the Fab fragments are able to act as powerful TSH agonists [7]. These observations provide compelling evidence that TSH receptor antibodies bind to the same region of the TSH receptor A subunit as TSH itself.

TSH receptor antibodies with TSH antagonist activity

TSH receptor antibodies are nearly always able to act as TSH agonists [8]. However, occasional patients with autoimmune hypothyroidism or hypothyroidism following 131-I ablative treatment for Graves' hyperthyroidism do have TSH receptor antibodies which can act as TSH antagonists [4, 19]. The blocking antibodies appear to be IgG class and their ability to bind to the TSH receptor and act as TSH antagonists can be demonstrated in Fab fragments prepared from the patients IgG [13].

Studies on the binding of TSH receptor antibodies with blocking activity to the TSH receptor indicate that they bind to the same region of the TSH receptor A subunit as TSH and TSH receptor antibodies with thyroid stimulating activity [10].

The difference between the ability of a receptor antibody from one patient to act as an agonist and a receptor antibody from another patient to act as an antagonist cannot be explained readily therefore in terms of the 2 antibodies acting at different sites on the receptor. It would seem far more likely that the difference in properties of the 2 types of receptor antibody is similar to the differences between agonists and antagonists in more conventional systems such as the beta receptor. In this situation the agonists and antagonists interact with the same region of the receptor but subtle differences in binding characteristics are probably responsible for differences between agonists and antagonists [18].

Charge – charge interactions and the TSH receptor

Several studies have shown that the isoelectric point (pI) of TSH receptor antibodies is in the region of 8 – 10 irrespective of whether the antibodies act as TSH agonists or antagonists [6]. Furthermore, the pI of TSH is about 9. Analysis of TSH receptor A subunit preparations by isoelectric focusing indicates that the free TSH receptor A subunit has an isoelectric point of about pH 5.

Consequently, at physiological pH, the TSH receptor A subunit on the outside surface of the thyroid cell will have a negative charge whereas TSH and TSH receptor antibodies will have a positive charge. This indicates that charge-charge interactions will be of major importance in the binding of hormone or antibody to the TSH receptor A subunit.

TSH receptor on $FRTL_5$ cells

Recently, Ambesi-Impiombato and his colleagues [1] have developed a continuously growing line of rat thyroid cells known as $FRTL_5$. This cell line is of considerable value in studying many aspects of thyroid disease. In particular, the cells contain functional TSH receptors and these can be studied by affinity labelling with 125-I labelled photoactive derivatives of TSH. Figure 1 shows the release by reduction of the $FRTL_5$ TSH receptor A subunit crosslinked to labelled TSH. These studies emphasize the similarity in the structure of TSH receptors in $FRTL_5$ cells and thyroid tissue from other species.

Analysis of the TSH receptor under non-denaturing conditions

Most studies of TSH receptor structure have been carried out in the presence of the denaturing detergent sodium dodecyl sulphate (SDS). Consequently, these investigations were unable to assess whether the A and B subunits were associated non-covalently with additional subunits. In order to investigate this possibility, we have used the non-denaturing detergent sodium deoxycholate (DOC) to solubilize TSH receptors photoaffinity labelled with 125-I TSH and then analysed the crosslinked complexes by gel filtration and sucrose density gradient centrifugation. The results obtained are summarised in table 1 and indicate that in the presence of 1% DOC the crosslinked TSH-TSH receptor has an $s_{20}w$ of 6.4 S and frictional ratio $\left(\frac{f}{fo}\right)$ of 1.8. These values are consistent with those which might be expected from an elongated protein complex with mol. wt. of about 100 k (the value obtained by SDS-PAGE) and suggest therefore that additional subunits are not associated with the TSH receptors A and B subunits.

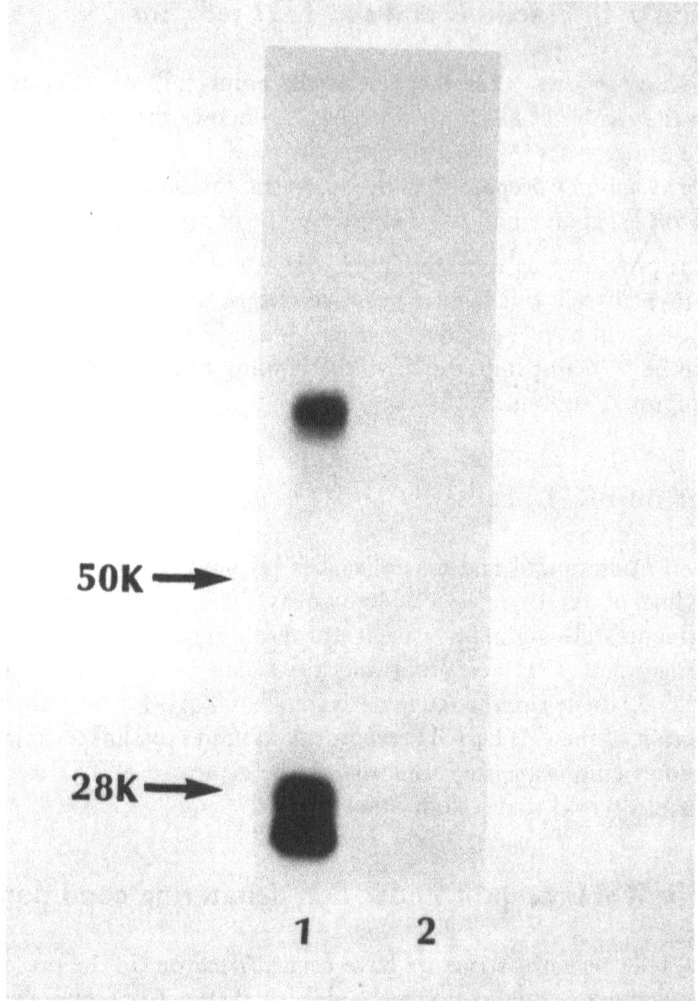

Fig. 1 Release by reduction of TSH receptor A subunit from $FRTL_5$ cells. $FRTL_5$ cells were removed from their plastic supports by treatment with EGTA and suspended (30×10^6 per ml) in Earles' balanced salt solution. Equal volumes (2 ml) of cell suspension and 125-I labelled HSAB-TSH (20 µCi) [5] were incubated (20 min; 37°) photolysed and washed. A crude membrane pellet was then obtained from a homogenate of the cells and treated with dithiothreitol (DTT) as described previously [15–16]. After centrifugation at 100000 g for 60 minutes the supernatants were analysed by SDS-PAGE and autoradiography.
Lane 1 = $FRTL_5$ cells treated with DTT in the absence of unlabelled TSH; Lane 2 = $FRTL_5$ cells incubated with an excess (5 µg; 300 mU) of unlabelled TSH prior to addition of 125-I labelled HSAB-TSH.
The Band with Mr = 80 k is the TSH receptor A subunit crosslinked to 125-I labelled HSAB-TSH.

Table 1 Summary of data obtained by sucrose density gradient centrifugation and gel filtration

	Sedimentation coefficient ($s_{20,w}$)	Stokes' radius	M_r by SDS-PAGE	Mol. wt. from S.	Frictional Coefficient
Intact TSH receptor crosslinked to TSH	6.4 ± 0.5S	55 ± 2A	100 k	131 k (range 108 – 150 k)	1.8
TSH receptor A subunit crosslinked to TSH	4.6 ± 0.4S	52 ± 2A	70 k	78 k (range 64 k – 89 k)	1.8
TSH receptor A subunit alone[a])	3.6S	34.5A	47 k	47 k	1.4
TSH alone[b])	2.6S	33 ± 1A	28 k	28 k	1.6
Microsomal antigen	6.0 ± 0.5S	42 ± 2A	110 k	125 k (range 99 k – 145 k)	1.3

[a]) Data from [11, 15];
[b]) Data (s_{20w} and M_r) from [3].

Comparison of the data obtained for the various components of the TSH-TSH receptor complex (tab. 1) allows assessment of the shapes and sizes of these components. It is possible to conclude that when TSH, which has an elongated structure, combines with TSH receptor A subunit (which has a compact structure) the 2 proteins do not fold into each other extensively but form a structure with an ever greater degree of elongation.

The TSH receptor and other thyroid autoantibodies

Patients with Graves' disease often, in addition to TSH receptor antibodies have serum autoantibodies to thyroglobulin and to thyroid microsomal antigen. Thyroglobulin is the major thyroid protein; it is water soluble and contains 2 identical subunits each with a mol. wt. of 320 k [20]. Thyroid microsomal antigen is an amphiphilic single chain glycoprotein with a mol. wt. of 110 k [17]. Recent studies suggest that thyroid microsomal antigen is the enzyme thyroid peroxidase [9]. Some of our own observations confirm this suggestion. For example, antibodies prepared against highly purified human microsomal antigen (giving a single 110 k band on SDS-PAGE) bind to highly purified water soluble fragment (prepared by trypsin digestion) of porcine thyroid peroxidase. In addition, some autoantibodies to human thyroid microsomalantigen bind to the highly purified porcine thyroid peroxidase fragment.

Autoantibodies to the 3 different thyroid antigens are quite distinct as are the antigens themselves. Thyroglobulin autoantibodies can be present in high concentrations in serum and can even form precipitin lines against thyroglobulin in gel diffusion studies. Microsomal antibodies can also be present in relatively high concentrations but there is far less microsomal antigen present in the thyroid than thyroglobulin [9].

In contrast to the microsomal/thyroglobulin antigen-antibody system, TSH receptor antibodies are present in serum in minute amounts probably of the order of ng per ml (This rough estimate is based on the concentration of TSH in human serum which is of the order of 0.1 ng per ml).

Are there major thyroid specific autoantigen-antibody systems in addition to those involving thyroglobulin, thyroid microsomal antigen and the TSH receptor?

In addition to the major systems described above, autoantibodies to a second (water soluble) colloid antigen have been described [2]. In order to investigate whether autoantibodies to additional thyroid membrane antigens exist in the serum of patients with autoimmune thyroid diseases we have analysed the interaction of different sera with crude human thyroid membrane preparations.

Preliminary experiments were carried out using plastic tubes coated with thyroid membranes or microsomes. After addition of test sera (diluted in an excess of thyroglobulin to neutralize any thyroglobulin autoantibodies) followed by washing, 125-I Protein A was added to assess the binding of serum antibodies to the membranes or microsomes. These studies showed a highly significant correlation between antibody binding to microsomes and membranes ($r = 0.82$; $P < 0.001$; $n = 82$). This suggested that the interaction between membranes and serum was principally due to microsomal antibodies binding to microsomal antigen contaminating the membrane preparations. However there were some clear discrepancies indicating that an additional antigen-antibody system might be present.

Consequently, human thyroid membranes were solubilized with 1% DOC, immunoprecipitated with test sera from patients with autoimmune thyroid disease and analysed by SDS-PAGE and autoradiography. Typical results are shown in figure 2 and indicate the presence of an autoantigen with mol. wt. 54 k. However, this antigen could also be immunoprecipitated from 125-I labelled DOC solubilized membranes prepared from human placenta or human skeletal muscle. Our studies indicated therefore that immunoprecipitation of labelled DOC solubilized thyroid membranes was unable to detect the presence of a thyroid specific autoantibody directed towards a thyroid membrane protein other than thyroid microsomal antigen.

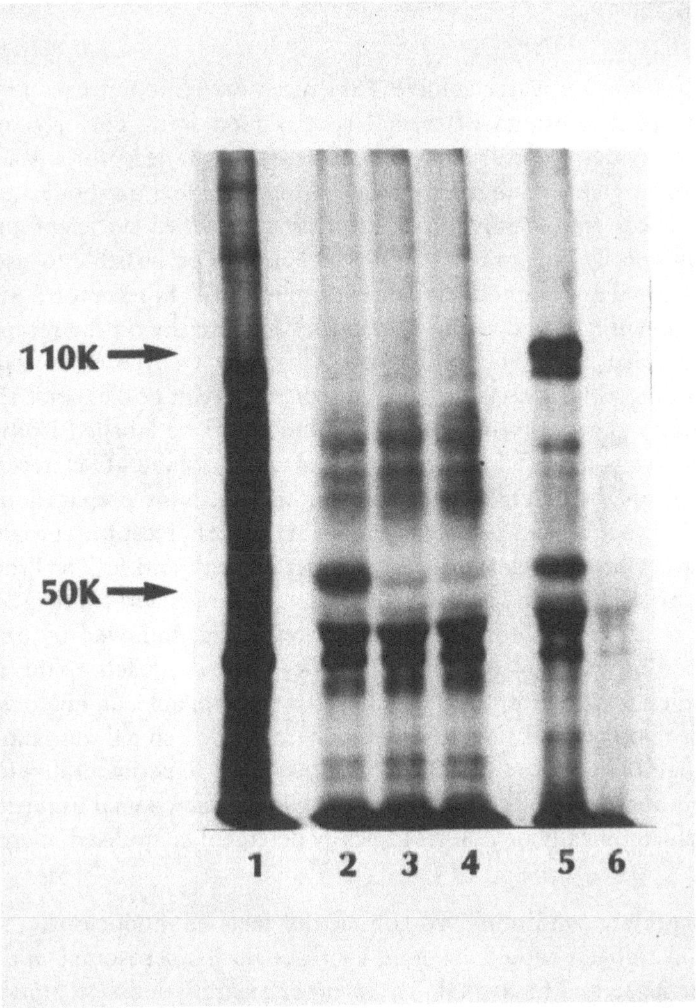

Fig. 2 Immunoprecipitation of DOC solubilized 125-I labelled thyroid and placenta membranes. Analysis by SDS-PAGE and autoradiography.
Lane 1 = Untreated 125-I labelled human placental membranes; lanes 2, 3, 4 = immunoprecipitation of labelled placental membranes with 2 different Graves' sera (lanes 2 and 4) and normal pool serum (lane 3); lanes 5, 6 = immunoprecipitation of labelled human thyroid membranes with a Graves' serum (lane 5) and normal pool serum (lane 6).
For full experimental details see [15 – 17].

The thyroid membranes used contained TSH receptors and some of the sera contained TSH receptor antibody activity as assessed by receptor assay. However, the concentrations of both these components were far too low to be detected by immunorecipitation under the conditions used.

Future developments

The ability to release the water soluble TSH receptor A subunit crosslinked to TSH from thyroid membranes of several species (and from TSH receptors in guinea pig fat) provides a useful approach to purifying the receptor's A subunit. In particular, affinity chromatography based on monoclonal antibodies to TSH can be used as a key step in this purification process. When sufficient amounts a purified A subunit-TSH complex are available it will be possible to use them to prepare polyclonal and monoclonal antibodies to the TSH receptor A subunit. These antibodies will not be directed at the TSH binding site on the receptor (as this will be occupied by TSH) and as such they may well be of considerable value in developing new assays for TSH receptor autoantibodies and TSH. In particular, the experimentally induced antibodies could be labelled isotopically or non-isotopically and then interacted with a water soluble TSH receptor A subunit preparation (or detergent solubilized intact receptor preparation). The resulting complex should then be able to bind TSH or TSH receptor autoantibodies and the amount bound determined by interaction with anti IgG or Protein A. Alternatively, the test serum could be allowed to interact with anti IgG (on a solid support) or Protein A (on staph aureus cells) first followed by antibody labelled receptor or receptor A subunit. This type of approach could also be used if antibodies to the receptor's B subunit were available. It might also be useful in the development of new assays for thyroid microsomal autoantibodies (or even thyroglobulin autoantibodies). For example experimentally induced monoclonal antibodies to different regions of thyroid microsomal antigen could be used to label isotopically or non-isotopically detergent solubilized microsomal antigen.

Under the appropriate conditions this complex of labelled monoclonal antibody and microsomal antigen would be able to react with microsomal antibodies present in patients sera. The availability of experimentally induced monoclonal and polyclonal antibodies to the TSH receptor A subunit will be of value in purifying the intact TSH receptor. In addition, such antibodies could be used in expression screening of thyroid DNA libraries for TSH receptor synthesing clones. The autoantibodies to the TSH receptor found in Graves' sera are present at very low concentrations and are directed to a region of the receptor (TSH binding site) which is readily and irreversibly rendered inactive (eg by gentle heating or treatment with SDS). Consequently the autoantibodies are unlikely to be useful in studies involving expression screening for the receptor.

Recently, the insulin receptor [24] and the beta receptor [12] have been cloned. Both laboratories involved approached the problem by using nucleotide probes constructed from a knowledge of the partial amino acid sequence of purified insulin receptor or beta receptor. It would seem therefore that a similar approach starting with a partial sequence of the TSH receptor A subunit will be the most likely to succeed in determining the structure of the TSH receptor gene and the primary structure of the receptor.

References

[1] Ambesi-Impiombato, F. S., L. A. M. Parks, H. G. Coon: Proc. Natl. Acad. Sci. USA **77** (1980) 3455–3459.
[2] Balfour, B. M., D. Doniach, I. M. Roitt, et al.: Brit. J. Exp. Pathol. **42** (1961) 307–316.
[3] Bates, R. W., P. G. Condliffe: Recent. Progr. Res. **16** (1960) 309–352.
[4] Beck K., H. Bliddal, K. Siersbaek-Nielsen, et al.: Clin. Endocrinol. **17** (1982) 395–402.
[5] Buckland, P. R., C. R. Richards, R. D. Howells, et al.: Biochem. J. **235** (1986) 879–882.
[6] Creagh, F. M., R. D. Howells, S. Williams, et al.: Clin. Endocrinol. **24** (1986) 79–88.
[7] Creagh, F. M., A. B. Parkes, E. Tunn, et al.: Clin. Endocrinol. **23** (1985 a) 175–183.
[8] Creagh, F. M., M. Teece, S. Williams, et al.: Clin. Endocrinol. **23** (1985 b) 395–404.
[9] Czarnocka, B., J. Ruf, M. Ferrand, et al.: FEBS Letts **190** (1985) 147–152.
[10] Davies Jones, E., F. A. Hashim, F. M. Creagh, et al.: Mol. Cell. Endocrinol. **41** (1985 a) 257–261.
[11] Davies Jones, E., F. A. Hashim, Y. Kajita, et al.: Biochem. J. **228** (1985 b) 111–117.
[12] Dixon, R. A. F., B. K. Kobilka, D. J. Strader, et al.: Nature **321** (1986) 75–79.
[13] Hashim, F. A., F. M. Creagh, A. El Hawrani, et al.: Clinical Endocrinology (in press).
[14] Ji, T. H.: Biochim. Biophys. Acta **559** (1979) 39–69.
[15] Kajita, Y., C. R. Rickards, P. R. Buckland, et al.: FEBS Letts **181** (1985 a) 218–222.
[16] Kajita, Y., C. R. Rickards, P. R. Buckland, et al.: Biochem. J. **227** (1985 b) 413–420.
[17] Kajita, Y., D. Morgan, A. B. Parkes, et al.: FEBS Letts **187** (1985 c) 334–338.
[18] Kenakin, T. P.: Pharmacol. Rev. **36** (1984) 165–214.
[19] Konishi, J., Y. Iida, K. Endo, et al.: J. Clin. Endocrinol. Metab. **57** (1983) 544–549.
[20] Lissitzky, S.: J. Endocrinol. Invest. **7** (1984) 65–76.
[21] Parkes, A. B., Y. Kajita, P. R. Buckland, et al.: Clin. Endocrinol. **22** (1985) 511–520.
[22] Rees Smith, B.: Receptors and Recognition, Series B. Vol. 13 p. 217–244. Chapman and Hall, London 1981.
[23] Rees Smith, B., C. R. Rickards, E. Davies Jones, et al.: J. Endocrinol. Invest. **8** (1985) 175–182.
[24] Ullrich, A., J. R. Bell, E. Y. Chen, et al.: Nature **313** (1985) 756–761.

TSH-receptor antibodies

P. Vitti, G. F. Fenzi, L. Chiovato, C. Marcocci, A. Pinchera

Introduction

Autoantibodies directed to different components of the thyroid cell are present in sera of patients with thyroid autoimmune disorders [1]. Among the thyroid cell structures, the TSH receptor has been implicated as the putative antigen of autoantibodies having different biological effects. Indeed, autoantibodies able to mimic TSH in its ability to stimulate thyroid hormone production and cell growth have been found in sera of patients with Graves' disease and in a minority of those with other thyroid autoimmune disorders [2]. The observation that the IgG fraction from the same patients inhibit the binding of radiolabeled TSH to its receptor suggested that these thyroid autoantibodies are directed to the TSH receptor itself. More recently, in sera of patients with idiopathic myxedema autoantibodies were described that inhibit some biological effects of TSH on the thyroid cell and may be important in the pathogenesis of thyroid atrophy and hypothyroidism [3, 4]. The clinical relevance of TSH receptor releated antibodies will be discussed in the present review.

Thyroid adenylate cyclase stimulating antibodies (TSAb)

TSAb historically was detected by LATS bioassay, but a consistent number of Graves' patients were negative by this test even after concentration of the IgG fraction. This relatively low incidence of LATS positive responses has been attributed to the species-specificity of TSAb, so that only those antibodies cross-reacting with the murine thyroid could be detected by LATS bioassay [1]. Results of assays directly assessing thyroid stimulating activity in human thyroid plasma membranes or slices have been reported by several investigators. The average positivity obtained with Graves' IgG is about 80% in different laboratories. In a series of 49 Graves' patients with untreated Graves' disease studied in our laboratory using human thyroid membranes we found 71.4% positivity with the IgG fraction. No adenylate cyclade (AC) activity was detectable in IgG preparations from 28 normal subjects and 12 patients with Hashimoto's thyroiditis or idiopathic myxedema [5]. Cultured human thyroid cells have also proved to be

Thyrotropin

a sensitive system for assessing TSAb [6]. More recently, a new very sensitive method for the measurement of TSAb was developed using a continuous line of rat thyroid cells (FRTL-5 cells) [7]. The ability of these cells to be grown under standard and highly reproducible conditions allowed easy optimization of the assay. Intracellular cAMP was measured by RIA after challenge of cells with the IgG specimens from patients with various thyroid disorders, or from normal subjects. In our series 90% of IgG preparations from hyperthyroid Graves' patients exhibited stimulating activity, thus the sensitivity of this assay is comparable with results reported using human thyroid cells or slices [8]. Essentially similar results can be obtained with a different methodological approach. In a series of 24 patients with Graves' disease, all IgG with positive values in the FRTL-5 cell cAMP assays, were able to stimulate ^{125}Iodide uptake in the same cells [9]. Since this activity is known to be a cAMP dependent phenomenon stimulated by TSH, this gives further proof of the ability of TSAb to mimic the TSH action. Furthermore, the iodide uptake assay may be used as an alternative method for the measurement of TSAb, and appears to be simpler, less expensive and less time-consuming than assays needing a cAMP radioimmunoassay.

Comparison between TSAb and TSH binding inhibiting IgG (TBIAb)

IgG from patients with Graves' disease not only are able to stimulate thyroid function, but also to inhibit the binding of radioiodinated TSH to particulate or solubilized receptor [10], suggesting an interaction through the same receptor site. The question of whether TSAb and TBIAb activities were confined in the same antibody is controversial. Parallel measurements of TSAb and TBIAb in IgG from patients with untreated Graves' disease resulted in a lack of correlation between these two parameters [5]. Moreover, it was possible to show that few IgG preparations derived from patients with Hashimoto's thyroiditis and idiopathic myxedema similarly inhibited the binding of TSH but were devoid of thyroid stimulating activity. The discrepancy between inhibition of TSH binding and stimulation of AC might be due to the occurrence of autoantibodies directed to different domains of the TSH receptor complex. Alternatively, it may be postulated the presence of a family of autoantibodies having different biological activities and coexisting in the same patient. This latter hypothesis seems to be confirmed by studies performed with monoclonal antibodies obtained by fusing Graves' lymphocytes with mouse myeloma cells. In fact, two groups of monoclonal antibodies were identified: some of them were potent inhibitors of TSH binding and action, others behaved as partial agonist of the hormone [11].

Autoantibodies inhibiting the TSH stimulation of thyroid AC

Hypothyroidism is observed in patients with idiopathic myxedema and less frequently with Hashimoto's thyroiditis. In these two conditions autoantibodies to different thyroid cell components have been described [1]. More recently it was proposed that hypothyroidism may result from antibodies blocking the effect of TSH on the thyroid in the absence of cell damage [12]. Two cases of transient neonatal hypothyroidism in newborns of a mother with idiopathic myxedema were described. In both cases it was possible to demonstrate the transplacental transfer of an antibody that was able to block TSH binding and TSH activated adenylate cyclase in human thyroid membranes. The occurrence of neonatal transient hypothyroidism due to TSH receptor blocking antibodies has been subsequently confirmed by other laboratories [13, 14]. The observation that hypothyroidism was transient and that the time of recovery of thyroid function in newborns was strictly related to the disappearance from the circulation of maternal antibody, indicates that clinical hypothyroidism may be produced by antibodies reacting with the TSH receptor. Furthermore, a different thyroid autoantibody was described in a patient with idiopathic myxedema who gave

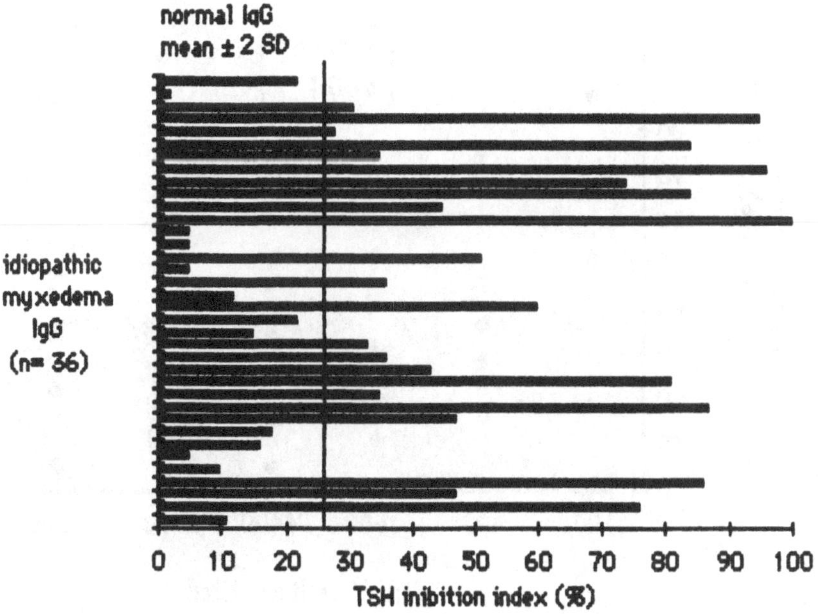

Fig. 1 Effect of IgG preparations from 36 patients with idiopathic myxedema on TSH stimulation of cAMP accumulation in FRTL-5 cells. The vertical dashed line represents the mean ± 2 SD of the effect produced by IgG from normal subjects. The amount of TSH used for the stimulation was 40 μU/ml.

birth to a neonate with transient hypothyroidism [13, 15]. This maternal antibody was able not only to inhibit TSH binding and TSH stimulated adenylate cyclase, but it also inhibited iodide uptake and organification at a post receptor level. However, the precise mechanism of this post receptor effect is still unclear and requires further investigation.

Autoantibodies blocking the TSH stimulated adenylate cyclase were also reported in several patients with adult idiopathic myxedema [3, 16]. A correlation with the ability by the antibody to inhibit the TSH binding to its receptor was also reported [16, 17]. At variance with neonates with transient immunogenic hypothyroidism, it is still unclear whether these antibodies blocking the TSH stimulation of thyroid function are the primary cause of hypothyroidism in adult patients with thyroid atrophy.

The incidence in idiopathic myxedema of autoantibodies blocking the TSH induced cAMP accumulation has been studied in our laboratory by a sensitive technique that employs a line of rat thyroid cells that grow in continuous culture (FRTL-5 cells). Twenty-three out of 36 patients with idiopathic myxedema had circulating autoantibodies able to significantly inhibit the TSH activation of adenylate cyclase in FRTL-5 cells (fig. 1). When the results obtained in this inhibition assay were compared with the titer of M antibody, as assessed by

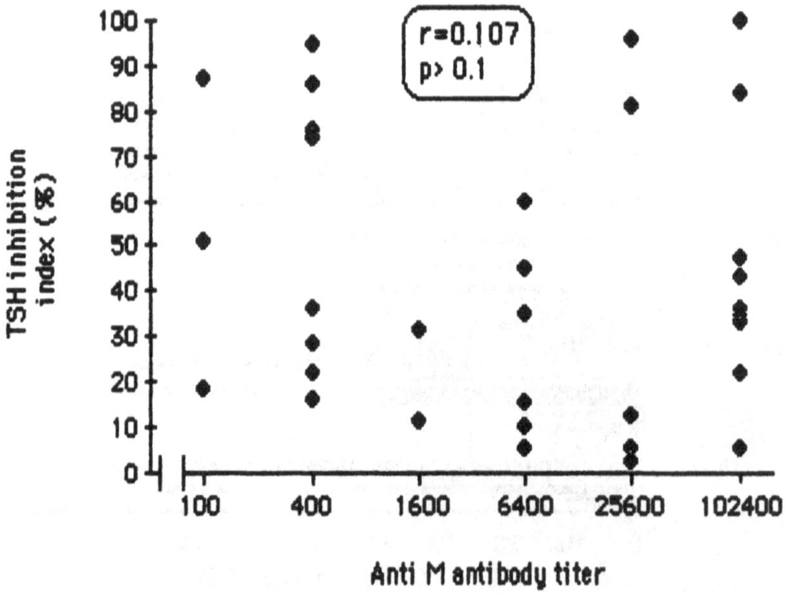

Fig. 2 Correlation between the inhibition of TSH-stimulated adenylate cyclase activity and M antibody titers in 21 IgG preparations from patients with idiopathic myxedema. Adenylate cyclase activity was assayed in FRTL-5 cells and M antibody titer (reported as reciprocal values) was assessed by passive hemagglutination.

passive hemagglutination, no correlation was found, indicating that a different type of autoantibody was involved (fig. 2).

Although preliminar, these data suggest that autoantibodies blocking the TSH stimulation of the AC may have a pathogenetic role in the development of hypothyroidism in some patients with thyroid autoimmune disorders.

Thyroid growth promoting antibodies (TGAb)

Recently, several reports have suggested that goiter may be linked to the presence of growth stimulating antibodies that may act through the TSH receptor but not necessarily involving the stimulation of the AC [2]. FRTL-5 cells can also be usefully employed for the measurement of TGAb. Using this assay we have found that IgG from patients with active Graves' disease and Hashimoto's thyroiditis can increase thyroid cell growth as measured by ^{3}H-thymidine incorporation [18, 19]. While several reports [19, 20] indicate that in sera of patients with Hashimoto's thyroiditis or nontoxic goiter may be present TGAb in the absence of TSAb, it is still unclear whether these two thyroid stimulating activities may exist separetely in Graves' disease. To answer this question, peripheral lympho-

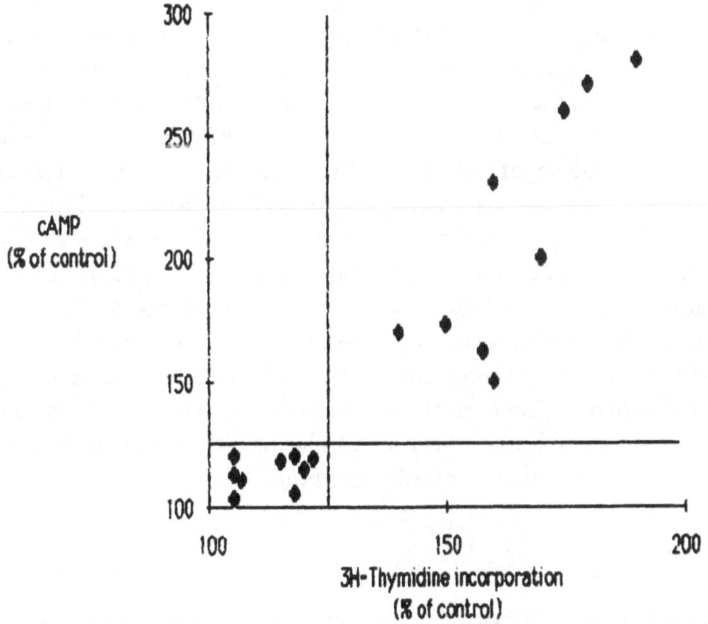

Fig. 3 Correlation between the stimulation of cAMP accumulation and 3H-thymidine incorporation by monoclonal antibodies to human thyroid membranes in FRTL-5 cells. The vertical and horizontal lines represent the upper limit of normal controls.

cytes from a goitrous patient with active Graves' disease were fused with mouse myeloma cells NS1. Eighteen out of 150 (12%) hybridoma supernatants showed a significant binding to solubilized human thyroid membranes. After appropriate subcloning and expansion, IgG was prepared from spent media using DEAE-Sephadex. The biological activity of these monoclonal antibodies was tested in two different functional assays using a continuous strain of rat thyroid cells (FRTL-5). A clear-cut increase of cAMP was produced by 9 out of 18 mAb. The same mAb were also able to stimulate ^{3}H-thymidine incorporation. Negative results in both assays were obtained with the remaining mAb (fig. 3).

These data indicate that, at least in these patients, the TSAb and TGAb activities coexist in the same IgG indicating that the adenylate cyclase-cAMP system may be one of the pathways of the signal transmission resulting in the growth of thyroid cells. However, the existence of different mechanisms of thyroid growth not involving cAMP production is also suggested by the observation that TGAb are present in sera from patients with no detectable TSAb activity [18–20] and by studies using mAb to the TSH receptor [2, 11].

Conclusive remarks

TSH receptor related antibodies may possess multiple biological activities, mimicking or interfering with the TSH function. The inhibiting and stimulating activities may coexist in the same patient with Graves' disease; however, the lack of correlation between these two activities, when measured in a large series of patients, suggest that they are elicited by different antibodies. This hypothesis is strenghtened by the finding of autoantibodies blocking the TSH function but devoid of thyroid stimulating activity in patients with autoimmune hypothyroidism. The question of whether in Graves' disease thyroid adenylate cyclase and growth are stimulated by the same autoantibody is still unsolved. In the Graves' patient with goiter we have selected in order to prepare mAb, the ability to stimulate thyroid adenylate cyclase and growth were simultaneously present in the same antibody molecule, suggesting that cAMP may be one of the signals mediating thyroid growth. However, the results obtained with mAb from different patients showed that growth and cyclase stimulating activities can be separated [11]. Further studies are needed to clarify this point.

References

[1] Pinchera, A., G. F. Fenzi, L. Bartalena, et al.: In: Autoimmune Aspects of Endocrine Disorders (A. Pinchera, D. Doniach, L. Baschieri, eds.), p. 57. Academic Press, London 1980.

[2] Kohn, L. D., S. M. Aloj, D. Tombaccini, et al.: In: Biochemical Actions of Hormones (G. litwack, ed.), vol. XII, p. 457. Academic Press, New York 1985.

[3] Konishi, J., Y. Iida, K. Endo, et al.: J. Clin. Endocrinol. Metab. **57** (1983) 544.
[4] Drexhage, H. A., G. F. Bottazzo, L. Bitensky, et al.: Nature **289** (1981) 594.
[5] Macchia, E., G. F. Fenzi, F. Monzani, et al.: Clin. Endocrinol. (Oxf.) **17** (1981) 175.
[6] Pinchera, A., G. F. Fenzi, L. Bartalena, et al.: In: Thyroid Research VIII (J. R. Stockigt, S. Nagataki, eds.), p. 707. Australian Academy of Science, Canberra 1980.
[7] Vitti, P., W. A. Valente, F. S. Ambesi,-Impiombato: J. Endocrinol. Invest. **5** (1982) 179–182.
[8] Vitti, P., C. M. Rotella, W. A. Valente, et al.: J. Clin. Endocrinol. Metab. **57** (1983) 782.
[9] Marcocci, C., W. A. Valente, A. Pinchera, et al.: J. Endocrinol. Invest. (1983) **6** 463.
[10] Pinchera, A., G. F. Fenzi, E. Macchia, et al.: Horm. Res. **16** (1982) 317.
[11] Kohn, L. D., C. M. Rotella, C. Marcocci, et al.: In: Monoclonal Antibodies 84: Biological and Clinical Applications (A. Pinchera, G. Doria, F. Dammacco, A. Bargellesi, eds.), p. 169. Editrice Kurtis, Milano 1985.
[12] Matzuura, N., Y. Yamada, Y. Nohara, et al.: N. Engl. J. Med. **303** (1980) 738.
[13] Takasu, N., T. Mori, Y. Koizumi, et al.: J. Clin. Endocrinol. Metab. **59** (1984) 142.
[14] Iseki, M., M. Shimizu, T. Oikawa, et al.: J. Clin. Endocrinol. Metab. **57** (1983) 384.
[15] Takasu, N., M. Naka, T. Mori, et al.: Clin. Endocrinol. **21** (1984) 345.
[16] Arikawa, K., Y. Ichikawa, T. Yoshida, et al.: J. Clin. Endocrinol. Metab. **60** (1985) 953.
[17] Konishi, J., Y. Iida, K. Kasagi, et al.: Ann. Int. Med. **103** (1985) 26.
[18] Chiovato, L., L. J. Hammond, T. Hanafusa, et al.: Clin. Endocrinol. (Oxf.) **19** (1983) 581.
[19] Valente, W. A., P. Vitti, C. M. Rotella, et al.: N. Engl. J. Med. **309** (1983) 1028.
[20] Drexhage, H. A., G. F. Bottazzo, D. Doniach, et al.: Lancet **2** 287.

TSH-binding analysis and TSH-receptor distribution pattern in thyroid disease

H.-W. Müller-Gärtner, G. Wasmus, A. Merx, C. Schneider, W. Rehpenning, V. Bay, U. Engel

Introduction

In analogy to other receptor models [1, 2] it can be presumed that thyrotropin-(TSH)receptor affinity for TSH or changes in TSH receptor concentration have an influence on or are influenced by thyroid cell metabolism. In a first attempt to elucidate the presumed mutual influence of TSH-receptors and cell metabolism we evaluated the TSH-binding to thyroid cell membranes in comparison with histological and metabolical features of the investigated tissue specimens.

Methods

To evaluate TSH-binding to thyroid gland membranes radioreceptor-assay-procedures (RRA) were employed. To determine the TSH-receptor distribution pattern *receptor autoradiography* in cryostatic specimens (−80 °C) of human thyroid tissue was used (3 sections from each tissue). Biologically active 125-I-TSH (Henning Co., Berlin), was dissolved in 1 ml Tris-HCl and dialysed against this buffer for 12 h at 4 °C immediately prior to use. The cryostatic specimens of thyroid tissue was fixed in acetone, dried and rehydrated with PBS (pH 7.4). They were incubated in a 111 µl 125 I-TSH solution for 3 h at 37 °C within a humid atmosphere. In order to effect separation of the bound and unbound 125-I-TSH molecules the material was then rinsed in PBS and treated twice with a chromalaune gelatine solution. This enabled stripping film procedures to be applied for autoradiography. As a means of semiquantitative evaluation of 125-I-TSH binding reflection photometry [3] or silver microparticle counting in defined areas of thyroid epithelium were employed.

To determine *TSH-binding to thyroid tissue homogenates* tissue samples were frozen in liquid nitrogen and stored at −80 °C. The tissue was thawed and homogenized in 200 µl 10 mM-Tris/HCl, pH 7.5. A crude membrane preparation was sedimented (15 000 g, 15 min., 4 °C). The membranes were resuspended in 200 µl 50 mM-NaCl/10 mM-Tris/HCl, pH 7.5, containing BSA 1 mg/ml and

Thyrotropin

incubated with 125 iodine labeled TSH (125-I-TSH, 90 min., 37 °C), which is a biologically active bovine pituitary TSH (Henning Co., Berlin). The tubes were centrifuged twice (each time 15 000 g, 20 min.) and the pellets were counted for receptor-bound 125 I-TSH. The intraassayvariation of this procedure amounted to 8.4%, the interassayvariation was 11.5%. Unspecific 125-I-TSH binding as measured by unlabeled-TSH excess was subtracted from the total binding results. To estimate the number of epithelial cells in tissue samples under investigation morphometrical analysis of corresponding tissue sections was conducted using the method of point counting [4]. Binding analysis was standardized by the estimated cell number.

For *Scatchard analysis* unlabeled TSH (Sigma) was used. The binding results were corrected for non specific binding as described by Rosenthal [5]. In the computer analysis use was made of the least square parameter fitting to resolve curvilinear Scatchard plots into one or two classes of binding sites with different affinities and capacities [6].

Results

125-I-TSH receptor autoradiography: Determination of TSH-receptor distribution pattern

125-I-TSH binding was inhibited in a dose-dependent manner by unlabeled TSH (fig. 1).

Human thyroid follicles dipicted a more pronounced 125-I-TSH binding as compared with porcine thyroid follicles which are known to have a lower concentration of TSH-receptors. Epididymal fat pat tissue from guinea pigs known to have TSH-receptors also depicted a specific 125-I-TSH-binding. There was no specific 125-I-TSH binding to human liver tissue, thyroid colloid or thyroid interstitium. Additional proves of specificity have previously been described in detail [3].

Reflection photometry as a semiquantitative means of measuring TSH-receptor density on thyroid cells revealed a significantly lower receptor density for 4 out of 5 investigated thyroid malignancies (follicular carcinoma n = 2, medullary carcinoma n = 1, anaplastic carcinoma n = 1) whereas one case of papillary carcinoma revealed a TSH-receptor density within the normal range. TSH-receptor density was significantly higher in 3 cases of diffuse colloid goiter.

TSH-receptors were usually homogeneously distributed (fig. 2) with the exception of tissue specimens (n = 6) from toxic nodular goiters.

This exception revealed regional 125-I-TSH binding variations (fig. 4 a) as measured by reflection photometry (fig. 3).

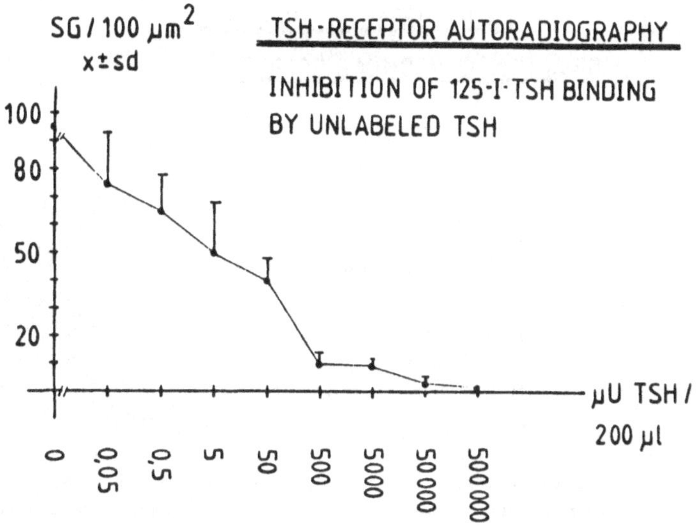

Fig. 1 125-I-TSH binding to thyroid gland tissue sections as determined by stripping film autoradiography was inhibited according to the given dose of unlabeled TSH. For each point (x ± sd) blackened silvery microparticles (SG) were counted from 10 different epithelial regions, each measuring 100 µm. Background activity as measured over the colloid compartement was subtracted.

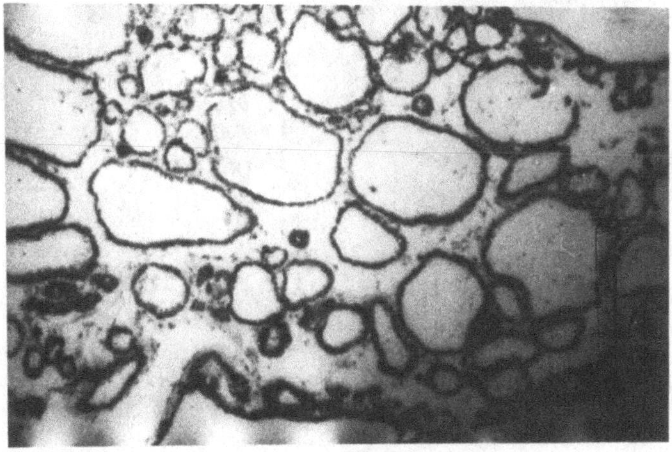

Fig. 2 125-I-TSH binding to normal human thyroid tissue. TSH-receptors are homogeneously distributed over the follicular epithelium.

This inhomogenicity could also be observed in the distribution pattern of epidermal-growth-factor-(EGF-)receptors (fig. 4 b).

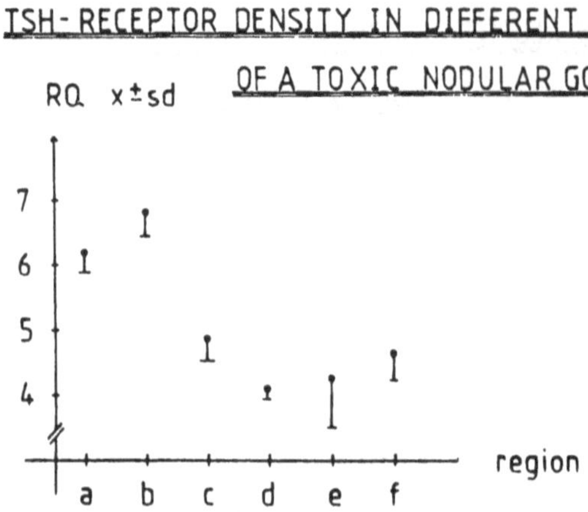

Fig. 3 125-I-TSH binding to tissue sections from toxic multinodular goiter showed a regionally variable receptor density. 6 different regions of the same tissue specimen were evaluated by 50 individual reflection photometry measuremtns (x ± sd): A reflectionquotient (RQ) correlated the epithelium reflection with the homogeneous background reflection.

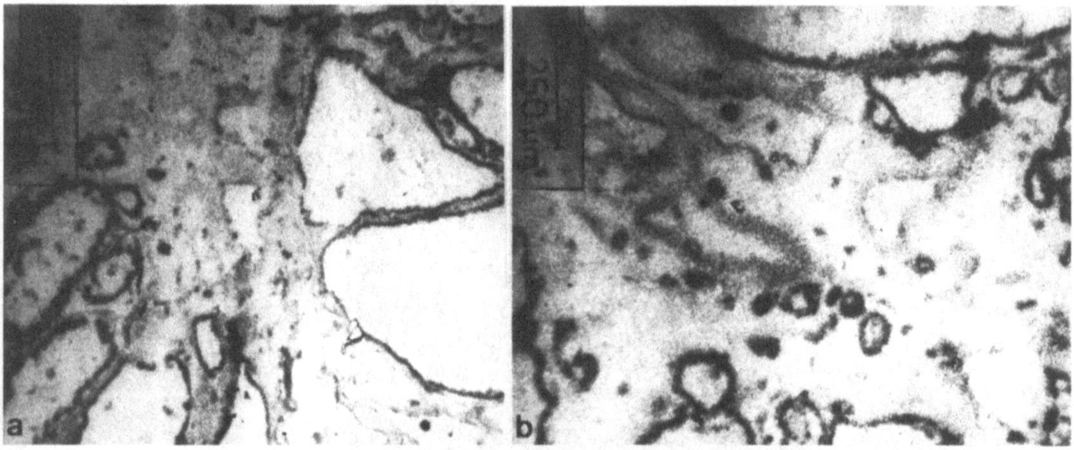

Fig. 4 a, b Inhomogeneous distribution of TSH- (fig. 4 a) and EGF- (fig. 4 b) receptors in toxic nodular goiter. Apart from follicles showing a regular TSH- or EGF-receptor density, single follicles or follicle groups lack any TSH- or EGF binding (specimen from fig. 4 a does not correspond to the specimen from fig. 4 b).

Quantitative 125-I-TSH binding analysis

Since quantitative determination is hardly possible using traditional methods of autoradiography, 125-I-TSH binding to thyroid membranes had to be measured using a RRA on homogenized membranes. 63 human thyroid glands (fig. 5 a – c) were investigated.

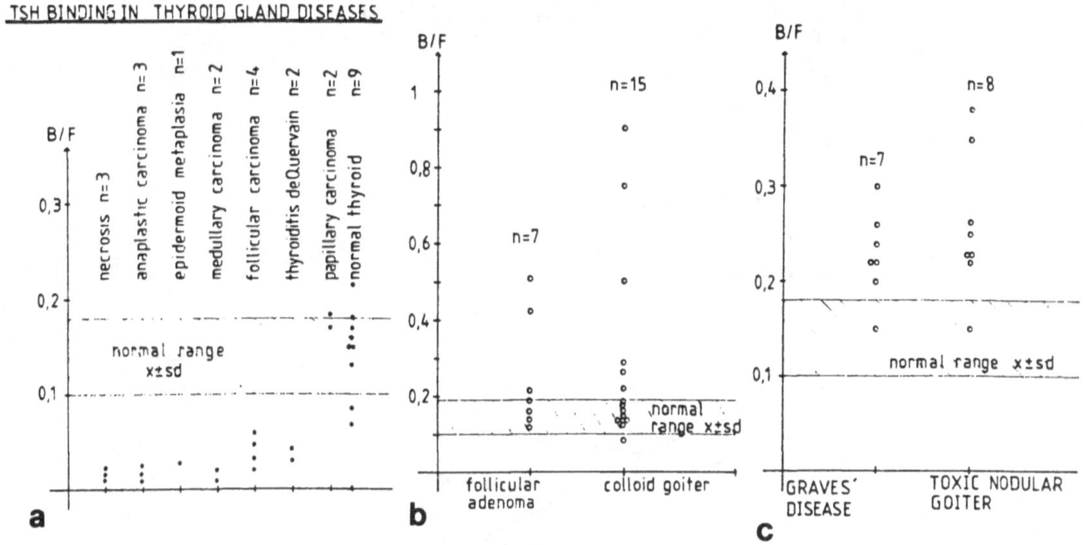

Fig. 5 a – c Bound-TSH/Free-TSH-ratio (B/F) for various thyroid diseases using 0.025 nU 125-I-TSH.

The application of RRA to medullary (n = 2), anaplastic (n = 3), and follicular (n = 4) carcinomas as well as one case of epidermoid metaplasia of a papillary carcinoma and two cases of thyroiditis de Quervain showed a significantly ($p < 0.05$) lower B/F ratio as compared with normal thyroid tissue (fig. 5 a). 125-I-TSH binding in two thyroid papillary malignancies was found to be at the uppermost point of the upper normal range (fig. 5 a).

Scintigraphically cold, follicular adenomas as well as diffuse colloid goiters had a remarkably variable B/F ratio from one specimen to the other. Although never appearing below the normal range some of them had a higher B/F ratio (fig. 5 b). Such measurements taken in Graves' disease- and autonomous nodular goiter-tissues were slightly higher than those expected in the normal range and clustered together on the border between the uppernormal and paranormal ranges (fig. 5 c).

When comparing the B/F ratios of follicular adenomas with the B/F ratios of the surrounding thyroid tissue as a reference specimens from 4 out of six patients revealed a significantly increased 125-I-TSH binding in follicular adenoma tissue ($p < 0.05$, fig. 6).

For detailed analysis of binding parameters (binding-affinity and -capacity) Scatchard plot analysis was additionally performed in 14 different tissue specimens (normal thyroid tissue, n = 5; Graves' disease tissue, n = 4; multinodular goiter with autonomy, n = 5). 11 out of 14 specimen showed two different TSH-

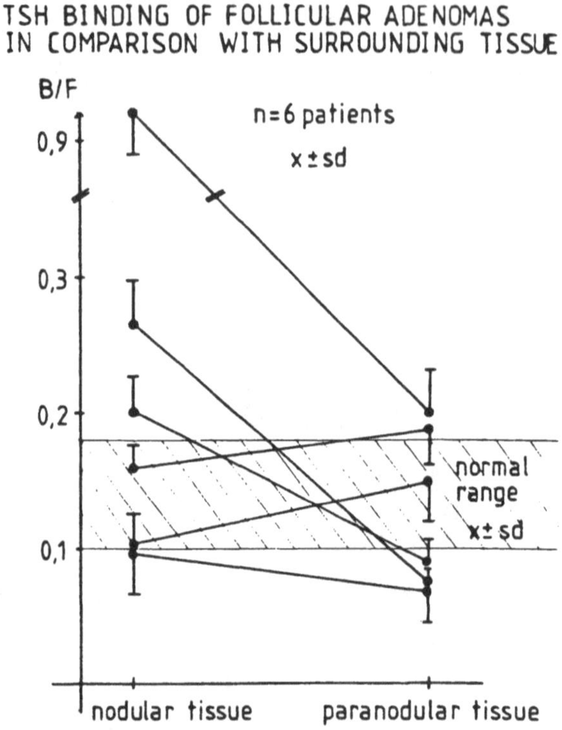

Fig. 6 Bound-TSH-ratio (B/F) in 6 uninodular goiters (histological diagnosis: follicular adenoma) using 0.025 nU 125-I-TSH. B/F ratios of the nodules are compared with the corresponding perinodular tissue.

binding sites, whereas in 3 specimens (macrofollicular adenoma n = 2, colloid goiter n = 1) a second binding site was undetectable. Normal thyroid tissue was found to have a high affinity binding site, for which the range of TSH-binding affinity was from 0.066 to 0.215 l/nMol and for which the range of TSH-binding capacity was from 0.956 to 4.09 nMol/l. The spread of TSH-binding affinity and capacity of the low affinity binding site was 0.055 to 4.33 l/pMol and 3.38 to 7.76 nMol/l respectively. As compared with normal thyroid tissue TSH affinity of the high-affinity binding site was increased whereas TSH-binding capacity was decreased in tissue samples taken from hyperthyroid patients caused by Graves' disease or toxic nodular goiter (fig. 7).

In this regard there was no obvious difference between samples from Graves' disease- or toxic nodular goiter tissue. A significant difference of TSH-receptor characteristics for the low-affinity/high capacity binding site could not be detected.

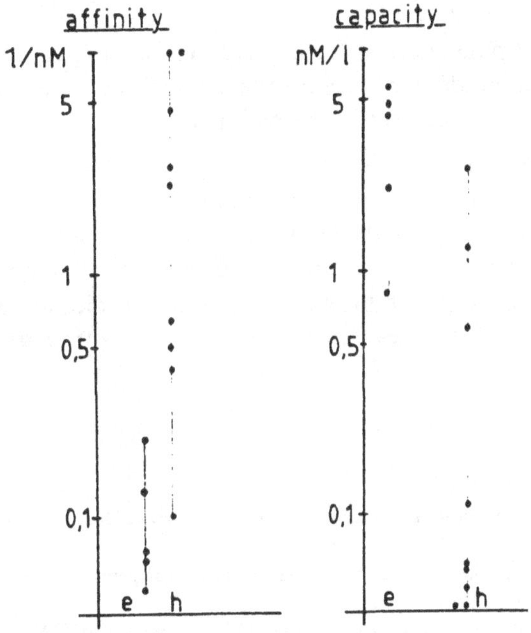

Fig. 7 Scatchard plot analysis showing a different TSH-binding affinity and TSH-binding capacity of the high-affinity-binding-site in euthyroid (n = 5) and hyperthyroid patients (Graves' disease n = 4, nodular toxic goiter n = 5); e = euthyroid, h = hyperthyroid.

Summary and conclusions

- TSH-receptor autoradiography as a means of semiquantitative measure of TSH-receptor density revealed a mostly homogeneous TSH-receptor distribution in normal and diseased thyroid glands. Exceptionally some toxic nodular goiters displayed regional differences in TSH-receptor density. Analogous results were obtained for EGF-receptors.
- The incidence of an increased TSH-binding of follicular adenomas in comparison with their surrounding tissue and the increased TSH-binding of some colloid goiters supports the hypothesis, that an increased TSH-sensitivity could be an explanation for accelerated proliferation of thyroid gland tissue.
- Quantitative TSH-binding analysis to thyroid gland membranes confirm previous reports [7 – 9] that malignant transformation of thyroid gland tissue results usually in a decreased ability to bind the TSH-molecule (exception: 2 cases of papillary carcinoma).

- Scatchard analysis of TSH-binding-affinity and -capacity applied to tissue samples from hyperthyroid patients revealed a decreased binding capacity in the presence of an increased binding affinity for the high-affinity binding sites as compared to tissue samples from euthyroid patients.

These results indicate that TSH-receptors of diseased thyroid glands in a functional and proliferative sense show remarkable quantitative and qualitative alterations of TSH-receptor characteristics. However, this does not proof of causal connection between TSH-receptor alterations and thyroid cellular metabolism. One should be aware of the possibility that TSH-receptor alterations are just epiphenomena of cellular disturbances which arrise at a very different point of cellular metabolism.

References

[1] Roth, J.: Insulin binding to its receptor: Is the receptor more important than the hormone? Diabetes Care **4** (1981) 27 – 32.

[2] Catt, K. H., J. P. Harwood, G. Aquilera, et al.: Hormonal regulation of peptide receptors and target cell responses. Nature **280** (1979) 109 – 116.

[3] Müller, H.-W., S. Schröder, G. Wasmus, et al.: Autoradiographical portrayal of TSH receptors in human thyroid gland tissues. Horm. Metab. Res. **17** (1985) 619 – 620.

[4] Weibel, E. R.: Stereological Methods. Practical Methods for Biological Morphometry, vol. 1. Academic Press, London – New York – Toronto – Sydney – San Francisco.

[5] Rosenthal, H. E.: A Graphic Method for the Determination and Presentation of Binding Parameters in a Complex System. Anal. Biochem. **20** (1967) 525 – 532.

[6] Scatchard, G.: The attraction of protein for small molecules and ions. Ann. NY. Acad. Sci. **51** (1949) 660 – 672.

[7] Clark, O. H., P. L. Gerend, T. C. Cote, et al.: Thyrotropin binding and adenylate cyclase stimulation in thyroid neoplasms. Surgery **90** (1981) 252 – 261.

[8] Carayon, P., C. Thomas-Morvan, E. Castanas, et al.: Human Thyroid Cancer: Membrane Thyrotropin Binding and Adenylate Cyclase Activity. J. Clin. Endocrinol. Metab. **51** (1980) 915 – 920.

[9] Abe, Y., Y. Ichikawa, T. Muraki, et al.: Thyrotropin (TSH) Receptor and Adenylate Cyclase Activity in Human Thyroid Tumors: Absence of High Affinity Receptor and Loss of TSH Responsiveness in Undifferentiated Thyroid Carcinoma. J. Clin. Endocrinol. Metab. **52** (1981) 23 – 28.

Clinical significance of antibodies to the TSH-receptor (stimulating and blocking thyroid function)*

H. Schleusener, G. Holl, A. Stadler, P. Kotulla, U. Bogner, K. Badenhoop, R. Finke, J. Hensen

Introduction

It is now clear that Graves' hyperthyroidism is an autoimmune disease. In 1956 Adams and Purves [1] found a factor in sera of thyrotoxic patients that caused delayed release of 131-iodine by guinea pig thyroid gland cells. This factor was named the long-acting thyroid stimulator (LATS). It could be identified as an antibody to the TSH receptor within the thyroid cell membrane which stimulates thyroid hormone synthesis/secretion via the adenyl cyclase system [5 – 7]. The first assay widely used for detection of LATS was the McKenzie bioassay [2]. It is based on the in vivo stimulation of 131-iodine secretion by the thyroid glands of mice. Using this method, LATS was only found in about 30 – 40% of patients with untreated Graves' hyperthyroidism. Other assays measure the rise of cyclic AMP, thyroxine and/or triiodothyronine [3 – 8] by isolated human thyroid cells, slices or membrane fragments. Depending on the sensitivity of these methods, 40 to 90% positive antibody results have been reported [3, 7, 9 – 12]. Thereupon the term LATS was confined to the antibody determination by the McKenzie bioassay; the term LATS protector was used for the detection of these antibodies with a technique developed by Adams et al. [13]. The terms thyroid-stimulating antibody (TSAb) or thyroid-stimulating immunoglobulins (TSI) have been given to the antibodies which can be detected by the other methods mentioned above.

---

* 33 West German Clinician's participate in the multicenter prospective study mentioned in this paper:
Althoff (Frankfurt), Badenhoop (Mannheim), Benker (Essen), Beyer (Mainz), Börner (Würzburg), Bogner (Berlin), Fiek (Berlin), Finke (Berlin), Gräf (Berlin), Grebe (Gießen), Hengst (Münster), Hensen (Berlin), Holl (Berlin), Hopf (Berlin), Hüfner (Heidelberg), Joseph (Marburg), Kahaly (Mainz), Koppenhagen (Berlin), Kotulla (Berlin), Müller-Eckhardt (Gießen), Pickardt (München), Raue (Heidelberg), Reiners (Würzburg), Reinwein (Essen), Schatz (Gießen), Schleusener (Berlin), Schöffling (Frankfurt), Schumm (Frankfurt), Schwedes (Mannheim), Seif (Tübingen), Usadel (Mannheim), Witte (München), Ziegler (Heidelberg).
Own data presented in this paper are from investigations supported by the Deutsche Forschungsgemeinschaft and the Bundesministerium für Forschung und Technologie (FRG).

Thyrotropin

For clinical purposes, all these tests are too difficult to handle. Therefore several groups developed a radioligand receptor assay [14–16, 41, 42]. It depends on the inhibition of the binding of ^{125}iodine to thyroid membrane fragments or solubilized TSH receptor material. The antibodies detected with this assay are called TSH-receptor-binding-inhibiting immunoglobulins (TBII) or TSH-binding-inhibiting antibodies (TBIAb). For the clinical routine laboratory, several commercial kits are now available (fig. 2).* Most recently, Shinozawa et al. reported on a receptor assay using guinea pig fat cell membranes [53]. Dr. R. B. Smith will give a lecture on the methodological aspects in the course of this meeting. Here in this paper, the following will be discussed: 1. whether the TBIAb measurements with a radioligand receptor assay are useful for a) the prediction of the clinical course of Graves' disease, and b) the differentiation between Graves' disease and autonomous goiter, and 2. whether TBIAb is also of importance in other thyroid diseases.

Clinical Results

Graves' disease

As in other autoimmune diseases, the rate of recurrences is also rather high in Graves' disease. In a retrospective study we found a relapse rate of 50% six months after the end of antithyroid therapy and a relapse rate of about 72% one year thereafter (fig. 1).

With the radioligand receptor assay mentioned above most authors could detect TBIAb in about 70–90% of their untreated Graves' disease patients (tab. 1).

Table 1 Incidence of TBIAb in Graves' disease

Author	Year	Incidence	%
Smith et al.	1974	22/25	88
Mukhtar et al.	1975	58/58	100
Davies et al.	1977	22/30	73
O'Donnell et al.	1978	32/42	76
Schleusener et al.	1978	55/110	50*
McGregor et al.	1979	41/55	76
Bliddal et al.	1981	76/116	66
Borges et al.	1982	47/50	94
Biro et al.	1982	81/104	78
Creagh et al.	1985	58/62	94

* The low value is caused by heterogeneity of patients. New investigations show an incidence of TBIAb in 90 of 107 (84.1%) Graves' disease patients with opthalmopathy.

* Trac/Fa. Henning, Thybia/Mallinckrodt, RSR Ltd., Cardiff, Wales

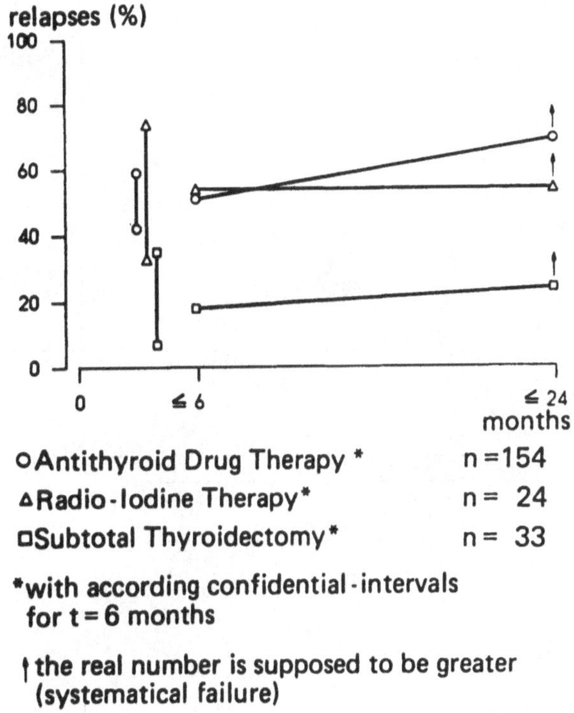

Fig. 1 Rate of relapses of Graves' Thyrotoxicosis, treated with antithyroid-drug-therapy, radio-iodine-therapy or subtotal thyroidectomy as second therapeutical try, 6 month and up to 24 months after end of the therapy (from A. Stadler, dissertation in preparation, 1985).

Table 2 TSH-receptor-antibodies at the end of antithyroid drug treatment and clinical outcome of Graves' disease

Author	Year	Patients (n)	TBIAb pos. (n)	Relapse (%)	TBIAb neg. (n)	Relapse (%)
Davies	1977	30	23	52	7	0
O'Donnell	1978	16	9	89	7	0
Schleusener	1978	49	15	87	34	29
Teng	1980	60	9	100	51	39
McGregor	1980	65	25	96	40	40
Docter	1980	17	7	57	10	60
Bliddal	1981	13	8	100	5	0
Hardisty	1981	52	24	88	28	29
Finke	1981	69	18	89	51	43
Gossage	1982	27	4	100	23	30
Creagh	1985	37	23	96	14	21

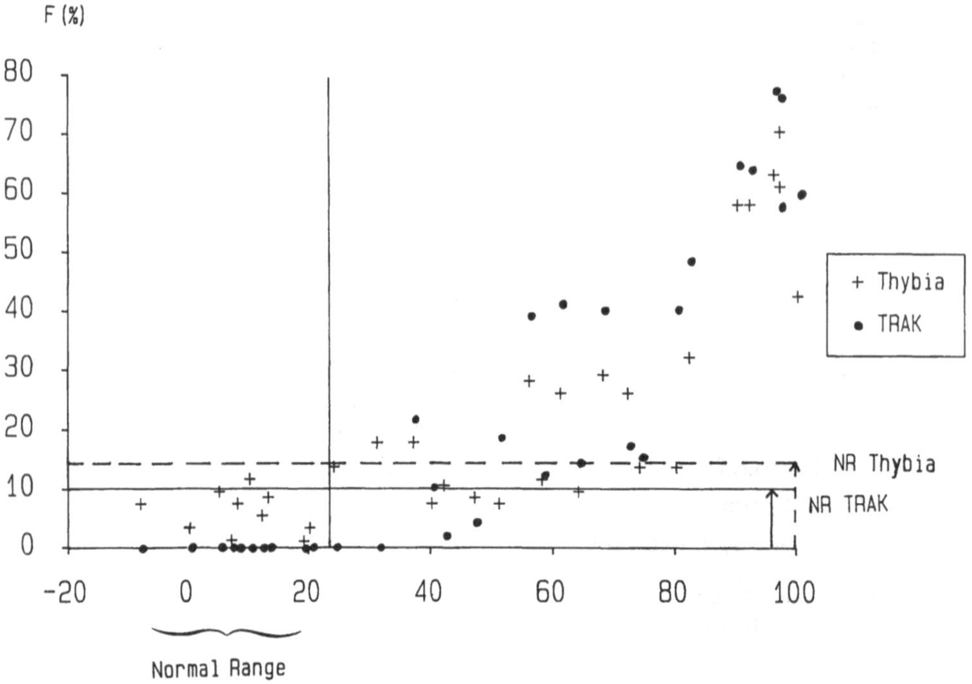

Fig. 2

Comparison of our radioligand receptor assay with membrane fragments (52) and two commercially available test kits in the measurements of TBIAb (THYBIA: Fa. Mallinckrodt, TRAK: Fa. Henning). Thirty-two sera were tested. The F-values [F = 100 x (1-B pat./B norm.)] were shown in the figure. The results obtained with our own methods were given on the x-axis, and those obtained with the two kits on the y-axis (THYBIA + TRAK).

A result was regarded as positive, if F > 23 for our own assay, F > 10 for TRAK and F > 15 for THYBIA. This was marked in the figure. Correlation coefficients were r = 0,81 for the method applied by us versus THYBIA, r = 0,89 for our method versus TRAK and r = 0,93 for THYBIA versus TRAK.

Discrepancies were only found in the range of borderline values. Some sera were positive in our assay and negative in one or both kits. In no case did we find the opposite situation.

This may be due to a higher sensitivity of our own method. To exclude the possibility of false positive values we have tested 116 healthy people. Less than 5% showed "positive" results.

Numerous groups investigated the question whether or not TBIAb measurements are a reliable tool to predict the further clinical course after cessation of antithyroid drug treatment. Some of the controversial findings are listed in table 2.

Some of these controversies can be explained – apart from methodological reasons – by the following points:

a) With the RRA one can measure stimulating *and* blocking antibodies to the TSH receptor. This might explain why TBIAb can also be detected in Graves' disease patients who are in remission at the time of measurement (tab. 3 and 4). Several investigators compared the RRA- and cAMP-assay and obtained different results. While Hensen et al. [17], Borges et al. [9], Bliddal et al. [18], Biro [19] and Creagh et al. [20] found a good correlation between these two methods, other investigators failed to find any correlation at all [3, 21–25].

Aside from methodological differences, there might be another explanation. Hensen et al. [17] speculated about separate locations of the TSH-binding site and the adenylate cyclase stimulation site on the TSH receptor complex. This theory was supported by findings of Valente et al. [26] who described monoclonal antibodies with either stimulatory or binding inhibiting properties.

Table 3 TBIAb and TSAb in 119 patients with Graves' disease and ophthalmopathy [17]

	Untreated hyperthyroidism (n = 42)	During treatment with thionamide drugs (n = 38)	In remission after anti-thyroid drug therapy (n = 39)
TBIAb positive TSAb positive	20 (48)	10 (26)	3 (8)
TBIAb positive TSAb negative	10 (24)	7 (18)	6 (15)
TBIAb negative TSAb positive	4 (9)	2 (5)	0 (0)
TBIAb negative TSAb negative	8 (19)	19 (50)	30 (77)
TBIAb prevalence (%)	71	45	23
TSAb prevalence (%)	57	32	8

Percentages are shown in parentheses.

Table 4 Clinical data from three patients with regained thyroid suppressibility in presence of persistent TBIAb-activity [52]

Patients	FT_4 Indexes[a]	TT_3 Levels[b]	TSH-levels (μU/ml)		Thyroid^{99n} Tc O_4 uptake (cpm/mCi^{99m} Tc O_4^-)[c]	
			Pre-TRH	Post-TRH	Pre-T_4	Post-T_4
1	59	1.36	0.8	3.3	56,000	14,000
2	61	1.50	3.0	28.0	150,000	62,000
3	82	1.54	1.3	8.0	12,207 (33%)	4,262[d] (9%)

[a] normal range, 32–113

[b] normal range, 1–3 mcl/liter

[c] normal range, 40000–80000 cpm/mCi

[d] performed with ^{131}I (24 h-uptake) instead of $^{99m}Tc\ O_4^-$. Normal range, 20–40%.

b) Since the studies of McLachlan et al. in 1983 [27], which showed that B-cell suspensions of thyroid glands of Graves' disease patients spontaneously produce IgG, intrathyroidal B-cells have been believed to be the origin of autoantibodies against microsomal antigen and thyroglobulin. These results could be confirmed by Weetman et al. [28] and Canonica et al. [29]. The latter expanded his findings on the T cells, indicating that the I a subgroup was elevated within the thyroid gland. The site of antibody production against the TSH receptor has not yet been located, but one might speculate that intrathyroidal B and T lymphocytes are involved in the production of the other two antibodies, too. Thus the TBIAb measurement seems to register an overflow of the antibody production by intrathyroidally located lymphocytes (fig. 3, tab. 5). These findings might explain that – as described most recently by Weetman et al. [54] – even TSAb measurements do not predict the course of the disease.

To reevaluate the problem of predicting the course of disease after therapy we started a multicenter prospective study. So far 162 patients with Graves' disease who were treated with methimazole for one year were followed up for another year. The starting dose mostly lay between 20 – 40 mg/day, the maintenance dose

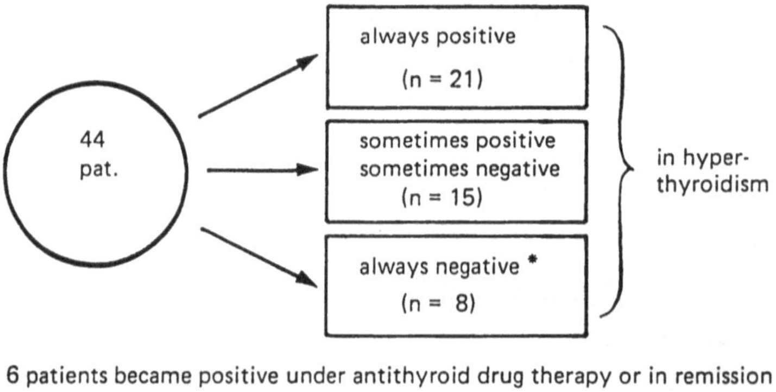

Fig. 3 Varying results on TBIAb in 44 Graves' disease patients with ophthalmopathy and repeated incidences of hyperthyroidism [31].

Table 5 Frequency (cumulative) of TBIAb in 44 Graves' disease patients (with ophthalmopathy) with several hyperthyroid episodes 31

A)	First hyperthyroidism	70% positive	
B)	Second hyperthyroidism	77% positive	
C)	Third hyperthyroidism	82% positive	cumulative
D)	6 patients (13%) were positive only during therapy or in remission	95% positive	

Table 6a Graves' disease patients with more than two positive measurements of TBIAb. Relapserate 1 year after therapy according to the TBIAb status at the end of therapy

	TBIAb neg.	TBIAb pos.	total
remission	37	12	49 (30%)
relapse	47	66	113 (70%)
total	84	78	162 (100%)

Sensitivity 0.58 (confidence int. 0.48 – 0.67)
Specificity 0.75 (confidence int. 0.61 – 0.87)
(Preliminary results from the multicenter study)

Table 6b Graves' disease patients with pretherapeutic detection of TBIAb. Relapserate 1 year after therapy according to the TBIAb status at the end of therapy

	TBIAb neg.	TBIAb pos.	total
remission	35	7	42 (35%)
relapse	34	45	79 (65%)
total	69	52	121 (100%)

Sensitivity 0.57 (confidence int. 0.45 – 0.68)
Specificity 0.83 (confidence int. 0.69 – 0.93)
(Preliminary results from the multicenter study)

was about 5 – 10 mg/day. The recurrence rate so far is about 70%. Table 6 a and 6 b demonstrate that the TBIAb measurement at the end of antithyroid drug treatment is of no clinical value.

In 152 patients, an "Alexander test" could be compared with the outcome of the antibody determination at drug withdrawal. Table 7 confirms earlier results showing that regained suppressibility is not significantly correlated to a loss of antibody activity. Altogether, the Thyroid Section of the German Endocrine Society does not recommend at the moment TBIAb measurements in the follow-up of Graves' disease [55].

Table 7 Relation between TBIAb and suppressiontest at the end of a 1 year drug therapy of Graves' disease patients (n = 152)

	Suppressiontest	
	normal	abnormal
TBIAb positive	28 (19%)	37 (24%)
TBIAb negative	49 (32%)	38 (25%)

(Preliminary results from the multicenter study)

Differentiation between Graves' disease and autonomous goiter

The autonomous adenoma and the disseminated thyroid autonomy are variations of the same disease. According to Studer et al. [43, 44] there are cell clones with different grades of function and growth ability in every thyroid. Some cells possess both faculties. In iodine-deficient goiters, not only 'normal' thyrocytes but also autonomous cells increase, especially in later stages of the disease. The term 'autonomously' can include both autonomous function and autonomous growth. There are also clones in which only function and others in which only growth is autonomous. This explains why one can find 'cold' areas in thyroid scintigraphy that go on growing under thyroxine suppression therapy (fig. 4). In

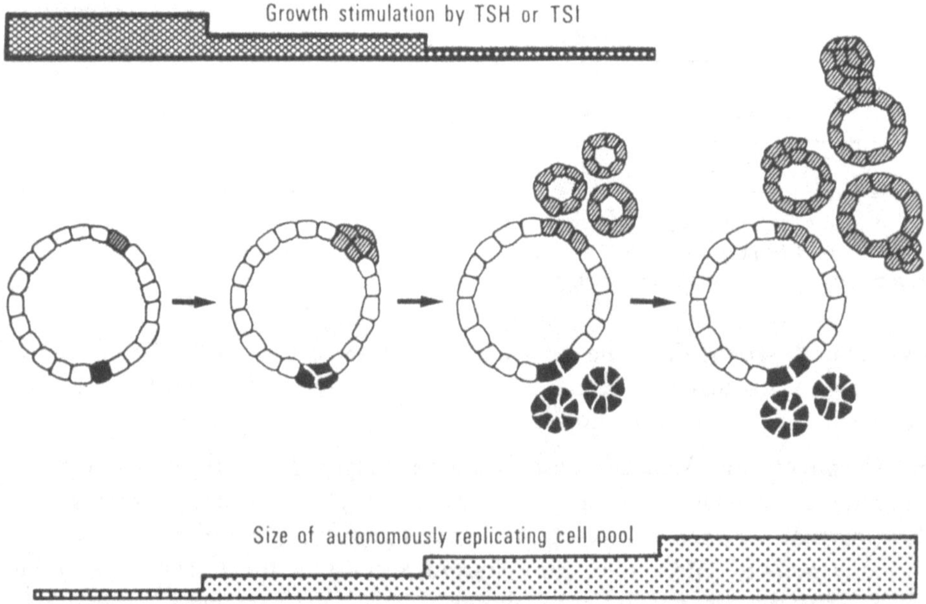

Fig. 4 Pathogenesis of Autonomous Goiter Growth

Diagrammatic representation of the sequence of TSH (or TSI) depending and autonomous goiter growth. The follicle is assumed to contain two clones of epithelial cells with high intrinsic growth potential (shaded cells). The clone shown in the upper part of the follicle is assumed to possess inborn growth potential high enough to maintain cell replication and, hence, follicle neogeneration, even in the absence of exogenous stimuli, while the cell clone in the lower segment of the follicle multiplies only in response to exogenous growth factors. Any goitrogen will enhance growth of both cell clones and gradually lead to an increase of the total cell mass. Upon cessation of the goitrogenic stimulus, the clone with the highest spontaneous replication rate will multiply at the initial rate but, since its total size has increased, considerable autonomous goiter growth is now apparent. (Reproduced with permission from Studer et al. [43].)

later stages of the disease, nodules develop in the autonomous goiter and, to a lesser extend, in Graves' goiters as well. The main reason for this development is an insufficient arterial supply to the areas with fresh growth which is followed by necrosis and vegetation of connective tissue.

As autonomous goiters usually develop from euthyroid goiters by increase of autonomous cell clones after a long enough period of time, the clinician can often observe that a patient with a goiter may have normal levels of thyroxine and triiodothyronine together with a positive response of TSH or TRH. Later on, this response diminuishes until it becomes undetectable, although the hormone levels remain within normal range. Finally the patient might become hyperthroid, especially after iodine exposure.

Most recently, some investigators have suggested that the development of 'autonomous' follicles can be accelerated not only by TSH but also by thyroid growth immunoglobulins (TGI). Drexhage et al. [30] found TGI in all of his 10 'colloid' goiter patients. Other groups reported about TGI in 27% [46], 62% [47], and 63% [48] of their nontoxic goiter patients. Recently Wiener and van der Gaag [49] found TGI activity in seven of nine patients with Plummer's disease. Additionally, histological and immunohistochemical data give support to the hypothesis that there might be some immunological background in the development of autonomous goiter [50, 51].

Generally spoken, a positive TBIAb assay confirms the diagnosis of Graves' disease, a negative finding, however, does not exclude its presence. From clinical observation alone it can be difficult, especially in patients without ophthalmopathy, to differentiate between the two types of toxic goiter. As Hensen et al. [31] was able to show, the TBIAb frequency differs among the subgroups of hyperthyroidism. While "cumulative" TBIAb positivity is 98% in Graves' disease

Table 8 TBIAb frequency in 230 patients* with a history of hyperthyroidism [31]

with ophthalmopathy (n = 104)		without ophthalmopathy (n = 126)	
diffuse thyroid (n = 77)	diffuse-nodular thyroid (n = 27)	diffuse thyroid (n = 78)	diffuse-nodular thyroid (n = 48)
92%	93%	74%	52%

* A patient was classified as TBIAb positive when he had antibody activity at least once in 1 – 10 years.

patients with endocrine ophthalmopathy regardless of the presence of a diffuse or a nodular goiter, TBIAb could be found in 74% of patients without eye signs and a diffuse goiter and in 52% of patients without eye signs and a nodular goiter. From these results one can conclude that also Graves' disease can be accompanied by both types of goiter (tab. 8). However, the presence of TSH-receptor antibodies seems to be very rare in patients with autonomous goiter. In agreement with others [45] we find TBIAb activity in about 5% of patients with uninodular autonomous adenomas (tab. 9).

Table 9 Frequency of elevated titers of microsomal antibodies (MAB ≥ 1:1600) and thyrotropin displacing activity (TBIAb) in various groups of euthyroid and hyperthyroid patients. Reproduced with Kind permission by Schicha et al. [45]

	N	TBIAb	MAB ≥ 1:1600
Normal	45	0 (0%)	10 (22%)
Euthyroid goiter	126	5 (4%)	29 (23%)
Autonomous adenoma	112	6 (5%)	21 (19%)
– euthyroid	69	4 (6%)	14 (20%)
– hyperthyroid	43	2 (5%)	7 (16%)
Autonomous goiter	63	2 (3%)	14 (22%)
Graves' disease	57	45 (79%)	55 (96%)

TSH receptor antibodies in hypothyroidism

In 1960 Sutherland et al. [32] described hypothyroid children without goiter. Further case reports were given by Goldsmith et al. [33] and Matsuura et al. [34]. The latter speculated that maternal blocking antibodies against the TSH receptor crossed the placenta and caused neonate hypothyroidism which gradually resolved when the antibodies were cleared. Zakarija et al. [35] reported about a mother whose IgG was stimulatory in cAMP assay at low – not at high concentrations – and was biphasic in its ability to affect ^{125}J-TSH binding. Her neonate had hyperthyroidism at the age of 4 months. Its IgG showed enhanced binding at lower concentrations and inhibition of binding at higher concentrations in the radioligand receptor assay. The authors concluded that the sera contained both stimulatory and inhibiting antibodies. Studies performed by Takasu et al. [36–37], Konishi et al. [38], Steel et al. [39], Endo et al. [40], and Drexhage et al. [41] revealed blocking antibodies in about 15 to 25% of hypothyroid patients, adults and children, indicating that several autoimmune thyroid diseases, including Graves' disease, produce a heterogeneous population of antibodies against the TSH receptor which could have stimulatory and inhibiting faculties.

Summary

In 1956, Adams and Purves described the presence of a thyroid-stimulating factor in sera of patients with Graves' disease. A few years later, it became evident that this factor is an autoantibody to the TSH receptor and acts via the adenyl cyclase system. By this pathway, the antibody ultimately leads the uncontrolled secretion of T4 and T3 by the thyrocytes. More recently, it became evident that there exist TSH receptor antibodies with both stimulating properties and with blocking properties. Such blocking antibodies, for example, might be found in patients with Graves' disease who are in remission after antithyroid drug treatment or in patients with the atrophic form of immune thyroiditis. The most widely used assay system for the measurement of TSH receptor antibodies is the radioligand receptor assay (RRA), which is based on the inhibition of the binding of radiolabelled TSH to TSH receptor material. Because of this technique, the widely accepted nomenclature is TSH-binding-inhibiting antibodies (TBIAb); only this method, for which commercial kits are available, can be used in routine laboratories.

Highly controversial data have been published on whether or not the measurement of TBIAb with the RRA gives reliable information predicting remission or recurrence of the disease in an individual patient after stopping antithyroid drug treatment. To reevaluate the problem, we started a multicenter prospective study in which 13 West German clinics participate. Preliminary results in 162 patients indicate that the RRA provides no help in the prediction of the clinical outcome (specificity: 0.8, sensitivity: 0.5). These disapointing results can be explained by the following: 1. Most, if not all, of the antibodies are synthesized by lymphocytes located within the thyroid gland, but not by peripheral lymphocytes. Presumably the antibody activity measured in the serum represents only an overflow from the thyroid. These findings are – apart from methodological problems – the reason why the antibodies are only detectable in about 80% of patients with active Graves' hyperthyroidism. 2. As mentioned above, the RRA detects stimulating *and* blocking antibodies. 3. Even more important, the results of antibody determinations can at most describe the immediate state of the immune status. The risk of recurrence of this disease is high. In the multicenter study mentioned above, the relapse rate after one year is in the order of about 70%. Other retrospective data from our group indicate that, after 2 years, the relapse rate is in the order of about 80%. These clinical observations alone would greatly limit the clinical significance of the TBIAb measurements. The Thyroid Section of the German Endocrine Society does not recommend the determination of TBIAb in the follow-up of Graves' thyrotoxicosis. The antibody determination is only useful in the differentiation of the two major forms of hyperthyroidism (Graves' disease and autonomous goiter) in patients who have no other signs of an autoimmune process such as Graves' ophthalmopathy. Of course, it is clear from the above that only a positive result, not a negative one, is meaningful.

References

[1] Adams, D. D., H. D. Purves: Abnormal responses in the assay of thyrotropin. Proc. Univ. Otago Med. School **34** (1956) 11.

[2] McKenzie, J. M., A. Williamson: Experience with the bioassay of the long-acting thyroid stimulator. J. Clin. Endocrinol. Metab. **26** (1966) 518.

[3] Kuzuya, N., S. C. Chiu, H. Ikeda, et al.: Correlation between thyroid stimulator and 3, 5, 3-triiodothyronine suppressibility in patients during treatment for hyperthyroidism with thionamide drugs: Comparison of assays by thyroid-stimulating and displacing activities. J. Clin. Endocrinol. Metab. **48** (4) (1979) 706.

[4] Kendall-Taylor, P.: Effects of long-acting thyroid stimulator (LATS) and LATS protector on human thyroid adenyl cyclase activity. Br. Med. J. **3** (1973) 72.

[5] Yamashita, S., M. Izumi, K. Sato, et al.: Spezific stimulatory effects of Graves' IgG on release of T3 from their own thyroids. 59th Meeting of the American Thyroid Assoc. New Orleans, LA (abstr 1) 1983.

[6] Orgiazzi, J., D. E. Williams, I. J. Chopra, et al.: Human thyroid adenyl cyclase-stimulator in immunoglobulin G (IgG) of patients with Graves' disease. In: Thyroid Research (J. Robbins, et al., eds.). Excerpta Medica, Amsterdam 1976.

[7] Bech, K., S. Nistrup Madsen: Human thyroid adenylate cyclase in non-toxic goiter: Sensitivity to TSH, fluorids and thyroid stimulating immunoglobulins. Clin. Endocrinol. (Oxf.) **8** (6) (1978) 457.

[8] Hensen, J., P. Kotulla, H. Schleusener: Comparison of TSH binding inhibiting and thyroid adenylate cyclase stimulation in sera of hyperthyroid patients. Acta Endocrinol. **99**, Suppl. 246 (1982) 73 (abstr).

[9] Borges, M., J. C. Ingbar, K. Endo, et al.: A new method for assessing the thyrotrophin binding inhibitory activity in the immunoglobulins and whole serum of patients with Graves' disease. J. Clin. Endocrinol. Metab. **54** (1982) 552.

[10] Kleinmann, R. E., L. E. Braverman, A. G. Vagenakis, et al.: A new method for measurement of human thyroid-stimulating immunoglobulins. J. Lab. Clin. Med. **95** (1980) 581.

[11] Karlsson, F. A., P. A. Dahlberg: Thyroid stimulating antibodies (TSAb) in patients with Graves' disease undergoing antithyroid drug treatment: Indicators of activity of disease. Clin. Endocrinol. (Oxf.) **14** (1981) 579.

[12] Feldt-Rasmussen, U., K. Bech, J. Date, et al.: Thyroid stimulating antibodies, thyreoglobulin antibodies and serum proteins during treatment of Graves' disease with radioiodine or propyl thiouracil. Allergy **38** (1982) 49.

[13] Adams, D. D., T. H. Kennedy: Occurrence in thyrotoxicosis of a gamma globulin which protects LATS from neutralization by an extract of thyroid gland. J. Clin. Endocrinol. Metab. **27** (1967) 173.

[14] Smith, B. R., R. Hall: Thyroid-stimulating immunoglobulins in Graves' disease. Lancet **II** (1974) 427.

[15] Mehdi, S. Q., S. S. Nussey: A radio-ligand receptor assay for LATS-inhibition by the long-acting thyroid stimulator of the binding of radio-iodinated thyroid stimulating hormone to human thyroid membranes. Biochem. J. **145** (1975) 105.

[16] Manley, S. W., J. R. Bourke, R. W. Hawkes: The thyrotrophin receptor in guinea-pig thyroid homogenate: Interaction with the long-acting thyroid stimulator. J. Endocrinol. **61** (1974) 437.

[17] Hensen, J., P. Kotulla, R. Finke, et al.: Methodological aspects and clinical results of an assay for thyroid-stimulating antibodies: Correlation with thyrotropin binding-inhibiting antibodies. J. Clin. Endocrinol. Metab. **58** (1984) 980.

[18] Bliddal, H., K. Bech, P. H. Peterson, et al.: Evidence of a correlation between thyrotrophin receptor binding inhibition and thyroid adenylate cyclase activation by immunoglobulins in

Graves' disease before and during longterm antithyroid treatment. Acta Endocrinol. (Copenh.) **101** (1) (1982) 35.

[19] Biro, J.: Thyroid-stimulating antibodies in Graves' disease and the effect of thyrotrophin-binding globulins on their determination. J. Endocrinol. **92** (1982) 175.

[20] Creagh, F., M. Teece, S. Williams, et al.: An analysis of thyrotrophin receptor binding and thyroid stimulating activities in an series of Graves' sera. Clin. Endocrinol. (Oxf.) **23** (1985) 395.

[21] Zakarija, M., A. Sato, J. M. McKenzie: Thyroid-stimulation versus inhibition of thyrotropin (TSH)-binding comparison of assays for thyroid-stimulating antibodies (TSAB) of Graves' disease. 53rd Meeting of the American Thyroid Association, Cleveland OH (Abstract T-6) 1977.

[22] Sugenoya, A., A. Kidd, V. V. Row, et al.: Correlation between thyrotropin-displacing activity and human thyroid-stimulating activity by immunoglobulins from patients with Graves' disease and other thyroid disease. J. Clin. Endocrinol. Metab. **48** (3) (1979) 398.

[23] Macchia, E., G. F. Fenzi, F. Monzani, et al.: Comparison between thyroid stimulating and TSH-binding inhibiting immunoglobulins of Graves' disease. Clin. Endocrinol. (Oxf.) **152** (1981) 175.

[24] Hardisty, C. A., P. Kendall-Taylor, S. Atkinson, et al.: The assay of Graves immunoglobulins: A comparison of different methods. Clin. Endocrinol. (Oxf.) **18** (1983) 637.

[25] Grant, S. J. B., B. M. Luttrell, J. B. Hales: The assay for thyroid stimulating immunoglobulins using cultured human thyroid cells. Clin. Endocrinol. **23** (1985) 325.

[26] Valente, W. A., Z. Yavin, E. Yavin, et al.: Monoclonal antibodies to the thyrotropin receptor: The identification of blocking and stimulating antibodies. J. Endocrinol. Invest. 5 (1982) 293.

[27] McLachlan, S. M., A. M. Dickinson, A. Malcolm, et al.: Thyroid autoantibody synthesis by cultures of thyroid and peripheral blood lymphocytes. I. Lymphocyte markers and response to pokeweed mitogen. Clin. Exp. Immunol. **52** (1983) 45.

[28] Weetman, A. P., A. M. McGregor, J. H. Lazarus, et al.: Thyroid antibodies are produced by thyroid-derived lymphocytes. Clin. Exp. Immunol. **48** (1982) 196.

[29] Canonica, G. W., M. Bagnasco, M. E. Cosulich, et al.: Why thyroid is major site of thyroid auto antibody synthesis in autoimmune thyroid disease. Lancet **I** (1983) 1163.

[30] Drexhage, H. A., G. F. Bottazzo, L. Bitensky, et al.: Thyroid growth-blocking antibodies in primary myxoedema. Nature **289** (1981) 594.

[31] Hensen, J., P. Kotulla, R. Finke, et al.: 10 years experience with consecutive measurement of thyrotropin binding inhibiting antibodies (TBIAb). J. Endocrinol. Invest. 7 (1984) 215.

[32] Sutherland, J. M., V. M. Esselborn, R. S. Burket, et al.: Familial nongoitrous cretinism apparently due to maternal antithyroid antibody. N. Engl. J. Med. **263** (1960) 336.

[33] Goldsmith, R. E., A. J. McAdams, P. R. Larsen, et al.: Familial autoimmune thyroiditis: Maternal-fetal relationship and role of generalized autoimmunity. J. Clin. Endocrinol. Metab. **37** (1973) 265.

[34] Matsuura, N., Y. Yamada, Y. Nohara, et al.: Familial neonatal transient hypothyroidism due to maternal TSH-binding inhibitor immunoglobulins. N. Engl. J. Med. **303** (1980) 738.

[35] Zakarija, M., J. M. McKenzie, D. S. Munro: Immunoglobulin G inhibitor of thyroid-stimulating antibody is a cause of delay in the onset of neonatal Graves' disease. J. Clin. Invest. **72** (1983) 1352.

[36] Takasu, N., T. Mori, Y. Koizumi, et al.: Transient neonatal hypothyroidism due to maternal immunoglobulins that inhibit thyrotropin-binding and postreceptor processor. J. Clin. Endocrinol. Metab. **59** (1984) 142.

[37] Takasu, N., M. Naka, T. Mori, et al.: Two types of thyroid function-blocking antibodies in autoimmune atrophic thyroiditis and transient neonatal hypothyroidism due to maternal IgG. Clin. Endocrinol. **21** (1984) 345.

[38] Konishi, J., Y. Iida, K. Endo, et al.: Inhibition of thyrotropin-induced adenosine 3'5'-monophosphate increase by immunoglobulins from patients with primary my edema. J. Clin. Endocrinol. Metab. **57** (1983) 544.
[39] Steel, N. R., D. R. Weightman, J. J. Taylor, et al.: Blocking activity to action of thyroid stimulating hormone in serum from patients with primary hypothyroidism. Br. Med. J. **288** 1559.
[40] Endo, K., K. Kasagi, J. Knoshi, et al.: Detection and properties of TSH binding inhibitor immunoglobulins in patients with Graves' disease and Hashimoto's thyroiditis. J. Clin. Endocrinol. Metab. Y6 (1978) 734.
[41] Kotulla, P., H. Schleusener: Solubilized TSH-receptor: Its usefulness for the radioligand receptor assay for TSH and TSH-displacing antibody. J. Endocrinol. Invest. **4** (1981) 155.
[42] Kotulla, P., Ch. Kostner, H. Schleusener: Radioligand receptor assay for TSH and TSH-binding-inhibiting antibodies using solubilized TSH-receptor. J. Endocrinol. Invest. **6** (1983) 135.
[43] Studer, H., H. J. Peter, H. Gerber: Morphologic and functional changes in developing oiters. In: Thyroid Disorders Associated with Iodine Deficiency and Excess (R. Hall, J. Köbberling, eds.), Serono Symposia, vol. 22, p. 227. Raven Press, New York 1985.
[44] Studer, M., H. J. Peter, H. Gerber: Toxic nodular goitre. Clin. Endocrinol. Metab. **14** (1985) 351.
[45] Schicha, H., D. Emrich, I. Schreivogel: Hyperthyroidism due to Graves' disease and due to autonomous goiter. J. Endocrinol. Invest. **8** (1985) 399.
[46] Schatz, H., R. Bär, F. Müller, et al.: Thyroid growth stimulating immunoglobulins in euthyroid goiter patients from an iodine deficient endemic goiter area (abstr. No. 43). International Symposium Thyroid and Autoimmunity, Amsterdam 1986.
[47] Rotella, C. M., C. Mavilia, L. D. Kohn: Thyroid growth promoting antibody in patients with non toxic goiter (abstr. No. 42). International Symposium Thyroid and Autoimmunity, Amsterdam 1986.
[48] Smyth, P. P. A., B. Grubeck-Loebenstein, T. J. McKenna: Possible significance of IgG thyroid stimulators in nontoxic goitre (abstr. No. 41). International Symposium Thyroid and Autoimmunity, Amsterdam 1986.
[49] Wiener, J. D., R. D. van der Gaag: Autoimmunity and the pathogenesis of localized thyroid autonomy (Plummer's disease). Clin. Endocrinol. **23** (1985) 635.
[50] Lawerenz, J. U., K. Badenhoop, G. Jautzke, et al.: Histological and immunohistochemical investigation of the inflammatory infiltrate in euthyroid goiter, hyperthyroid autonomous goiter and Graves' disease. Workshop on "Current topics in Thyroid Autoimmunity" (Henning Symposion) 5. Oktober 1983 (D. Doniach, H. Schleusener, B. Weinheimer, eds.), p. 209. Thieme Verlag, Stuttgart 1984.
[51] Grubeck-Loebenstein, B., K. Derfler, H. Kassal, et al.: Immunological features of nonimmunogenic hyperthyroidism. J. Clin. Endocrinol. Metab. **60** (1985) 150.
[52] Schleusener, H., P. Kotulla, R. Finke, et al.: Relationship between thyroid status and Graves' disease-specific immunoglobulins. J. Clin. Endocrinol. Metab. **47** (1978) 379.
[53] Shinozawa, T., M. C. Villadolid, S. H. Ingbar: A new serum-based assay for fat cell-binding immunoglobulins: Application to the detection of the thyrotropin receptor antibodies of Graves' disease. J. Clin. Endocrinol. Metab. **62** (1985) 10.
[54] Weetman, A. P., S. Ratanachiyavong, G. W. Middleton, et al.: Prediction of Outcome in Graves' Disease after Carbimazole Treatment. Q. J. Med., New Series **59** (1986) 228.
[55] Scriba, P. C., W. Börner, D. Emrich, et al.: Schilddrüsenfunktionsdiagnostik und die Diagnose von Schilddrüsenkrankheiten. Der Nuklearmediziner **8** (1985) 67.

Autoantibodies reacting with thyroid plasma membranes in Graves' disease: importance of multiple plasma membrane antigens

J. Nauman, A. Gardas, B. Czarnocka

Introduction

It is almost generally assumed [1, 2, 3] that autoantibodies present in serum of patients with hyperthyroid Graves-Basedow disease almost exclusively bind to the TSH receptor and react with the same receptor epitopes as does thyrotropin itself [2].

By using data collected during last two years both in our experimental and clinical studies we intend to show that autoantibodies circulating in the bloodstream of untreated hyperthyroid patients with Graves-Basedow disease in addition to the TSH receptor react also with other thyroid plasma membrane components. Although, the nature of these multiple thyroid plasma membrane antigens remains unknown we would present evidence which exclude the role of thyreoglobulin and suggest that the microsomal antigen (which can be present in thyroid plasma membranes) is of limited importance for our assay. We will also attempt to answer the question whether estimation of autoantibodies against thyroid plasma membrane antigens (ATMA) is useful in an early diagnosis of Graves-Basedow disease, helpful in the choice of appropriate anti-thyroid therapy and its termination and important in prognostic study.

Material and methods

Thyroid tissues were obtained during surgical treatment of patients with thyroid disease, serum samples were collected from 168 patients with untreated hyperthyroid Graves-Basedow disease, from 120 patients with hyperthyroid Graves-Basedow disease in early stage of anti-thyroid treatment, 79 patients with Hashimoto disease, 116 patients with toxic nodular goiter and 124 patients with non-toxic nodular goiter. Serum samples were also obtained each month during 6 months treatment of 43 hyperthyroid Graves-Basedow patients with methimazol, as well as from 16 Graves-Basedow patients treated with ^{131}-Iodide and

Thyrotropin

followed for 6 months and from 34 patients with Graves-Basedow disease who were euthyroid but ATMA "positive" when qualified for subtotal thyroidectomy. These patients were also followed for 6 months after surgery. Finally material consisted also 114 patients with Graves-Basedow disease treated previously with methimazol, or radio-iodide, or by subtotal strumectomy and examined 3 to 9 months after termination of respective therapy. Serum samples from patients with non-thyroidal autoimmune diseases were kindly donated by National Rheumatological Institute, Warsaw, and Department of Dermatology, Medical College, Warsaw. 120 healthy blood donors served as controls. Thyroids were homogenized and crude plasma membrane fractions obtained as previously described [4]. Methods of thyroid plasma membrane proteins solubilization and further purification as well as method of bovine TSH (kindly donated by prof. J. Pierce, USA) ^{125}I labelling and purification by affinity chromatography were also previously published [5]. Autoantibodies against thyroid plasma membrane antigens were estimated by RIA [4] and recently by more specific and sensitive ELISA [6]. Some results shown here were also previously presented [6, 7].

Results and discussion

Methods used led to the solubilization of 65% of proteins and approximately 75% of autoantigens present in thyroid plasma membranes which react with autoantibodies from serum of patients with hyperthyroid Graves-Basedow disease. Solubilized proteins were further purified by column chromatography on Ultrogel AcA-34 and these with molecular weight of about 70 000 daltons were found to be most active in inhibiting autoantibodies binding to crude thyroid plasma membranes in our RIA ATMA assay or to solid phase bound purified plasma membrane antigens in ELISA procedure. Solubilized and purified thyroid plasma membrane proteins were able to bind bovine TSH and this binding could be in dose dependent manner inhibited by native human TSH or by purified thyroid plasma membrane proteins. The preincubation of thyroid plasma membranes (prior to the solubilization) with pooled serum from hyperthyroid Graves-Basedow patients almost complitely abolished the ability of solubilized proteins to inhibit binding of autoantibodies to solid phase bound thyroid plasma membrane proteins, however, these proteins were still able to bind TSH-^{125}I.

Enrichment of serum samples from untreated Graves-Basedow patients with purified thyreoglobulin (1 mg/ml) have had no effect on ATMA estimation thus providing evidence that our method does not determine antibodies against thyreoglobulin (tab. 1). Enrichment of the same serum samples with TSH (1 mU/ml) had no effect on ATMA estimation in some patients but in others inhibited the reaction between autoantibodies and antigens from 5 to 39% thus suggsting

Table 1 Influence of human thyreoglobulin and thyrotrophin Ambinon on binding of autoantibodies to human thyroid plasma membrane antigenes in the ELISA

Patient no.	Serum titre	% of inhibition	
		TSH 1 mU/ml	thyreoglobulin 1 mg/ml
1	1/ 16 000	37	0
2	1/256 000	34	0
3	1/ 64 000	14	0
4	1/ 16 000	0	0
5	1/ 64 000	0	0
6	1/ 16 000	5	0
7	1/ 64 000	0	0
8	1/ 64 000	10	0
9	1/ 16 000	0	0
10	1/ 64 000	14	0
11	1/ 16 000	12	0
12	1/ 64 000	0	0
13	1/ 64 000	19	0
14	1/ 64 000	0	0
15	1/ 4 000	27	0
16	1/ 64 000	0	0

polyclonal character of autoantibodies and participation of multiple thyroid plasma membrane antigens in the reaction with these autoantibodies (tab. 1).

The possibility that in addition to TSH receptor also other thyroid plasma membrane components react with autoantibodies present in serum of patients with hyperthyroid Graves-Basedow disease was further supported by experiments in which we attempted at least indirectly calculate maximal binding capacity (MBC) of thyroid plasma membrane proteins for autoantibodies. Values of MBC obtained were at least 10 times higher than well known [5, 8] MBC values for TSH binding.

The polyclonal character of autoantibodies was also suggested by results of experiments in which we calculate the amounts of thyroid plasma membrane proteins which were needded to produce 50% inhibition of the reaction between autoantibodies and solid phase bound antigens. This amount varied from 3.39 μg/ml to 12.03 μg/ml. It was of interest that at least 10 times more of thyroid microsomal membrane proteins have to be used to obtain similar 50% inhibition (tab. 2). This shows that the participation of Microsomal antigens in ATMA estimation although possible is of minor significance.

Polyclonal character of autoantibodies has been also shown by results of clinical study in which we estimated ATMA (by ELISA), antibodies against microsomal antigen (TMS, Serono RIA) antibodies a against TSH receptor (TRAK, Henning)

Table 2 Amounts of soluble thyroid plasma membrane and soluble microsomal membrane proteins required to obtain 50% inhibition of autoantibodies binding to solid phase bound plasma membrane antigen in the ELISA

Patient no.	Serum titre	μg/ml of protein required to obtain 50% inhibition of autoantibodies binding	
		soluble plasma membrane	soluble microsomal membrane
1	1/ 64 000	5.25	55
2	1/ 64 000	4.37	48
3	1/ 4 000	3.37	29
4	1/ 4 000	3.12	24
5	1/256 000	12.03	100
Pooled serum from 20 Graves' patients	1/ 64 000	3.87	60

and antibodies against thyreoglobulin (ELISA) in 25 untreated hyperthyroid Graves-Basedow patients. Titer of ATMA shown no correlation with titer of other autoantibodies (TMS, TRAK, ATG). Moreover in few cases titer of ATMA was high while TMS and TRAK assays gave negative results (tab. 3).

In our study in which substantial number of thyroid patients were investigated antibodies against multiple thyroid plasma antigens (ATMA) were present in almost all (97% of cases by RIA and 95% of cases by ELISA) patients with untreated hyperthyroid Graves-Basedow disease. Different patients were studied by both methods. It seems important to add that the titer of Abs were high or very high ATMA were also present in patients with Hashimoto disease (in 25% of cases estimated by RIA anf 62% of cases estimated by ELISA). Here again different patients were investigated and these with ATMA present have the titer of Abs lower than in Graves-Basedow patients. ATMA were also present in few cases with toxic nodular goiter (5% of patients when ATMA was estimated by RIA and 6.7% when ELISA was used) and absent in all patients with other thyroid diseases or in healthy blood donors. The ATMA were identified in serum samples of some patients with non-thyroidal autoimmune diseases. When less specific RIA method has been in use ATMA were found to be positive in 6% of cases with Lupus erythematodes (SLE), 2% of cases with sclerodemia and 2% of patients with rheumatoid arthritis. With the use of more specific ELISA method ATMA were identified only in 2 cases with SLE and patients with other non-thyroidal autoimmune diseases were all found to be negative (tab. 4). It is possible that either these ATMA positive patients were likely to develop disease or that there is some similarity in the nature of autoantigens [9]. Estimation of ATMA during 6 months treatment with methimazol revealed that in majority of patients with hyperthyroid Graves-Basedow disease this treatment produce

Table 3 Levels of autoantibodies in Graves' patients sera estimated by different methods

Patient no.	ATMA titre	TMS IU/ml	TRAK %	antithyreoglobulin titre
1	1:64000	58	70	1: 400
2	1:16000	200	42	1:1600
3	1:16000	240	neg.	1: 400
4	1:16000	350	17	neg.
5	1:16000	112	60	1:6400
6	1:16000	240	neg.	1: 400
7	1:16000	201	60	1:1600
8	1:16000	neg.	12	1: 400
9	1:16000	neg.	neg.	neg.
10	1:16000	210	22	1:1600
11	1:16000	107	57	1:1600
12	1: 4000	220	59	neg.
13	1: 4000	78	31	neg.
14	1: 4000	86	26	1: 100
15	1: 4000	192	51	1: 400
16	1: 4000	150	64	1: 400
17	1: 4000	70	20	neg.
18	1: 4000	260	30	1: 400
19	1: 4000	108	neg.	neg.
20	1: 4000	124	neg.	1: 400
21	1: 4000	78	32	neg.
22	1: 4000	168	16	1: 100
23	1: 1000	neg.	neg.	1: 100
24	neg.	neg.	76	neg.
25	1: 1000	102	39	neg.

Table 4 Presence of antithyroid plasma membrane antibodies (ATMA) in serum from patients with thyroid diseases, some nonthyroid autoimmune diseases and healthy blood donors estimated by the ELISA

	No. of patients	No. of patients with positive ELISA and % of total	Mean value of titre for ELISA positive patients
Untreated Graves'	90	86 (95%)	1/84000
Treated Graves'	120	82 (68%)	1/32000
Hashimoto' thyroiditis	35	22 (62%)	1/30000
Toxic nodular goiter	67	6 (8.9%)	1/45000
Non-toxic nodular goiter	57	0 (0%)	–
Lupus erythematosus	34	2 (5.8%)	1/ 4000
Scleroderma	18	0 (0%)	–
Rheumatoid arthritis	12	0 (0%)	–
Healthy blood donors	80	0 (0%)	–

progressive decrease of ATMA titer and this correlate with decrease in levels of serum T_4 and T_3 and with improvment of clinical state. In minority of cases, however, the effect to treatment of ATMA titer is not seen and these patients represent "poor or non-responders to anti-thyroid therapy. We have also shown as some others [10] that there is different ATMA "profile" during successful anti-thyroid, ^{131}I and surgical therapy.

Finally follow up study of 114 patients after termination of different anti-thyroid treatment revealed that among 14 patients who became again ATMA "positive" 11 patients relapsed during next 2 months. Contrary to that only in 1 case of ATMA "negative" the relapse of the hyperthyroidism has been observed (tab. 5).

Table 5 Prognostic significance of ATMA estimation

Type of therapy and number of patients	Time after termination of therapy (months)	Patients ATMA "positive"			Patients ATMA "negative"		
		total	remission	relapse	total	remission	relapse
Mathimazole 64 patients	6–9	7	1	6	57	56	1
Radio-iodide 16 patients	6–9	4	2	2	12	12	0
Thyroidectomy 34 patients	3–4	3	0	3	31	31	0

Summary and conclusions

Our clinical study revealed that anti-thyroid plasma membrane autoantibodies (ATMA) are detectable in almost all untreated hyperthyroid patients with Graves-Basedow disease and that during treatment with methimazol the titer of ATMA decrease and after 4–6 months Abs become undetectable in patients positively responding to the therapy. In minority of patients who are ATMA positive the response to the treatment is poor and these patients if treated with methimazol should be refered to radio-iodide therapy. We also shown that the presence of ATMA after termination of respective therapy might indicate that patient is likely to relapse. Results of clinical study permit us to conclude that determination of ATMA helps to make appropriate diagnosis, control treatment regimen and predict stable remission or risk of relapse in Graves-Basedow disease.

From both experimental and clinical studies we conclude that TSH receptor antibody binding to thyrotropin receptor does not represent the only means of modulating thyroidal secretion in hyperthyroid Graves-Basedow disease.

It seems likely that autoantibodies to other thyroid plasma membrane components which are present in hyperthyroid Graves-Basedow disease are also important for the clinical course of the disease.

These Abs might either modulate TSH receptor – autoantibodies interaction or affect the thyroid function by other unknown yet mechanism.

References

[1] Rees-Smith, B., C. R. Rickards, E. Davies-Jones, et al.: J. Endocrinol. Invest. 8 (1985) 175.
[2] Farid, N. R., G. Fahraeus van Ree, R. Briones-Urbina: In: Autoimmunity and the Thyroid, pp. 249–271ess, New York 171. Academic Press, New York 1985.
[3] Kohn, L. D., S. M. Aloj, D. Tambaccini, et al.: In: Biochemical Actions of hormones, vol. XII, pp. 466–512. Academic Press, New York 1985.
[4] Gardas, A., B. Czarnocka, M. Faryna, et al.: Acta Endocrinol. (Copenh.) 105 (1984) 492.
[5] Czarnocka, B., J. Nauman, G.Adler, et al.: Acta Endocrinol. (Copenh.) 92 (1979) 512.
[6] Gardas, A., H. Domek: In: Thyroid and Autoimmunity, Elsevier, Amsterdam, in press.
[7] Nauman, J., A. Gardas, H. Domek, et al.: Nucl. Med. Cummun. 6 (1985) 582.
[8] Dawes, P. J., V. B. Petersen, B. Rees-Smith, et al.: J. Endocrinol. 78 (1978) 89.
[9] Weetman, A. P., A. M. Mc Gregor: Endocrine. Rev. 5 (1984) 309.
[10] Mc Gregor, A. M., M. M. Petersen, R. Capiferi, et al.: Clin. Endocrinol. 11 (1979) 437.

Thyroid growth stimulating immunoglobulins: Clinical significance in euthyroid goitre and relationship to thyrotropin-binding inhibiting antibodies

H. Schatz, H. Stracke, R. G. Bretzel, H. Müller, S. F. Grebe

Introduction

^{3}H-thymidine incorporation during culture of thyroid follicles isolated from porcine glands [12, 13] can be taken for estimating thyroid growth stimulating immunoglobulins [1, 3, 10, 15]. Using thyroid follicles isolated by a modified technique which are more pure than those taken for our first experiments the stimulatory action of TSH was found less pronounced or sometimes even lacking. Therefore, it should be tested whether addition of thyroglobulin to the culture medium (thyroglobulin from disrupted follicles was present to some extent in our first series using more impure follicles) might increase the responsiveness of the follicles against TSH.

Furthermore, the effect on ^{3}H-thymidine incorporation of TSH and epidermal growth factor [4, 7, 17] should be tested both without and with anti-TSH serum or anti-EGF serum present in the medium. Having established such a test system, TGI was assayed in sera of goitrous patients for evaluating the incidence and clinical significance of TGI in our iodine-deficient endemic goiter region [11].

Material and methods

Thyroid follicles were isolated from porcine glands as described elsewhere [13] using a modified technique: For mechanical disruption, Pasteur pipettes with a minimal diameter of 600 (instead of 200) µm were used [8], and washing was performed with 3 × 300 ml medium (instead of 2 × 50 ml). This technique resulted in much cleaner and better preserved follicles.

The follicle cells were estimated in a Neubauer haemocytometer chamber and 20 000 thyroid cells per well were cultivated in 180 µl of minimal essential medium (MEM (Earle), Boehringer/Mannheim, containing 10% fetal calf serum (Gibco) together with 1 mg per ml thyroglobulin (porcine, Type II, Sigma) in the wells

Thyrotropin

of an agar-gel coated microtiter plate for 24 hours. Afterwards, ^{3}H-thymidine (0,4 uCi, Amersham, 5 Ci/mmol) was added together with either standard TSH (0.01, 0.1, 1, 10 and 100 mU/ml, from bovine pituitary, Sigma) or epidermal growth factor (EGF, from mouse submaxillary glands, Digma 10^{-9} to 10^{-6} mol), both alone or together with anti-TSH serum (final concentration 1:200, from the rabbit, obtained from Paesel, Frankfurt/Main), or with anti-EGF serum (final concentration 1:100, 1:200 and 1:20000), from the rabbit, obtained from Immuno Biological Laboratories GmbH, Hamburg. For estimating TGI, ammonium sulphate-precipitated and dialysed immunoglobulins from patients' serum (and normal controls) were added yielding final concentrations of 0.01, 0.1, 1, and sometimes also 10 mg per ml. After another 48 hours of cultivation the cells were harvested with a cell harvester (Titertek, Flow Laboratories) and incubated for 24 hours with a tissue solubilizer (Soluene 350, Packard). Each concentration of TSH and EGF was tested in all wells of one row of the microtiter plate, i. e. 8 or 12 fold.

For the clinical studies the normal range (mean $\pm$ 2 SD) was established with immunoglobulins from healthy controls. Mean ^{3}H-thymidine incorporation in the presence of immunoglobulins from controls for all experiments was 93% (range 63 – 117%) of the „blank" value found with medium alone. This value for the normal immunoglobulins in each individual experiment was taken as 100%. Each serum sample was tested 6 fold and the points on the figures represent the mean values for each 6 determinations.

In the sera of all the patients with euthyroid goiter and, for comparison, also with hyperthyroid goiter, anti-microsomal and anti-thyroglobulin antibodies (MAb, TgAb) were estimated by the hemagglutination technique (Thymune M, Thymune T, Wellcome), TgAb also by radioimmunoassay (PEG-method, Serono). All sera were tested for TSH receptor antibodies (TbIAb) using the TRAK$^{(R)}$ assay (Henning). Goiter size was classified according to the WHO. Statistical evaluations were carried out using the Student's t-test.

Results

In our test system using 10% fetal calf serum, the "basal" incorporation of tritiated thymidine was high and reached values between 10000 and 15000 cpm. TSH responsiveness of the – highly purified – isolated thyroid follicles was significantly increased in the presence of thyroglobulin up to TSH concentrations of 1 mU/ml (fig. 1). The typical bell-shaped pattern was observed for the dose-response curve of TSH (figs. 1, 2): At the high concentration of 100 mU/ml, a decrease even below the zero value was found. Epidermal growth factor proved to be also a potent stimulator of thymidine incorporation (fig. 2). Anti-TSH

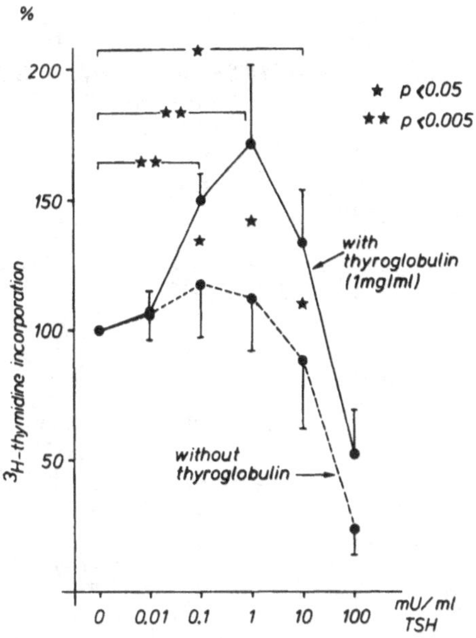

Fig. 1 Effect of thyroglobulin on TSH response of ^{3}H-thymidine incorporation into reconstituted isolated porcine thyroid follicles during culture for 48 hrs. Thyroglobulin was present in all following experiments (figs. 2–5), ($\bar{x} \pm SD$, n = 24).

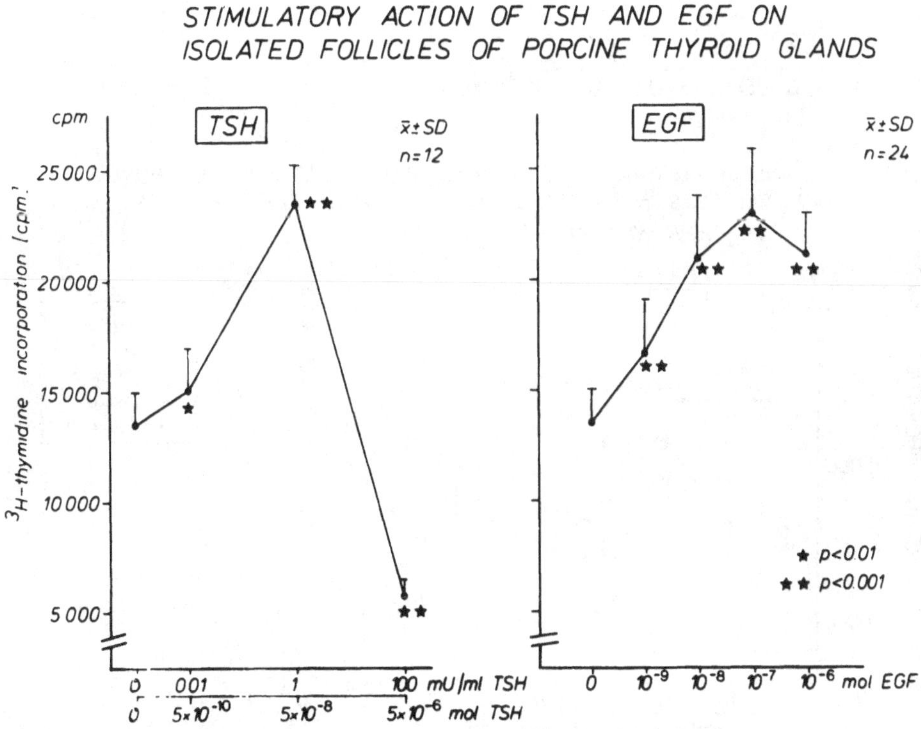

Fig. 2 Effect of TSH and EGF on ^{3}H-thymidine incorporation into reconstituted porcine thyroid follicles during culture for 48 hrs ($\bar{x} \pm SD$, n = 12 and 24, respectively).

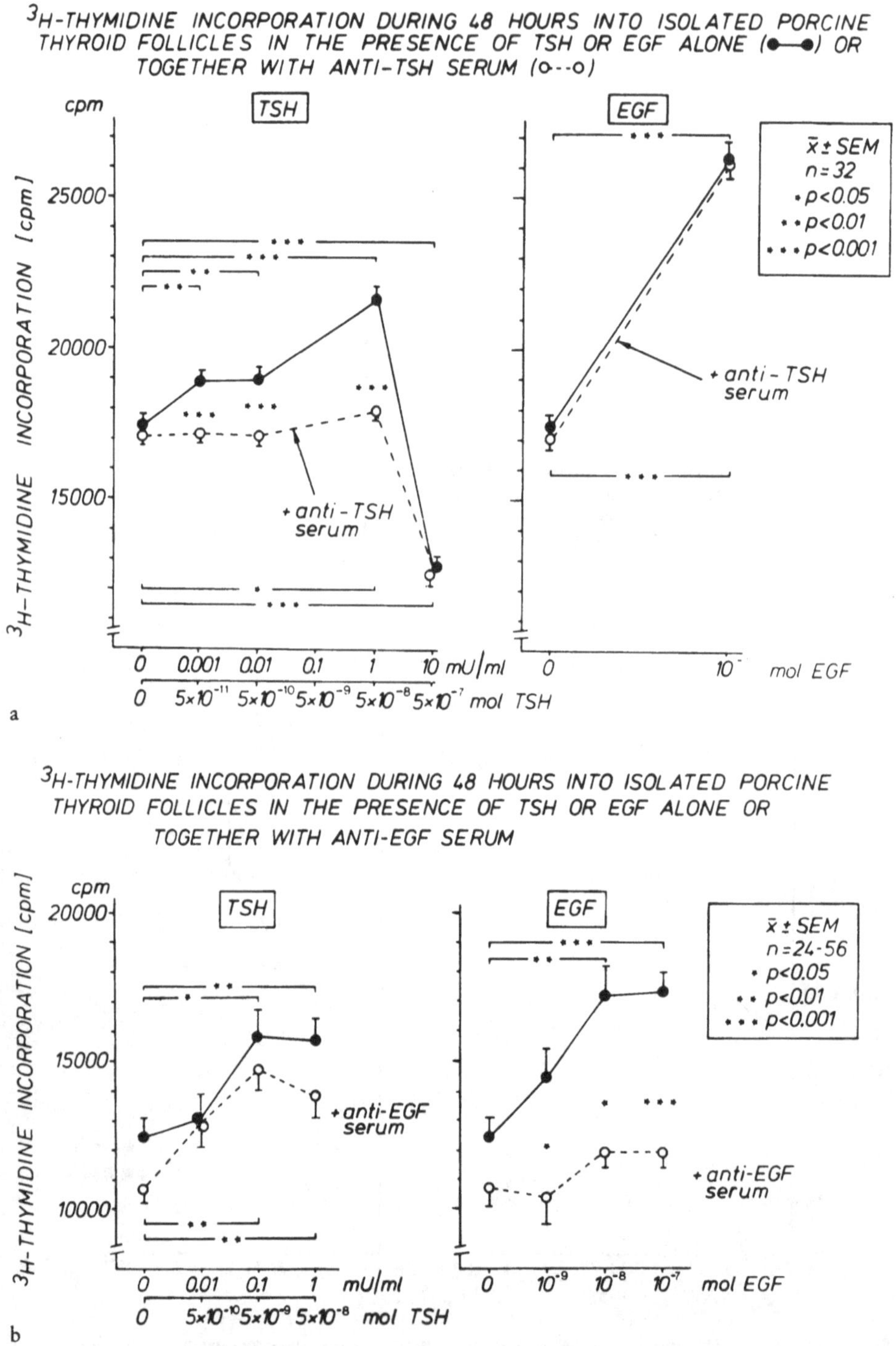

Fig. 3 a, b ³H-Thymidine incorporation during 48 hrs into isolated porcine thyroid follicles in the presence of TSH or EGF alone or together with anti-TSH serum (fig. 3 a) or anti-EGF serum (fig. 3 b), (final concentration 1 : 200).

serum abolished the stimulatory effect of TSH but not that of EGF (fig. 3 a). On the other hand, in the presence of anti-EGF serum (fig. 3 b), the "basal" thymidine incorporation was somewhat however not significantly depressed.

The stimulatory action of EGF on ^3H-thymidine incorporation was almost blocked by anti-EGF serum. TSH however still provoked a significant increase in thymidine incorporation also in the presence of anti-EGF serum at all concentrations tested.

Fig. 4: Twenty out of 72 patients (27 per cent) with euthyroid goiter (diffuse or nodular, without surgery) were TGI-positive. In patients with recurrent goiter after surgery TGI was found in 10 out of 26 patients (38 per cent). TGI was also detected in sera of untreated and in some of the treated patients with hyperthyroid goiter, mainly in cases positive for TBIAb and/or with E. O. (endocrine ophthalmopathy). There was no difference in the percentage of TGI-positive cases between diffuse and nodular euthyroid goiter (27 and 29 per cent, respectively).

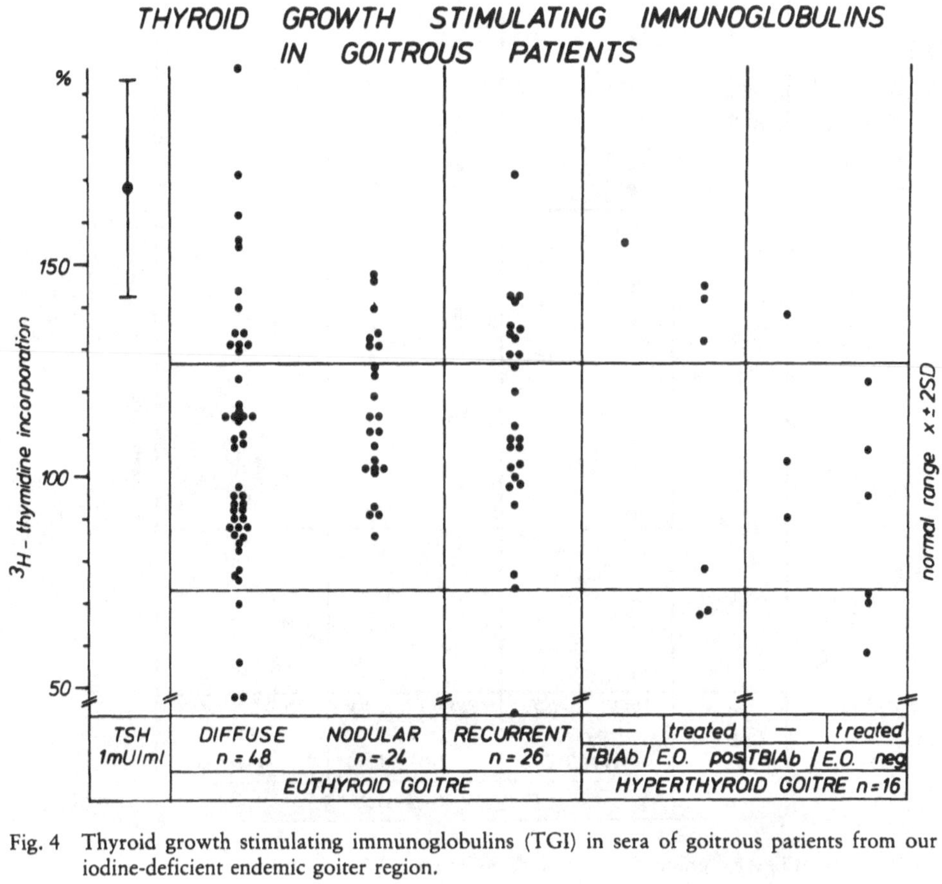

Fig. 4 Thyroid growth stimulating immunoglobulins (TGI) in sera of goitrous patients from our iodine-deficient endemic goiter region.

No significant increase of TGI was observed with increasing goiter size (fig. 5). The immunoglobulins were tested at various protein concentrations. TGI-positive results already at a low concentration of immunoglobulins (0.01 and 0.1 mg/ml, indicating a high antibody "titer") was quite often detected in sera of patients with recurrent goiter (in 4 and 3 patients, respectively, out of the 10 TGI-positive cases).

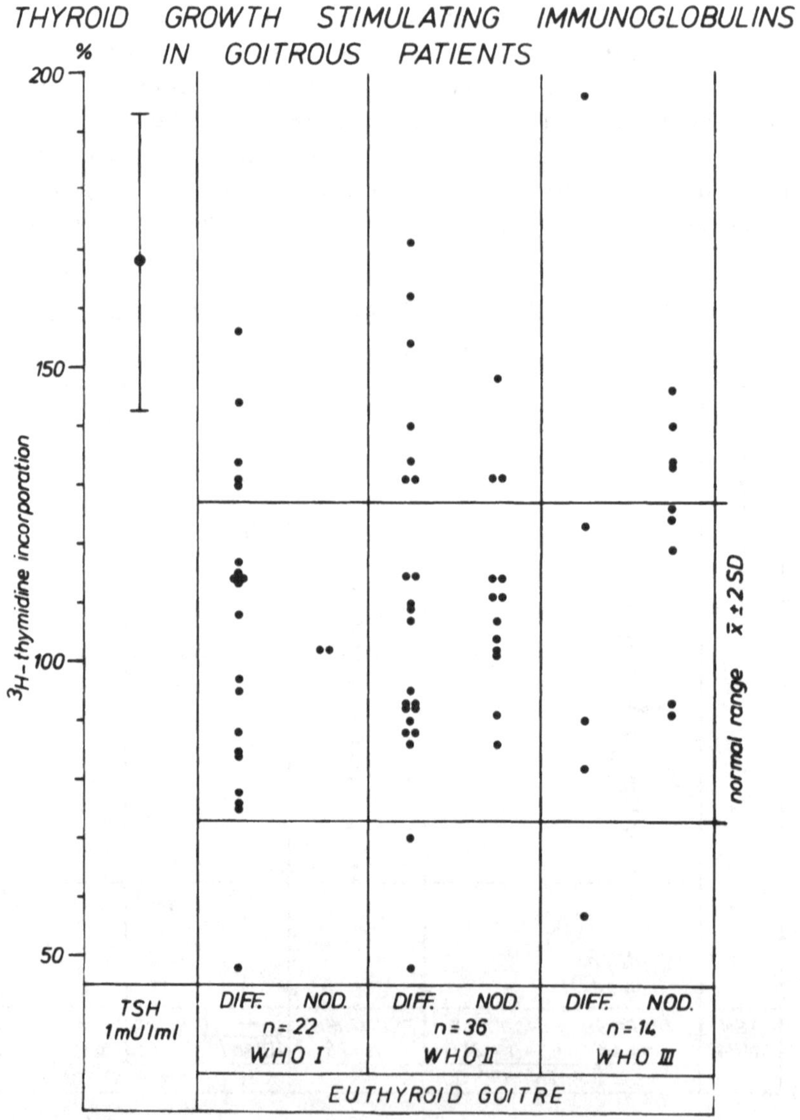

Fig. 5 Data of figure 4 grouped according to goiter size (WHO I–III).

Table 1 shows that, out of 80 patients with euthyroid goiter, 59 were negative for TgAb, MAb and TBIAb although 21 of these 59 patients were "TGI-positive" (positive at least at one of the immunoglobulin concentrations tested). From the patients exhibiting MAb and/or TgAb only few were also TGI-positive. From table 2 it can be seen that, altogether, TGI was not clearly related to the result of the TRH test. However, in patients without thyroxine treatment, TGI positivity was found in 5 patients with a positive and in no patient with a negative TRH test.

Table 1 TGI positivity in 80 patients with euthyroid goiter grouped according to the absence or presence of other thyroid antibodies

	MAb, TgAb, TBIAb neg.	MAb pos.	TgAb pos.	MAb, TgAb pos.	TBIAb pos.
n	59	4	9	8	–
TGI positive	21	1	2	1	–

Table 2 TGI and TRH test in 20 patients with euthyroid goiter with or without thyroxine (T_4) treatment (an increase of TSH more than 2.5 uU/ml was regarded as "positive")

	TGI positive		TGI negative	
	with T_4	without T_4	with T_4	without T_4
TRH test negative	3	–	4	1
TRH test positive	2	5	4	1

Discussion

In the first part of the study the previous own results were confirmed which had shown [12] that TSH can promote the growth of thyroid follicle cells isolated from porcine glands. Using highly purified follicles prepared according to Herzog [8], however, addition of thyroglobulin appears to facilitate cellular events resulting in increased thymidine incorporation. A bell-shaped dose-response curve for TSH like in this study has been found also in other systems [5, 10]. In our experiments thymidine incorporation became even depressed below the (relatively high) "blank" value (without TSH, in medium containing 10% fetal calf serum) at the high TSH concentration of 100 mU/ml. Other authors have also obtained an inhibition of thymidine incorporation below the Zero value by TSH [7, 16] however without any significant increase at lower TSH concentrations. These differences might be due to the experimental conditions, e. g. addition of thyroglobulin and/or differences in the content of fetal calf serum of the culture media.

Since the effect of EGF was blocked by anti-EGF serum, but not the effect of TSH, the growth promoting action of TSH does not necessitate the involvement of (locally produced) EGF. EGF, however, is certainly a potent stimulator of thyroid growth as demonstrated also in our follicle preparation.

In the second part of this study our previous findings were confirmed concerning the occurrence of TGI also in goitrous patients from an endemic goiter region with iodine deficiency.

The incidence in our region is, however, lower compared to other areas which are differing in nutritional iodine supply [1, 3, 6, 10, 15]. In cases of recurrent goiter, the incidence (fig. 4) and also the concentration of TGI appears to be relatively high. Which therapeutic consequences should be drawn if a goitrous patient exhibits a high concentration of TGI is still under discussion [2].

No major difference has been found in TGI between diffuse and nodular goiter [6] which would have corroborated the hypothesis put foreward by Studer and Ramelli [14]. No clear-cut relationship could be demonstrated between TGI and goiter size (fig. 5). It should be considered, however, that our study was a cross-sectional study so that the patients' immunoglobulins have been testet at different phases of goiter formation, i. e. in active and also in inactive periods.

From table 1 it can be seen that TGI represent a distinct class of thyroid antibodies. In euthyroid goiter, TGI have little relationship to other thyroid antibodies including TBIAb. This has been interpreted by others that, at least in euthyroid goiter, TGI does not represent an antibody against the TSH receptor. However, it might well be that this antibody recognizes other structures of the TSH receptor then those responsible for TSH binding. TGI did also not show a clear-cut relationship to the function of the pituitary-thyroid axis (tab. 2). The exact pathogenetic role and the clinical significance of thyroid growth stimulating immunoglobulins have yet to be established.

References

[1] Chiovato, L., L. J. Hammond, T. Hanafusa, et al.: Detection of thyroid growth stimulating immunoglobulins (TGI) by (^{3}H)-thymidine incorporation in cultured rat thyroid follicles. Clin. Endocrinol. (Oxf.) **19** (1983) 581–590.

[2] Doniach, D.: Discussion remark. In: Autoimmunity in Thyroid Disorders (H. Schatz, D. Doniach, eds.), p. 77. Thieme-Stratton, Stuttgart–New York 1984.

[3] Drexhage, H. A., G. F. Bottazzo, D. Doniach, et al.: Evidence for thyroid growth stimulating immunoglobulins in some goitrous thyroid disease. Lancet **2** (1980) 287–292.

[4] Eggo, M. C., L. K. Bachrach, G. N. Burrow: Growth and differentiation – two separate effects in cultured thyroid cells. Endocrinology **113** (1983) Suppl.: T 22.

[5] Van der Gaag, R. D., H. A. Drexhage: Time-dose related effects of TSH and TGI in the Feulgen densitometric method for measuring thyroid growth. Its clinical relevance. In: Current

topics in thyroid autoimmunity (D. Doniach, H. Schleusener, B. Weinheimer, eds.), pp. 179 – 186. Thieme-Stratton, Stuttgart – New York 1984.

[6] Van der Gaag, R. D., H. A. Drexhage, W. M. Wiersinga, et al.: Further studies on thyroid growth stimulating immunoglobulins in euthyroid non endemic goiter. J. Clin. Endocrinol. Metab. **60** (1985) 972 – 979.

[7] Gärtner, R., W. Greil, R. Demharter, et al.: Bovine thyrotropin inhibits DNA synthesis inversely with stimulation of cyclic AMP production in cultured porcine thyroid follicles. Mol. Cell Endocrinol. **42** (1985) 145 – 155.

[8] Herzog: Preparation of inside-out thyroid follicles for studies on transcellular transport (transcytosis). Methods in Enzymology, Vol. 98, pp. 447 – 458. Academic Press, New York 1983.

[9] Herzog, V., F. Miller: Membrane retrieval in epithelial cells of isolated thyroid follicles. Eur. J. Cell Biol. **19** (1979) 203 – 215.

[10] McMullan, N. M., P. P. A. Smyth: In vitro generation of NADPH as an index of thyroid stimulating immunoglobulins (TGI) in goitrous disease. Clin. Endocrinol. (Oxf.) **20** (1984) 269 – 280.

[11] Rotella, C. M., R. Toccafondi, W. Hoffman, et al.: Thyroid cell growth factors in the sera of patients with goiters. Endocrinology **115** (1984) Suppl.: T-9.

[12] Schatz, H., F. H. Beckmann, M. Floren: Radioassay for thyroid growth stimulating immunoglobulins (TGI) with cultivated porcine thyroid follicles. Horm. Metab. Res. **15** (1983) 626 – 627.

[13] Schatz, H., F. H. Beckmann, M. Floren: ^{3}H-Thymidine incorporation into porcine thyroid follicles for estimation of thyroid growth stimulating immunoglobulins. In: Current Topics in Thyroid Autoimmunity (D. Doniach, H. Schleusener, B. Weinheimer, eds.), pp. 200 – 207. Thieme-Stratton, Stuttgart – New York 1984.

[14] Studer, H., F. Ramelli: Simple goitre and its variants: Euthyroid and hyperthyroid multinodular goitre. Endocr. Rev. **3** (1982) 40 – 61.

[15] Valente, W. A., P. Vitti, C. M. Rotella, et al.: Antibodies that promote thyroid growth. A distinct population of thyroid stimulating autoantibodies. N. Engl. J. Med. **309** (1983) 1028 – 1234.

[16] Watanabe, Y., N. Amino, H. Tamaki, et al.: Bovine thyrotropin inhibits DNA synthesis inversely with stimulation of cyclic AMP production in cultured porcine thyroid follicles. Endocrinol. Jp. **32** (1985) 81 – 88.

[17] Westermark, K., F. A. Karlsson, L. E. Ericson, et al.: Epidermal growth factor: A regulator of thyroid growth and function in vitro. In: Thyroglobulin – The Prothyroid Hormone (M. C. Eggo, G. N. Burrow, eds.), pp. 255 – 262. Raven Press, New York 1985.

Detection of antibodies directed against bovine TSH in patients with and without endocrine ophthalmopathy*

R. Moncayo, R. Hoermann, E. F. Pfeiffer

Introduction

Up to date little is known about the pathogenesis of endocrine exophthalmos (EO). It can be observed associated with cases of Graves' disease but also with hypothyroidism and even euthyroidism [1]. Attempting to investigate the possible ethiology of this disease, a model was presented in 1975 by Bolonkin et al. [2]. It suggested that TSH degradation products obtained after pepsin digestion could be succesfully used as an immunogen in order to produce experimental exophthalmos. This data imparted TSH a central role in the pathogenesis of EO, however, after this experimental work no attempts had been made to try to confirm this observation in patients with EO. We therefore conceived this investigation in order to try to document this model by attempting to detect TSH antibodies in patients with EO and correlating the results with the duration of the eye involvement.

Materials and methods

Patients

37 patients with Graves' disease were studied. 20 patients presented with EO, 3 had a recent onset of EO and 14 had had EO for more than 2 years. All patients were in remission at the time of study.

Detection of antibodies to TSH

To try to demonstrate the existence of antibodies directed against TSH we chose an ELISA method. bTSH from Organon was used as the antigen. Microtiter plates (Immulon II, Dyantech) were coated overnight at room temperature with an antigen solution containing 5 μg/ml bTSH diluted in PBS. After incubation was completed the plates were washed three times with PBS-0.5% Tween. The sera to be investigated were prediluted 1:10 and added to the plates. On the plates 7 further 1:5 dilution steps were carried out. The plates were incubated

* This work was supported by the Deutsche Forschungsgemeinschaft.

for 60 minutes at 37 °C. After completing the incubation, the plates were washed again with PBS-Tween. In order to detect the bound immunoglobulins, an affinity chromatography purified goat anti-human antibody conjugated to alkaline phosphatase (TAGO) was added at a concentration of 1:3000 diluted with PBS-Tween and incubated for 60 minutes at 37 °C. The plates were again washed and phosphatase substrate (Sigma) was added at a concentration of 1 mg/ml and incubated also for 60 minutes at 37 °C. The intensity of the color reaction was measured with an automatical photometer (Dynatech MR600) at 410 nm. A reaction was called positive when it exceeded the mean plus three standard deviations of the optical density observed for the group of normals used as control.

Results

The results are summarized in table 1. It can be seen that none of the patients with EO of recent onset presented antibodies against bTSH, whereas both patients with long standing EO and patients without EO had such antibodies.

Table 1 Detection of antibodies directed against bovine TSH in patients with endocrine ophthalmopathy

	Duration of exophthalmos		
	Recent	Long standing	None
TSH Ab+	0	8	7
TSH Ab−	3	6	13

Discussion

We have attempted to document whether patients with EO of recent onset present antibodies directed against bTSH. Our results demonstrate the absence of such antibodies in patients with EO of recent onset. It appears thus that a previous immunological process aimed towards TSH does not precede the onset of EO. The involvement of TSH as a target for the humoral immune response appears not to be related with the EO since they can be found both in patients with long standing EO and in patients without EO. The role of such TSH antibodies awaits to be investigated.

References

[1] Kendall-Taylor, P.: The pathogenesis of Graves' Ophthalmopathy. In: Clinics in Endocrinology and Metabolism (A. D. Toft, ed.), vol. 14, No 2, pp. 331–349. W. B. Saunders Company, London 1985.

[2] Bolonkin, D., R. L. Tate, J. H. Luber, et al.: Experimental exophthalmos. J. Biol. Chem. 250 (1975) 6516–6521.

List of contributors

Blockx, P., Department of Nuclear Medicine, Antwerp University Hospital, B-2520 Edegem

Böttger, I. G., Medizinische Universitätsklinik, Abteilung für Nuklearmedizin, Albert-Schweitzer-Str. 33, D-4400 Münster

Bretzel, R. G., Medizinische Klinik III und Poliklinik der Universität Gießen, Rodthohl 6, D-6300 Gießen

Caldwell, G., University Departments of Medicine and Clinical Chemistry Royal Infirmary, Edinburgh EH3 9YW, U. K.

Chin, W. W., Laboratory of Molecular Genetics Georg W. Thorn 917 Brigham and Women's Hospital, 20 Shattuck Street, Boston, MA 02115 (617) 732-5856, USA

Faglia, G., Chair of Endocrinology School of Medicine, University of Milan, Via F. Sforza 35, I-20122 Milano

Földes, J., Semmelweis University, First Department of Medicine, H-1083 Budapest

Fritzsche, H., Landeskrankenhaus Feldkirch, Abteilung für Nuklearmedizin, A-6807 Feldkirch

Gallone, G., Mauriziano Hospital, Endocrine Division, I-10100 Turino

Goodman R. H., Associate Professor of Medicine, Endocrinology Division, Department of Medicine, 171 Harrison Avenue, 275 Boston, MA 02111, USA

Gräf, K.-J., Department of Internal Medicine, Klinikum Charlottenburg, Freie Universität Berlin, Paulinenstraße 24, D-1000 Berlin 19

Grebe, S. F., Leiter der Abteilung Nuklearmedizin im Zentrum für Radiologie des Klinikums der Justus-Liebig-Universität, Friedrichstraße 25 u. 27, D-6300 Gießen

Hadjidakis, D., Second Department of Internal Medicine-Propaedeutic, Athens University, P. O. Box 14127, 11510 Athens, Greece

Keck, S. F., Zentrum für Innere Medizin, Universität Ulm, Steinhövelstr. 9, D-7900 Ulm

Köhn, H., Wilhelminenspital der Stadt Wien, Institut für Nuklearmedizin, Montleartstr. 37, A-1171 Wien

Kusić, Z., Department of Nuclear Medicine and Oncology, „Dr. M. Stojanovic" Clinical Hospital, Vinogradska 29, YU-41000 Zagreb

Leicht, E., Medizinische Klinik und Poliklinik, Innere Medizin II der Universität des Saarlandes, D-6650 Homburg/Saar

Lind, P., Krankenhaus der Barmherzigen Brüder, Bergstr. 27, A-8020 Graz-Eggenberg

Loos, U., Department of Internal Medicine I, University of Ulm, D-7900 Ulm, Steinhoevelstr. 9

Moncayo, R., Department of Internal Medicine I, University of Ulm, D-7900 Ulm, Steinhoevelstr. 9

Müller-Gärtner, H. W., Universitätskrankenhaus Eppendorf, Radiologische Universitätsklinik und Strahleninstitut – Abteilung für Nuklearmedizin, Martinistraße 52, D-2000 Hamburg 20

Nauman, J., Department of Biochemistry, Medical Center of Postgraduate Education, P-01-813 Warszawa

Passath, A., Medizinische Universitätsklinik Graz, Auenbruggerplatz, A-8036 Graz

Pfannenstiel, P., Department of Nuclear Medicine, German Diagnostic Center, Aukammallee 33, D-6200 Wiesbaden

Pickardt, C. R., Medizinische Klinik Innenstadt der Universität München, Ziemssenstraße 1, D-8000 München

Rees Smith, B., Endocrine Immunology Unit, 7th Floor Medicine, University of Wales College of Medicine, Cardiff CF4, 4XN, U. K.

Schatz, H., Zentrum für Innere Medizin der Justus Liebig Universität, Rodthohl 6, D-6300 Gießen

Schemmel, K., Kreiskrankenhaus Heide/Holstein, Innere Abteilung, D-2240 Heide

Schleusener, H., Freie Universität Berlin, Universitätsklinikum Steglitz, Medizinische Klinik und Poliklinik, Abteilung für Innere Medizin mit Schwerpunkt Endokrinologie, Hindenburgdamm 30, D-1000 Berlin 45

Schnack, Ch., II. Medizinische Universitätsklinik, Alserstr. 4, A-1090 Wien

Schurz, B., I. Universitäts Frauenklinik,. Spitalgasse 23, A-1090 Wien

Swift, A. D., Department of Chemical Pathology, University of Manchester, Hope Hospital, Salford M6 8HD, U. K.

Szalbolcs, I., 1st Department of Internal Medicine, Postgraduate Medical School, H-1083 Budapest

Talbot, J. N., Services de Médicine Nucléaire de l'Hospital Saint-Antoine, 27, Rue de Chaligny, F-75012 Paris

Varl, B., University Clinic for Nuclear Medicine, Zaloska 7, YU-61000 Ljubljana

Vierhapper, H., Division of Clinical Endocrinology and Diabetes mellitus, I. Medizinische Universitätsklinik, Lazarettgasse 14, A-1090 Wien

Vitti, P., Instituo di Metodologia Clinica e Medicina del Lavoro, Cattedra di Endocrinologia, Viale del Tirreno 64, I-56018 Tirrenia/Pisa

Waldhäusl, W., I. Medizinische Universitätsklinik, Lazarettgasse 14, A-1090 Wien

Wolf, G., Universitätsklinik für Chirurgie, Graz, Auenbruggerplatz, A-8036 Graz

Wood, W. G., Klinische Laboratorien, Klinik für Innere Medizin, Medizinische Universitätsklinik zu Lübeck, Ratzeburger Allee 160, D-2400 Lübeck 1

Authors' index

Subject index

FSC
www.fsc.org
MIX
Papier | Fördert gute Waldnutzung
FSC® C083411

Kolibri 360 GmbH
Ferdinand-Jühlke-Straße 7
99095 Erfurt, Deutschland
produktsicherheit@kolibri360.de